PALAU PRIMARY HEALTH CARE MANUAL

Health Care in Palau: Combining Conventional Treatments and Traditional Uses of Plants for Health and Healing

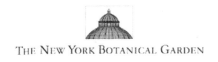

THE NEW YORK BOTANICAL GARDEN

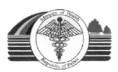

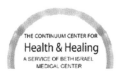

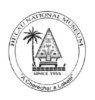

AUTHORS AND CONTRIBUTORS
Stephen Dahmer, M.D., Michael Balick, Ph.D., Ann Hillmann Kitalong, M.S., Christopher Kitalong, M.S., Katherine Herrera, Wayne Law, Ph.D., Roberta Lee, M.D., Van-Ray Tadao, Faustina Rehuher, M.A., Sholeh Hanser, Kiblas Soaladaob, M.A., Gemma Ngirchobong, Meked Besebes, M.A., Flora Wasisang, Daniel Kulakowski, and Irina Adam.

FOREWORD AND PREFACE
Stevenson Kuartei, M.D., and Victor Yano, M.D.

LOCAL EXPERTS
Obakradebkar Clarence Kitalong, Dirraurrak Ibul Ngiraibai, Ebilbachel Ngemelas Kitalong, Ebilradebkar Siabal L. Kitalong, Dilsechalraimul Ingas Spesungel, Dirratkelkang Dirraklang Merei Ngirametuker, Tomomi Watanabe, Dilchadelbai Raphaela Sumang, Dirrngerchemuul Hinako Takeo, Dirrabelluu Kerngel Tesei, Kerungil Augustin, Kosekesii Alfonsa Bintorio, Maria Kim, Dirrakerkur Nona Luii, Dirratesei Eriko Singeo, Dorothy Yukie Yano, Dirraidechor Oderai Beouch, Madrabelluu Tsuneo Tesei, Madrabars Tadashi Belchal, Iyechaderachodelomel Risao Bausoch, Ngirachitei Victor Yano, M.D., Ulengchong Scott Yano, Aderdei Gillian Johanes, Rufino Alii, Gloria Emesiochel, Bedebii Sechalboi Chiokai, Elin Rebluud, Dirradelangebiang Martha Nabeyama, Dirraiderecherech Kerengel, Linda Omekatel Belaiok, Rechiuang Demei Otobed, Subediang Ubedei, Johnson Emesiochel, Henry Yuri, Rubeang Hiromi Nabeyama, Ridep Emesiochel, Ucheldikes Ellabed Rebluud, Albino Etpison, and Oukeredeu Patrick Tellei, Ed.D.

Support for the publication of this work was provided by:

The Gildea Foundation

The V. Kann Rasmussen Foundation as the leadership funder of The New York Botanical Garden's Biodiversity and Human Health in Micronesia Program ·

Multi-year support for The New York Botanical Garden's Institute of Economic Botany has been provided by Pfizer Inc

Disclaimer

The information presented in this book is based on traditional knowledge of Palauan lore and belief and has been recorded as presented by the persons interviewed. This book should be used as a reference and is not intended to medically prescribe or promote any product or substance. It is not intended to replace professional medical care. Readers should first consult with a qualified physician or health care provider before administering or undertaking any course of medically related treatment. Even plants that are commonly consumed as food and reported to be generally recognized as safe may have adverse effects, including drug interactions, potential allergic reactions, and hypersensitivity in some individuals. The authors have checked with sources believed to be reliable to confirm the accuracy and completeness of the contents of this book; however, the authors, the editors, copyright holders, and the publisher disclaim all warranties, expressed and implied, to the extent permitted by law, that the contents are in every respect accurate and complete, and they are not responsible for errors, omissions, or any consequences from the application of this book's contents. New research is being released all the time, and this publication represents our best efforts at the time this manual was compiled.

CONTENTS

PREFACE

"Philosophies of one age have become the absurdities of the next, and the foolishness of yesterday has become the wisdom of tomorrow." – William Osler

Primary Health Care is disguised as such, when all along it is simply basic human development attempting to alleviate poverty. The current practice of providing health care has moved so far from traditional health practices. These traditional practices became suspect and were deemed archaic and obsolete amidst "modern" scientific discovery. Traditional medicine has been thought to be non-scientific and destined for the archives, when in fact these practices improved survival and social development.

The fact that these traditional medicines had improved survival and social development go along with what practitioners of allopathic medicine, in my view, must endeavor to make a habit of two things—to help, and/or at the least, do no harm. There have been significant changes in medicine through the course of my life and career in medicine. I feel that Primary Care availability and use has decreased in this generation. The practice of Primary Care was more prevalent when I returned as a young practitioner to Palau in 1980. The Trust Territory Government was well organized and had resources enough to carry out dramatic improvement in health indicators.

More recently the Primary Care and health access are fragmented because of the cash economy and the varied levels of family financial resources and educational background. For a better future, Primary Care and medicine in Palau needs to be redefined, and marketed to the new generations who have a much higher standard of living and different expectations from the last generation. There is much to be learned from the past but Palauan culture is being slowly, consistently eroded by modern culture and the dominance of the Western influence.

The *Palau Primary Health Care Manual* has been a collaborative effort between academics of Western knowledge and those of traditional knowledge, both with the objective of innovating the approach to health and to improve the "Klengar ma Klechad" (Life and Living) of the inhabitants of these lands. In conclusion, "Healing is a matter of time, but it is sometimes also a matter of opportunity. However, knowing this, one must attend to medical practice not primarily to plausible theories, but to experience combined with reason. For a theory is a composite memory of things apprehended with sense perception" (Precepts, Hippocrates translated by W. H. S. Jones 1923).

Victor M. Yano, M.D.
Local Practitioner
Republic of Palau

FOREWORD

Life in Belau is like a woven mat, with parts that transect under and overlay each other and are equally important in the mat's final functional integrity. Traditional healing is woven in such a manner, with many fabrics, guided by knowledge, experiences, beliefs, historical experimentation, and finally mysticism and spiritualism. There is also a fundamental difference between traditional and contemporary healing in the order of prioritization of the healing process. Traditional healing requires that a comprehensive evaluation of all the environments surrounding a patient, including the physical, social, mental, behavioral, spiritual and other environments, are performed and resolved before prescriptions of medicines given. The biomedical model utilized by contemporary medicine narrows the healing approach to the physical and psychosocial environments. Sometimes medications are given prematurely to implement interventions that mitigate environmental concerns and sometimes the problems are exacerbated when the process is tainted with economic concerns. However, a positive integral part of contemporary healing is the science that comes with formalized medical research. Weaving in this positive attribute of contemporary healing to the overall fabric of healing process in Belau will enhance the art and the science of healing in Belau.

From *Dirrairechuul* (Genesis) to *Ngirchobeketang* (Revelation), the mystical and spiritual fabric of Belauan society is woven together with an overlay of modern religions. It is through this mystical and spiritual fabric that we begin to understand all the different kinds of healing (natural, assisted, inner, improbable and ultimate) even when some of them are deemed to be "out of line" with modern religion (Gills 2004).

Progression of "disease" in Belau

In science many mutations are results of free radical ions; similarly, the health of the Neo-Belauan is affected by "social ions" that are the cause for many "social mutations" (evolution). These social mutations have resulted in increased negative health risk factors for the Neo-Belauan. The social ions I refer to include moderniza*tion*; migra*tion*; urbaniza*tion*; imperializa*tion* (food, media, language), commercializa*tion*; and altera*tion* (of our worldview). This results in social mutations that pry us away from those values and practices that have made us survive over the last 4,000 years. For example, moderniza*tion* through "plastica*tion*" of life in Belau and the world, or the introduction of chemicals (chemicaliza*tion*) and metallurgic products (metalliza*tion*) into mainstream consumption. These products have increased the quantity of persistent organic pollutants (POPs), heavy metals and other organic and inorganic pollutants in the environment. These pollutants are direct environmental and health threats.

The "medicalization" of health has gradually eroded the confidence of the Belauan society toward traditional medicine and healing. The changes over the last one and half century in Belau have gradually made the disease phenomenon the central feature of healing. This narrow approach to healing has led to the marginalization of our traditional healers and the disintegration of the confidence in traditional healing especially when it is coupled with the adoption of the "new" ways to address "new" illnesses (Rapaport 1999). It is ironic that while the diseases of modernity are lifestyle- related, most of the time contemporary healing resorts to the prescription of drugs, rather than the prescription of environmental and behavioral changes prior to drugs.

Genetic studies suggest that the "thrifty genes", mitochondrial genes present in Belauans, have helped them survive during the migration to Belau, especially during the time of famine

(Kagawa *et al.*, 2003). But now during the time of abundance, these once necessary genes are presently becoming the cause of many illnesses and in particular lifestyle-related diseases. Furthermore, urbanization and job competitiveness favors Western-educated individuals including Western medical practices, therefore pushing health education further away from the aforementioned traditional approach of prophylaxis.

Contemporary Approach to Traditional Medicine and Healing in the Pacific

The Yanuca Island Declaration (Dever & Finau 1995; World Health Organization (WHO) 1995) adopted a goal of "Healthy Islands" by the twenty-first century. The concept of Healthy Islands is articulated in the following basic principles: a) children are nurtured in body and mind, b) environments invite learning and leisure, c) people work and age with dignity, and d) ecological balance is a source of pride.

In August 1997, the Rarotonga Agreement recommended that the "use of traditional medicine should be encouraged where appropriate, and that steps should be taken to incorporate its use into the health care system." This posture portrays traditional medicine and healing as the "alternative medicine" that must be incorporated into the Western medical systems (WHO 1997).

The Palau Action Statement on Healthy Islands in March 1999 (WHO 1999) had six recommendations: a) healthy island initiative, b) human resources for health, c) pharmaceuticals, d) traditional medicine, e) non-communicable diseases, and f) health information. With regards to traditional medicine, the Palau Action Statement further stipulated four specific courses of action to be taken by each Pacific Island. These four areas were: 1) governments to develop policies in support of the proper use of traditional medicine, 2) commonly used local plants with medicinal value should be selected and their proper use should be assessed and promoted, 3) traditional medicine practitioners should be mobilized as community health providers in order to provide further training opportunities and pass the knowledge to other health workers, and 4) the potential contribution of scientifically proven traditional medicine should be fully explored (WHO 2002). The insensitivity of the Western medical system percolates through these recommendations toward traditional medicine and healing by framing them outside of its mystical and spiritual milieu.

The Apia Action Plan 2000 (WHO 2001) was put forth with the intention of facilitating the work of interested Pacific Island Communities (PICs) to initiate and further develop their traditional medicine programs. It provided a "step by step approach" for developing these programs. And while the intention was honorable, the essence of traditional healing was not integrated into the plan of action. The stakeholders such as those who practice the art should have been there to "salvationalize" the great efforts of the modern health systems. The incorporation of the practices (mystical and spiritual) and the sacredness of traditional medicine and healing would have brought the necessary credibility of the Apia Action Plan, especially if articulated by traditional healers.

The current knowledge of traditional healing in the Pacific is poorly documented because in large measure it is secretly orated. The documentation has been done by various disciplines, some of which are quite myopic with tunnel vision in their attempt to document traditional healing in the Pacific. The gradual desegregation of the traditional concept of health in the Pacific through the expatriate intrusion has given way to the separation of health from the culture, spiritual beliefs, foods, local herbs and magic. As a result, this has also led to some of the dismantling of the confidence in traditional medicine and healing. Traditional medicine and healing in the Pacific post contact years was considered to be less efficacious for "modern" diseases (Macpherson and Macpherson 1990).

The importance of this manual is to get Belauans to revert back to the positive fundamentals, *Klebelau* (Belauness) and *Klechibelau* (Belauism) of the Belauan society to address these negative social mutations. The practice of traditional healing holds us Belauans accountable for our actions before medication is given and is our best form of prophylaxis and prevention for diseases of modernity. Healing is not just about medicine, it is about food, sleep, relationships, beliefs, magic and sometimes even sorcery (although few would admit this).

Words of Acknowledgement for this Book

It takes courage and the sense of "community-ism" to divulge or share the knowledge that made this manual possible and so we thank those who have contributed to this body of knowledge. Obviously, this manual is made possible because of the foresight of those for whom this is their passion, their responsibility or their custody by which they would share their expertise and resources and we thank them. This is the initial step toward the preservation of this traditional knowledge and intellectual property of the equivalent of so called "over the counter" remedies in Belau and opens the door for those who will follow to develop ways to protect the hidden formulas—the "prescriptive" remedies—so that they can be shared for healing posterity in Palau. Healing does not always happen to those who seek healing but also to those who seek to heal.

Stevenson Kuartei, M.D.
Minister of Health
Republic of Palau

4

INTRODUCTION

The Republic of Palau is the westernmost archipelago of the Caroline Islands in Micronesia that lies within latitudes 8°12' to 2°48' and longitudes 131°07' to 134°44' (Map 1). Major study sites for the information presented in this manual included the village of Oikull, Airai State and the village of Ibobang, Ngatpang State, which are part of Babeldaob, the largest island in Palau. We interviewed many people from these villages as well as from villages elsewhere in Palau. Oikull is located in southeastern Babeldaob and consists of volcanic and limestone soils with mangrove forests and freshwater wetlands and grasslands. Oikull is very unique as a transitional habitat with a diverse assemblage of plants. Ibobang is located in southwestern Babeldaob and consists of similar habitats as Oikull but does not have limestone forests. These two study sites, Oikull and Ibobang, were chosen based on a number of considerations, including local interest, accessibility, the level of cultural knowledge, the presence of plant diversity and guidance from the Board of The Belau National Museum. A comprehensive literature review was conducted as part of the information gathering process that produced this manual, and many other plant uses were added.

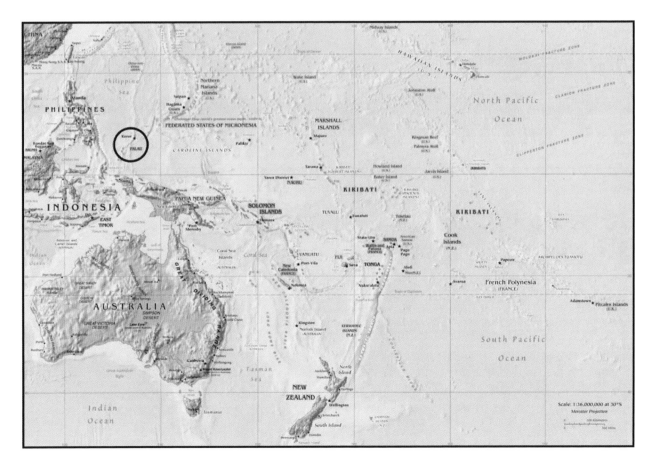

Map 1. Palau (encircled), showing its position within Oceania. Source: https://www.cia.gov/library/publications/the-world-factbook/maps/maptemplate_ps.html

The *Palau Primary Health Care Manual* documents indigenous knowledge of useful medicinal plants on the island of Palau. Traditional knowledge is reflected in the dynamic ways in which people identify with and relate to their natural environment as well as how they organize this knowledge (Semali & Kincheloe 1999).

This manual was developed as a reference for medical professionals and others knowledgeable about or interested in the use of plants for healing. It also serves as a resource for Palauans to address and understand selected medical conditions as well as document traditional plant knowledge. Organized into the following twelve chapters, this manual describes various health conditions and combines current Western medical knowledge with traditional Palauan botanical remedies; pharmacological efficacy and toxicity of each species are also included when available:

> Chapter One: Preventive Medicine in Palau
> Chapter Two: Chronic Disease
> Chapter Three: Bites and Stings
> Chapter Four: Gastrointestinal Disorders
> Chapter Five: Skin Disorders
> Chapter Six: Cuts, Wounds, and Broken Bones
> Chapter Seven: Stress
> Chapter Eight: Pain
> Chapter Nine: Women's Health
> Chapter Ten: Men's Health
> Chapter Eleven: Colds and Flu
> Chapter Twelve: Ear, Nose, and Throat (ENT)

The above health conditions were selected for inclusion in this manual based on the most frequent diagnoses reported by healers and by the volume of information available from data collected as part of the Plants and People of Micronesia Program during the years 2007 to 2011. In support of the data collected from local healers, interviews were also conducted with numerous health professionals in Palau.

Due to the many uses of either a single plant species or a combination of species for treating health conditions in Palau, selected "recipes" were based upon the frequency of use reported and documented from local expert healers. For example, if we received five reports of similar use the knowledge was valued differently than if we received only one report. Combination therapies are listed at the end of each section. Obtaining permission to use the commonly known botanical remedies in this manual was of utmost importance and necessary to protect the knowledge that is documented. Informed consent was obtained from each individual involved. In addition, we deliberately did not collect or report proprietary family recipes or sensitive "secret" knowledge. Thus, as many people on the island know, there are far more recipes for the conditions discussed in this manual. The information shared with us is common knowledge that has been passed down from generation to generation, independently discovered on their own or shared between families.

The importance of documenting traditional botanical knowledge is relevant to both conservation of biodiversity and enhancing public health. Roberta A. Lee, M.D., discussed the model of integrative medicine and how it blends traditional Pohnpeian medical practices with Western medicine in *Ethnobotany of Pohnpei: Plants, People and Island Culture* (Balick 2009, p. 213-214).

"Until Weil (1983, 1995) proposed the concept of integrative medicine and holistic care, there existed few models for bridging indigenous medical practices with conventional Westernized biomedical care. Integrative medicine includes indigenous medical systems and alternative modalities as part of conventional care. In this approach, judicious use of modalities from indigenous systems such as plants (in the form of botanical supplements), acupuncture, chiropractic or osteopathic manipulation, massage, and other treatments are embedded in primary care. This integrated model of Western and traditional practitioners has been attempted in a few countries—driven primarily by economic circumstances where limited resources for healthcare exist. In some situations, the integration has worked well; the Cuban medical system has been one system which has received acknowledgement for its efficient blending of Western and Traditional medical systems (Feinsilver 1993)." Lee, continues,

"An integrative medicine model advocates for the value of indigenous treatment in partnership with the best of conventional care—not because indigenous practices are less expensive but because they are potentially more efficacious and less harmful when compared to other biomedical treatments commonly used. The idea that an integrated medical system including indigenous healers can represent a more efficient use of healthcare resources is valuable for several reasons in environments where resources for healthcare are limited. Some of the potential benefits with an integrated healthcare system are:

- Conservation of financial resources using a mixture of conventional medicine and traditionally used botanical medicines.
- Establishment of a uniform and blended healthcare system with use of traditional healers formally communicating with conventional medical personnel.
- Establishment of best practices based on shared observation by conventional medical personnel and traditional healers.
- Minimization of adverse clinical outcomes through partnership between conventional medical personnel and traditional healers.
- Reinforcement of cultural knowledge through its inclusion in a modern medical format.

The effort in making this system a more effective provider of healthcare—as compared to a traditional biomedical Western model—lies in pooling the expertise of the healers and those delivering primary care—with each group helping to identify the techniques that are appropriate for each condition. Other components of an integrated system include how to structure medical evaluations to identify and properly treat conditions that are perceived as culture-bound syndromes."

The development of a variety of medical and educational resource materials for Palau, employing a multi-disciplinary approach, can be a first start. One example of a move towards this blending is our project to produce primary health care manuals of traditional plant uses on Micronesian Islands. The present publication, the second in a series (following the Pohnpei manual, Lee *et al.*, 2010), blends current conventional medical knowledge regarding specific medical conditions with the plants traditionally used in the treatment of each ailment.

Globalization and the deleterious effects of climate change are a threat to Palau's biodiversity, natural resources and traditional knowledge. "Traditional knowledge refers to the knowledge, innovations and practices of indigenous and local communities around the world. Developed from experience gained over the centuries and adapted to the local culture and environment, traditional knowledge is transmitted orally from generation to generation. It tends to be collectively owned and takes the form of stories, songs, folklore, proverbs, cultural values, beliefs, rituals, community laws, local language, and agricultural practices, including the development of plant species and animal breeds. Traditional knowledge is mainly of a practical nature, particularly in such fields as agriculture, fisheries, health, horticulture, and forestry" (Society for Ecological Restoration International 2009). Medicinal plants are but one component of the value of natural habitats. It is therefore imperative to document traditional ecological knowledge (TEK) before it disappears. Moreover, TEK can assist in finding sustainable solutions to protecting local biodiversity. By documenting plant species and their uses, we hope to encourage the conservation of plants and their habitat as well as promote sustainable management of medicinal plants.

In Palau, the banana species known locally as *cherasech* (*Musa troglodytarum* L.) has been shown to have some of the highest levels of pro-vitamin A carotenoids of all the bananas, over 100 times more than bananas regularly consumed in the United States (Englberger *et al.*, 2009). In a region where vitamin A deficiency is a significant public health concern, this local cultivar, if more widely consumed in the local diet, has the potential of addressing this serious issue. Vitamin A deficiency is linked to "...increased problems with infection (particularly, pneumonia, diarrhea, and respiratory and skin infections), night blindness, and total blindness" (Englberger *et al.*, 2009). As noted in that same reference, "epidemiological studies have shown that improving the vitamin A status of young children can decrease child mortality rates by 23% (McLaren & Frigg 2001)."

In this manual, we have interpreted medical information specifically to assist the general reader in determining whether a condition is severe enough to warrant immediate medical assistance. Oftentimes, traditional knowledge is used in a manner that is not part of conventional medical care; we aim to develop a "bridge" for medical personnel to obtain scientific information pertaining to non-prescriptive botanical medicines. Thus, this manual includes basic information on pharmacology, toxicity and adverse effects of the plants mentioned where known. We also encourage communication between health care providers, both conventional and traditional, in the hopes of improving overall health care.

Methodology

The *Palau Primary Health Care Manual* is based on numerous interviews (Hillmann Kitalong *et al.*, 2011) with local Palauan community members, collection of nearly 3,000 plant specimens during 2007-2011 and their associated knowledge when available, and the existing ethnobotanical literature for Palau. The list of representative voucher specimens (e.g. one per species) cited in this manual can be found in the Appendix. Composites and single image photographs that illustrate the species are presented with captions listing plant parts clockwise from the left, with the corresponding photographer in that same order. Plant collections were generated as part of the "Biodiversity and Human Health in Micronesia/Plants and People of Micronesia" program conducted by Michael J. Balick, Ph.D., Ann Hillmann Kitalong, M.S., Wayne Law, Ph.D., Stephen Dahmer, M.D., Roberta Lee, M.D., Christopher Kitalong, M.S., Katherine Herrera, Faustina Rehuher, Van-Ray Tadao, Meked Besebes, M.A., Kiblas Soaladaob, M.A., Sholeh Hanser, Gemma Ngirchobong, Flora Wasisang, and Daniel Kulakowski, along with the following local ethnomedical specialists: Dirratkelkang Dirraklang Merei Ngirametuker, Ebilbachel Ngemelas Kitalong, Obakradebkar Clarence Kitalong, Dirraurrak Ibul Ngiraibai, Ebilradebkar Siabal L. Kitalong, Dilsechalraimul Ingas Spesungel, Tomomi Watanabe, Dilchadelbai Raphaela Sumang, Dirrengerchemuul Hinako Takeo, Dirrabelluu Kerengel Tesei, Kerungil Augustin, Kosekesii Alfonsa Bintorio, Maria Kim, Dirrakerkur Nona Luii, Dirratesei Eriko Singeo, Dorothy Yukie Yano, Dirraidechor Oderai Beouch, Dirradechor Sariang Timulech, Ngiraichitei Victor Yano, M.D., Tsuneo Tesei, Madrabars Tadashi Belchal, Iyechaderachodelomel Risao Bausoch, Ulengchong Scott Yano, Aderdei Gillian Johanes, Oukeredeu Patrick Tellei, Ed.D., Rufino Alii, Gloria Emesiochel, Bedebii Chiokai, Elin Rebluud, Dirradelangebiang Martha Nabeyama, Dirraiderecherech Kerengel, Linda Omekatel Belaiok, Rechiuang Demei Otobed, Subediang Ubedei Johnson Emesiochel, Henry Yuri, Rubeang Hiromi Nabeyama, Ridep Emesiochel, Ucheldikes Ellabed Rebluud, and Albino Etpison.

The range and description data related to scientific plant names was largely based on published literature including *Flora Vitiensis Nova* Vol. 1-5 by A.C. Smith (1979, 1981, 1985, 1988, 1991); previous studies of Palau's flora including Kanehira's (1933) floristic work, and Fosberg and his colleagues' extensive floristic surveys and systematics research over a 45 year period (Fosberg 1946, 1947, 1953, 1960; Fosberg & Raulerson 1990; Fosberg & Sachet 1975a, 1975b, 1977, 1979, 1980a, 1980b, 1980c, 1981, 1984, 1987, 1991; Fosberg, Sachet & Oliver 1979, 1982, 1987, 1993; Fosberg *et al.*, 1980). Stemmermann (1981) described wetland communities including mangrove forests. Cole *et al.* (1987) conducted a vegetation survey. Canfield, Herbst, and Stemmerman (1992) did a rapid ecological study of the Ngeremeduu Bay Drainage. Raulerson *et al.* (1997) did a botanical reconnaissance in Babeldaob. Donnegan *et al.* (2007) conducted a systematic inventory of the forests of Palau. Studies of important forest areas, long term vegetation trends and species diversity (Hillmann Kitalong and Holm 2004; Costion and Kitalong 2006; Hillmann Kitalong 2008; Hillmann Kitalong, DeMeo & Holm 2008) were conducted; *Manual of the Flowering Plants of Hawaii* by Wagner, Herbst, and Sohmer (1990) was consulted; and, Robbin Moran provided determinations and plant descriptions of fern species where necessary. The plant collections are housed in The William and Lynda Steere Herbarium at The New York Botanical Garden, as well as at The National Tropical Botanical Garden Herbarium, Hawaii, The Belau National Museum Herbarium, and the University of Guam Herbarium.

Ethnobotanical studies in Palau have focused mainly on the medicinal uses of plants (Okabe 1941; Black 1968; Salsedo 1970; Salsedo and Smith 1987; DeFilipps, Maina & Pray 1988; Telmetang 1993; Friend and Tabak 1995; Machiko 2002; Palau Society of Historians 2000, 2001; Del Rosario and Esguerra 2003), documenting over 80 plant species with over 235 medicinal uses.

To save space and avoid repetition, when the range and/or the description have been cited earlier in a specific chapter, we have not included these paragraphs with the traditional plant remedy but refer the reader elsewhere in the chapter.

In Palau, traditional botanical therapies consist of utilizing a plant species or plant part, which may or may not use water as a solvent or medium. Additionally, throughout the manual, you will find that many recipes use *Cocos nucifera* L. (coconut) oil as the solvent and medium for remedies using other plants. Coconut oil contains a high concentration of vitamin E and it is an excellent emollient for the skin (Henson 2008). The chemical composition includes medium chain fatty acids, such as lauric acid (45-52%), myristic acid (16-21%), and palmitic acid (7-10%)—fats that have an 8-16 carbon chain. This property makes coconut oil an efficient vehicle for absorption through the skin and the intestinal walls, to ease the passage of medications into the blood stream (Temme, Mensink & Hornstra 1997). Moreover, coconut oil's antibacterial and antiviral properties have been extensively studied (Lewis & Elvin-Lewis 2003).

Pharmacology and toxicology are included for each traditional remedy because these sections are specific to the individual local use. A literature review of each species and its pharmacological properties and toxicity was conducted using the following online databases:

- HerbClip (http://abc.herbalgram.org/)
- NAPRALERT (www.napralert.org)
- PubMed (www.pubmed.gov)
- ScienceDirect (www.sciencedirect.com)
- Scopus (www.scopus.com)
- TOXNET (www.toxnet.nlm.nih.gov)

These online databases are important modern search tools that provide a comprehensive survey of published pharmacological and toxicological studies undertaken in laboratories around the world. Pharmacology, toxicity and adverse effects data for each of the plant species, when available, are specifically included to help inform medical personnel of current and pertinent information. However, this information often has significant limitations and may not relate to clinical use. There is a lack of good clinical data and *in vivo* studies that directly relate to the use of many of the plants discussed in this work, particularly when considering the dosage and preparation traditionally used on Palau. Therefore, this manual cannot be considered as a true evidence-based guide. Continued pre-clinical and clinical research on these herbal preparations remains to be done.

The following databases were used to cross-check facts, definitions and botanical nomenclature:

- The International Plant Names Index (http://www.ipni.org/)
- W³ TROPICOS (http://www.tropicos.org/)

Acknowledgments

The information in this book is based on ongoing ethnomedical and ethnobotanical research undertaken on Palau beginning in 2007. This research program is a collaborative effort of a number of organizations including the Continuum Center for Health and Healing at Beth Israel Medical Center, NY, The New York Botanical Garden, the National Tropical Botanical Garden, HI, the Belau National Museum, and The Ministry of Health, Republic of Palau. Discussions with colleagues from the Pacific Basin Medical Association, the University of Arizona College of Medicine Program in Integrative Medicine, and The Nature Conservancy have helped shape the content of this book. We at The New York Botanical Garden are very grateful to Martin S. Kaplan (former Managing Director), Lois E. H. Smith, M.D. (current Managing Director) and the Trustees of the V. Kann Rasmussen Foundation for their leadership gift and long term commitment to this project, as well as the MetLife Foundation, the Overbrook Foundation, Pfizer Inc, Edward P. Bass and the Philecology Trust, the Prospect Hill Foundation, the Marisla Foundation, The Germeshausen Foundation, The National Geographic Society, and the Belau National Museum, for their support and interest in this project and related Pacific Island programs at The New York Botanical Garden. We thank the Trustees of The Gildea Foundation for their long-term interest in the ethnobotanical and floristic work in Micronesia. Pfizer Inc is acknowledged for its multi-year support of The New York Botanical Garden's Institute of Economic Botany. We are grateful to the following NYBG staff: Sarah Bolson, Dale Brooks, Cindy Mooney, Lisa Synoradzki, Michelle Meesawan, Flávia Stoike, Stephan Chenault, Arthur Fairweather, and Patrick Maraj, and the following dedicated IEB volunteers: Nivedita Kaushal, Ph.D., Rachel Corey-Pacheco, R.N., and Gillian Stevens, who helped make this book possible. We are grateful to Temmy Temengiil and Mark Bauernfiend for contributing information about the status of public health in Palau, and to Drs. David H. Lorence and Diane Ragone as well as their colleagues at The National Tropical Botanical Garden for their ongoing support and collaboration.

About the collectors and photographers

In addition to the people listed above, the following people participated in fieldwork: McKnight MacArthur, Yadna Desmond, Dr. Cristina Llerena Law, Dr. Nathan Chin, Nicholas Penna, Dr. David H. Lorence, Clay Trauernicht, Steve Perlman, Dawnette Olsundong, Jesse Czeckanski-Moir, Dr. George and Mrs. Carol Milne, Yvonne Singeo, Sachi Singeo, Olympia Morei, and Jasmine Lim.

Photographers' initials are as follows: Ann Hillmann Kitalong [AK], Clay Trauernicht [CT], David Lorence [DL], Katherine Herrera [KH], Kiblas Soaladaob [KS], Michael Balick [MB], Roberta Lee [RL], Steve Pearlman [SP], and Wayne Law [WL]. Images from The William and Lynda Steere Herbarium of The New York Botanical Garden [NY] are indicated as such. Photo credits [in brackets] are listed under each photograph. Where there is more than one photo, the credits are listed from left to right as related to the top and bottom photos.

CHAPTER ONE: PREVENTIVE MEDICINE IN PALAU

Preventive medicine refers to measures taken to prevent diseases (or injuries) before an individual is affected rather than curing them or treating their symptoms after the fact. The goal of preventive medicine is to reduce the medical, psychological, financial, and occupational burdens of avoidable disease and injury through prevention, screening, and education.

An important part of preventive medicine is regularly scheduled well visit check-ups with a medical doctor and staying up-to-date on immunizations. Check-ups should include screening for chronic diseases such as high blood pressure, obesity, and diabetes, tests for cancer, determining tobacco, illicit drug, and alcohol use, and obtaining past individual and family medical histories. The United States Preventive Task Force issues updated recommendations for screening on a regular basis; their latest recommendations can be accessed at: http://www.uspreventiveservicestaskforce.org/recommendations.htm.

The Division of Primary and Preventive Health within the Ministry of Health (MOH) identifies primary health as its first and foremost service priority. These services include maternal health, prenatal care, infant care, immunization, physical check-up, and basic preventive health. All services are provided mainly through the community health center in the Belau National Hospital. Services are additionally made available through four super dispensaries as well as four additional satellite dispensaries. The Division of Primary and Preventive Health is led by highly qualified and dedicated personnel whose goal is to revitalize healthcare through a comprehensive and collaborative approach to primary and preventive health (MOH, Republic of Palau 2009).

Immunization has also long been an important part of preventive medicine in Palau, having achieved over 96% coverage rates for many years. Palau has also been at the forefront of accepting and administering new vaccines approved by the World Health Organization (WHO), which include Hepatitis A and B, childhood meningitis, influenza, and pneumonia. Hepatitis B has been the leading cause of death from infectious disease in Palau and will hopefully change in the future with the increase in vaccination and the focus on preventive medicine. A key part of the future of preventive medicine in Palau will be the continued support of community groups.

Non-communicable diseases (NCDs) were once considered by the WHO as a problem of only developed countries. In Palau, the Ministry of Health has followed this pandemic for many years, watching the increasing trends of key NCD indicators in the Palauan population. The Pacific Islands appear regularly at the top 20 health risk categories associated with NCDs (WHO, http://apps.who.int/gho/indicatorregistry)

Due to the small population of the islands, they are drowned out when compared to regional figures. Nevertheless, there has been increased recent attention through initiatives from individual countries and organizations focusing attention on NCDs in developing countries. This attention culminated earlier this year in *Executive Order 295* declaring a "state of emergency on NCDs" in Palau. Internationally, due to the high prevalence of NCDs in developing countries, especially Small Island Developing States, high-level meetings of the General Assembly on the prevention and control of non-communicable diseases were held on September 19th and 20th, 2011 in New York. This meeting addressed the prevention and control of non-communicable diseases worldwide, with a particular focus on developmental and other challenges as well as social and economic impacts, particularly for developing countries. The Ministries of Health as well as all islands in the Pacific have made NCD prevention a top priority.

During 2009, the Non- Communicable Disease Unit merged all the NCD programs such as Diabetes, Obesity, Cancer, Heart Disease, and Tobacco Use under one umbrella unit. The goal of this merger was to improve services to the community by creating more efficiency and consolidating resources to be shared by all programs. Two major community organizations were also realigned to improve efficiency and share resources for the common goal of reducing NCDs within the Republic of Palau. The NCD Strategic Plan has now been finalized. New and innovative NCD outreach programs were initiated for other Ministries as well as outlying states. A Program Evaluation Training to build MOH staff capacity was conducted. A series of community based workshops such as the "Palliative Workshop," "Healthy Workplace Workshop," and "Lifestyle and I: What Can I Do Workshop" were provided to the community and the MOH Staff. In addition, the Childhood Obesity Program has been enacted in schools and individual states to prevent increased rates of NCD's risk factors within the younger population. With support from the MOH, agencies and businesses have begun "The Greatest Loser" programs with incentives to live healthier lifestyles.

An integrated environmental approach to wellness has been taken at the Ministry of Health to incorporate all aspects surrounding a patient in order to treat the *state of illness* and not only to treat the illness itself. It incorporates a large scale approach to preventative medicine, which incorporates all the factors surrounding the population in Palau. The model aims to harmonize all the environments leading to health without focusing specifically on disease. This approach will help to eliminate risk factors that may be associated with the state of illness by assisting in improving outside factors and therefore acting as a first line preventative approach (Figure 1) (MOH, Republic of Palau 2009).

As mentioned in the foreword and validated by many traditional healers, "Traditional healing requires that a comprehensive evaluation of all the environments surrounding a patient, including the physical, social, mental, behavioral, spiritual and other environments, is performed and resolved before prescriptions of medicines is given," and in this way traditional medicine is a direct form of preventative medicine and an adjuvant in the prevention of disease progression.

In 2009, the overall life expectancy for Palauans was 72 years [females 77, males 66] (WHO 2011). Through preventive medicine, with the combined help of traditional healing and modern medicine as well as the implementation of Dr. Kuartei's Integrative Environmental Approach to Health supported by increased focus on NCD prevention, the hope is for both the number and quality of life years to increase for all Palauans.

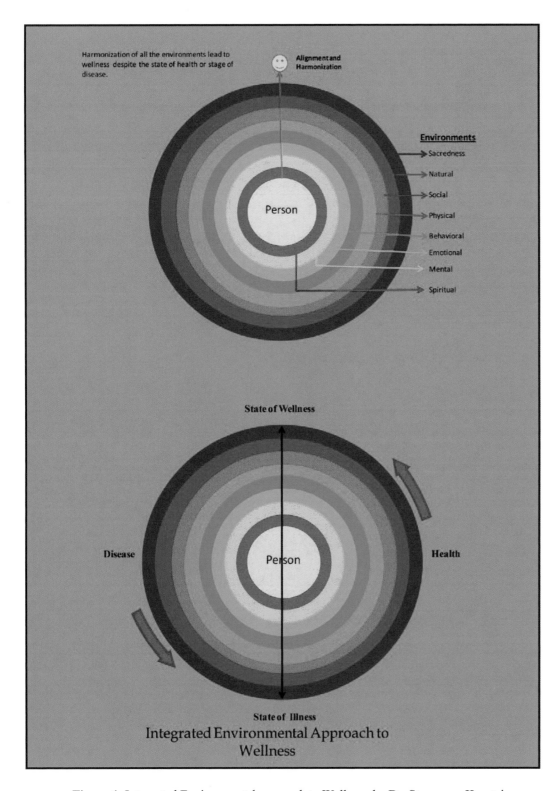

Figure 1. Integrated Environmental approach to Wellness by Dr. Stevenson Kuartei

CHAPTER TWO: CHRONIC DISEASE

Chuab is one of the most popular demigods in Palauan mythology[1]. She was a heavy eater, beyond comparison to others, and grew very quickly. People built an especially large house for her, but she soon grew too large for it. They carried abundant food to her every day to satisfy her appetite, but the food became scarce. Perplexed, they decided to kill her, and piled up firewood at her feet and set fire to it. Chuab struggled hard to escape from the fire, but eventually fell down and died (Machiko 2002).

Chronic diseases—such as heart disease, cancer, and diabetes—are leading causes of death and disability in Palau in addition to being major causes of limitations for many of its citizens. Combined into a single category, heart and cardiovascular disease is Palau's leading cause of death. While the mortality rates for these diseases have fallen in recent years, it still remains the leading cause of death, with an actual rate that is still significantly higher than Palau's national goal. Hypertension (high blood pressure) and diabetes mellitus are diseases that have emerged as health challenges for Palau as the result of changes in lifestyle and eating habits. Both of these conditions are closely associated with being overweight and obesity.

In 2008, 44.9% of males over 20 were obese and 56.3% of females (compared to regional averages of 5.1 and 6.8% respectively) (WHO 2011). Unwillingness or inability to participate in physical exercise is a related problem closely linked to obesity.

Chronic disease continues to become even more prevalent as the socioeconomic status of the Republic continues to boom.

Heart Disease

There are many forms of heart disease which can affect the heart in various ways. The ultimate problem with all varieties of heart disease is the disruption of the vital pumping action of the heart. The diseases that fall under the umbrella of heart disease include diseases of blood vessels such as coronary artery disease, heart rhythm problems (arrhythmias), heart infections, and congenital (from birth) heart defects.

The term "heart disease" is often used interchangeably with "cardiovascular disease." Cardiovascular disease generally refers to conditions that involve narrowed or blocked blood vessels that can lead to a heart attack, chest pain (angina) or stroke. Other heart conditions, such as infections and conditions that affect the heart's muscle, valves or rhythm, are also considered forms of heart disease. Most forms of heart disease can be prevented or treated with healthy lifestyle choices.

Cancer

Cancer refers to any one of a large number of diseases characterized by the development of abnormal cells that divide uncontrollably and have the ability to infiltrate and destroy normal body tissue. A simple way to explain cancer is an abnormal growth of cells. Normally, cells are created to replace those that die and to allow for growth. When cancer is present, cells reproduce at an unchecked rate. A tumor is a cluster of these cells that is capable of dividing uncontrollably. Because these cells do not function properly and often disrupt the normal function of healthy cells, they cause

---

[1] Chuab is discussed in various references as a male or female demigod. Many contemporary Palauans consider Chuab a male.

problems in the human body. A tumor can be malignant or benign. Benign tumors usually grow slowly and stay in one area, but malignant tumors spread rapidly and can destroy body tissue in the process. Cancer also has the ability to spread throughout the body (metastasize).

Diabetes

Diabetes is a disease that occurs when a person's body does not make enough of the hormone insulin or cannot use insulin properly. There are 2 types of diabetes. People with Type 1 diabetes are completely unable to produce insulin. People with Type 2 diabetes can produce insulin, but their cells do not respond to it. In either case, glucose cannot move into the cells and blood glucose levels increase. Over time, these high glucose levels cause serious complications.

Chapter Two discusses six botanical treatments for chronic disease in Palau.

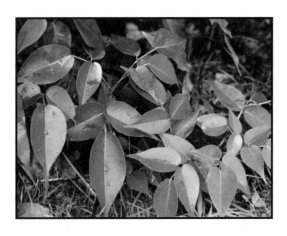

Figure 2. Leaves of *Derris trifoliata*. [MB]

Local names: *kemokem* (Palauan); common derris (English)
Scientific name: *Derris trifoliata* Lour.
Family: Fabaceae (Legume Family)

Description
Woody vine or liana, frequent near sea level, sometimes on limestone cliffs and on the edges of mangrove swamps. The calyx is pale green; the petals are pale pink or greenish white. The fruits are subreniform to oblong, usually 3-4.5 × 2-3.5 cm, with a wing 1-2 mm broad along the upper suture, and the 1 or 2 seeds are 1.5-2.5 cm long (Smith 1985).

Range
Eastern Africa to tropical Asia, eastward through Malaysia to Australia and into the Pacific as far as Tonga and Samoa, sometimes cultivated and naturalized elsewhere (Smith 1985). Native to Palau (Hillmann Kitalong, DeMeo & Holm 2008).

Traditional Uses
Medicine to treat diabetes. Seven young leaves are boiled in water and consumed every day [Kerengel Tesei, Eriko Singeo, Raphaela Sumang].

Pharmacological Properties
A dichloromethane/methanol root extract of the related plant, *Derris indica*, displayed antihyperglycemic activity in a glucose-tolerance test in a healthy rat model, and also displayed alpha-glucosidase inhibition (Ranga Rao *et al.*, 2009).

Toxicology
No cytotoxicity was reported for any of the rotenoids isolated from *Derris trifoliata* (Tewtrakul, Cheenpracha & Karalai 2009). No mortality or changes in behavior were observed with oral doses of the related species, *D. brevipes*, up to 600 mg/kg in rats, although antifertility effects were observed (Badami *et al.*, 2003).

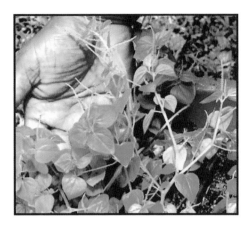

Figure 3. *Peperomia pellucida.* [MB]

Local names: *rtertiil*, *rtiil* (Palauan)
Scientific name: *Peperomia pellucida* (L.) Kunth
Family: Piperaceae (Pepper Family)

Description
A terrestrial or occasionally epiphytic herb usually 20-45 cm high. Occurs at elevations from sea level to about 400 m. As a weed, it grows along roadsides, in plantations, on damp ground in shady places near houses, and occasionally along forest trails. Flowering and fruiting throughout the year (Smith 1981).

Range
Tropical America, but now widely dispersed as a weed throughout tropical areas (Smith 1981). It was introduced to Palau (Hillmann Kitalong, DeMeo & Holm 2008).

Traditional Uses
Medicine for healing arthritis & gout. Gather 1 handful of leaves and stems, not the roots, then boil with 1 gal of water for 15-25 min. Drink 8 oz, morning and evening every day [Ingas Spesungel].

Pharmacological Properties
An aqueous extract of the aerial parts of *Peperomia pellucida* exhibited anti-inflammatory and analgesic activity in rats and mice, respectively, after oral administration (de Fatima Arrigoni-Blank *et al.*, 2004).

Toxicology
The LD_{50} was determined to be 5,000 mg/kg orally in rats and mice, indicating low toxicity (de Fatima Arrigoni-Blank *et al.*, 2004).

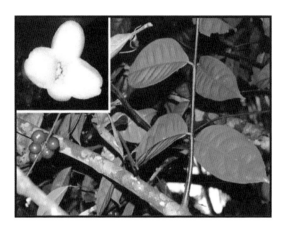

Figure 4. *Phaleria nisidai* fruits and leaves, with inset showing flower. [AK & CT]

Local names: *ongael*, *delalakar* (Palauan); mother of medicine (English)
Scientific name: *Phaleria nisidai* Kaneh.
Family: Thymelaeaceae (Mezereum Family)

Description
A ca. 15 m tall tree with opposite leaves, 15-20 cm long, 7-8 cm wide; the corolla tube is white, 15 mm long (Kanehira 1933). The drupe is red at maturity. It is native to Palau (Hillmann Kitalong, DeMeo & Holm 2008).

Range

Malaysia, New Britain, New Guinea, and the Western Carolines (van Steenis & van Steenis-Kruseman 1972). In Palau, it grows in volcanic lowland and freshwater swamp forests (Hillmann Kitalong, DeMeo & Holm 2008).

Traditional Uses

Medicine for serious internal problems such as liver/pancreatic cancers. Use leaves, mixed with other ingredients [Clarence Kitalong].

Medicine considered as mother of medicines (a panacea and energizing tonic). Boil 5-7 leaves in one gal of water for 3 min and let cool. Drink throughout the day. Make new concoction everyday [Eriko Singeo, Dirraklang Merei Ngirametuker].

Pharmacological Properties

A crude ethanolic extract of *Phaleria nisidai* inhibited a tumor-induced reduction of immunostimulatory cytokines and decreased tumor size in carcinoma-bearing mice (Matsuda *et al.*, 2005a).

Toxicology

No reports of toxicity were identified.

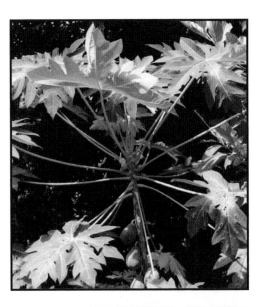

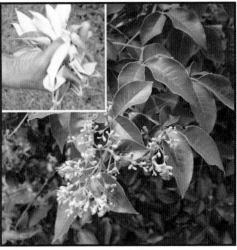

Figure 5. *Carica papaya* leaves, flowers, and fruits. [AK] (above); *Vitex trifolia* var. *trifolia* leaves and flowers, with inset showing four harvested branch tips [CT & AK] (below)

Local and scientific names:

bobai (Palauan); papaya (English) - *Carica papaya* L. (Caricaceae)
kelsechedui (Palauan); simple-leaf chastetree, Arabian lilac (English) - *Vitex trifolia* L. var. *trifolia* (Lamiaceae)

Descriptions

Carica papaya L.: A fast growing tree, reaching 2-10 m in height. The trunk is soft and fibrous with large leaf scars. The fruit is a fleshy berry, weighing up to 9 kg. The skin may be yellow or green when ripe and the flesh is orange. The seeds are numerous, black and wrinkled (Smith 1981).

Vitex trifolia L. var. *trifolia:* Small tree or shrub with leaves 3- or 5-foliolate; the central leaflets are petiolulate, the blades pubescent on both surfaces and oblong-elliptic to ovate-lanceolate. Flowers sessile; grayish to white, 2-4 mm long, 1.5-3 mm broad (Smith 1991).

Ranges

Carica papaya L.: Probably originated from Central America and spread to other tropical regions during the European colonial period. Currently, it is cultivated extensively throughout the tropical regions for its edible fruit (Smith 1981).

Vitex trifolia L. var. *trifolia*: Southeastern Asia to southern Africa and Indian Ocean islands and eastward through Malaysia and northern Australia to Polynesia (Smith 1991). Introduced to Palau and found growing in areas that typically have cultivated landscape with ornamental plants (Hillmann Kitalong, DeMeo & Holm 2008).

Traditional Uses

Medicine for reducing high blood pressure. Four branch tips of *kelsechedui* (*Vitex trifolia*) including flowers, fruits and leaves, four of the longest tips (opposite petiole) of *bobai* (*Carica papaya*) are boiled with 4 cups of water and consumed hot, 3× daily [Kerungil Augustin].

Pharmacological Properties

Carica papaya L.: Demonstrates antioxidant and anti-inflammatory properties that can reduce the severity of local inflammation (Mikhal'chick *et al.*, 2004) and has antimicrobial effects (Dawkins *et al.*, 2003; Starley *et al.*, 1999).

Vitex trifolia L. var. *trifolia*: An aqueous extract of the leaves of *V. trifolia* inhibited inflammatory cytokine expression and increased levels of the inflammatory regulator cytokine IL-10 in RAW 264.7 macrophages (Matsui *et al.*, 2009). Vitexicarpin, isolated from the hexane extract of this plant, was able to block the effects of histamine released from sensitized mast cells in isolated guinea pig trachea (Alam *et al.*, 2002).

Toxicology

Carica papaya L.: Due to the powerful effects of some of the compounds in *Carica papaya*, oral use should be avoided by young children and pregnant women. Use of *C. papaya* should also be limited to no more than 7 consecutive days (Germosen-Robineau 1998). *Carica papaya* may possess abortifacient activity (Anuar *et al.*, 2008). Allergic reactions to *C. papaya* are common, with anaphylaxis occuring in 1% of the patients studied (Iwu 1993). People allergic to latex may have an allergic reaction to papain, an enzyme that degrades polypeptides (Quarre *et al.*, 1995). Change in the structure or function of the esophagus in humans may occur with an oral dose of 71 mg/kg (Davis, Thomas & Guice 1987).

Vitex trifolia L. var. *trifolia*: No reports of toxicity were identified.

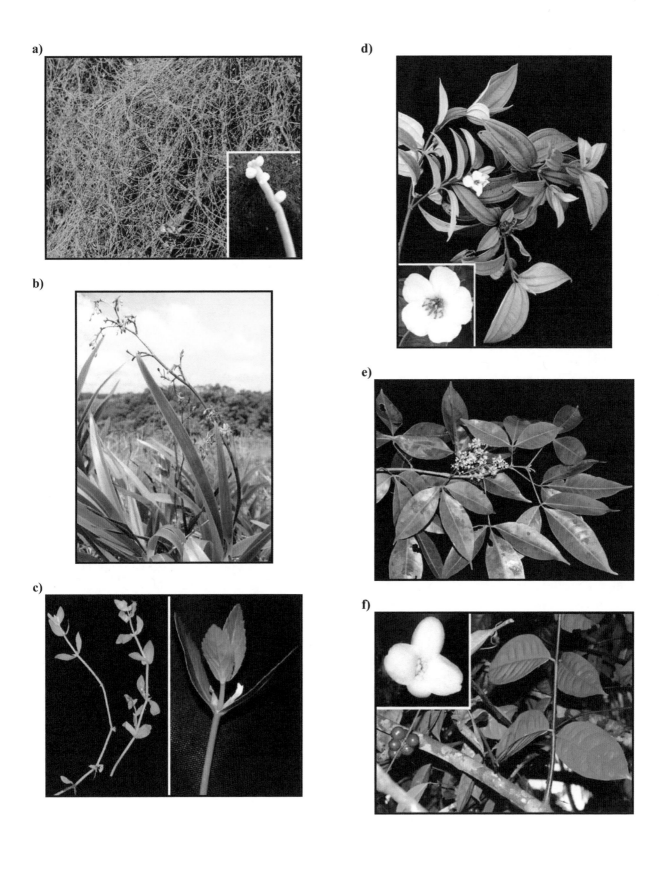

g)

Figure 6. **a)** *Cassytha filiformis* with inset showing flowers. [MB]; **b)** *Dianella carolinensis* leaves and flowers. [CT]; **c)** *Limnophila chinensis* subsp. *aromatica* leaves and close-up of flowers. [MB & WL]; **d)** *Melastoma malabathricum* L. var. *mariannum* leaves, flower, and fruit, with inset showing close-up of flower. [MB & AK]; **e)** *Melicope denhamii* leaves and flowers. [WL]; **f)** *Phaleria nisidai* fruits and leaves, with inset showing flower. [AK & CT]; **g)** *Phyllanthus palauensis* with inset showing flowers. [SP]

Local and Scientific names:
techellelachull (Palauan); laurel dodder (English) - *Cassytha filiformis* L. (Lauraceae)
kobesos (Palauan) - *Dianella carolinensis* Laut. (Xanthorrhoeaceae)
iaml (Palauan); rice paddy herb (English) - *Limnophila chinensis* (Osb.) Merr. subsp. *aromatica* (Lam.) Yamazaki (Scrophulariaceae)
matakui (Palauan) - *Melastoma malabathricum* L. var. *mariannum* (Naudin) Fosb. & Sach. (Melastomataceae)
kertub (Palauan) - *Melicope denhamii* (Seem.) T.G. Hartley (Rutaceae)
ongael, ***delalakar*** (Palauan); mother of medicine (English) - *Phaleria nisidai* Kaneh. (Thymelaeaceae)
dudurs, ***ukellelachedib*** (Palauan) - *Phyllanthus palauensis* Hosok. (Phyllanthaceae)

Descriptions
Cassytha filiformis L.: Herbaceous parasitic vine. (Hillmann Kitalong, DeMeo & Holm 2008). Tepals are white and the immature fruit is green, becoming yellow and then white (Smith 1981).

Dianella carolinensis Laut.: A coarse herb, 1 m tall, with a subterranean rhizome, the leaves linear, crowded on stem base (Smith 1979). Flowers with racemiform branches, petals are bluish-gray and anthers are yellow. The fruit is a purple berry.

Limnophila chinensis (Osb.) Merr. subsp. *aromatica* (Lam.) Yamazaki: Herb, 5-50 cm tall. Leaves opposite or in whorls of 3 or 4, sessile, ovate-lanceolate, 0.5-5.3 × 0.2-1.5 cm. Flowers solitary, purple-red or blue corolla, 1-1.5 cm. Capsule compressed, broadly ellipsoid, 5 mm (Wu & Raven 1994).

Melastoma malabathricum L. var. *mariannum* (Naudin) Fosb. & Sach.: Shrub or small tree to 2 m. Leaf blades entire, glossy green superior and pale green inferior side, 3-7 nerved, with conspicuous cross-veins. Solitary flowers, petals 4-5 white, pink to red carpels and stamens (Smith 1985). Red fruits.

Melicope denhamii (Seem.) T. G. Hartley: Understory tree up to 14 m tall, 33 cm dbh. Stipules absent; leaves opposite, tri-foliolate compound, leaflets glabrous to hairy. Flowers 4 mm diameter, greenish white, placed in panicles. Fruits 5 mm diameter, greenish, dehiscent capsules [T. Flynn 6410].

Phaleria nisidai Kaneh.: A ca. 15 m tall tree with opposite leaves, 15-20 cm long, 7-8 cm wide; the corolla tube is white, 15 mm long (Kanehira 1933). The drupe is red at maturity. It is native to Palau (Hillmann Kitalong, DeMeo & Holm 2008).

Phyllanthus palauensis Hosok.: Shrub to 1 m tall. Brown bracts; flowers and young fruits green. It is found growing in the savanna grassland (Hillmann Kitalong, DeMeo & Holm 2008).

Ranges
Cassytha filiformis L.: Cosmopolitan in tropical areas, occurring abundantly in most Pacific archipelagos (Smith 1981). Native to Palau, found growing in savannah, grassland, and freshwater swamp forest (Hillmann Kitalong, DeMeo & Holm 2008).

Dianella carolinensis Laut.: Species in this genus are found in tropical Asia to Australia, New Zealand, and the Pacific Islands (Smith 1979). There is only one species found in Palau, which is native and found growing in the savanna grasslands (Hillmann Kitalong, DeMeo & Holm 2008).

Limnophila chinensis (Osb.) Merr. subsp. *aromatica* (Lam.) Yamazaki: The genus is paleotropical (Smith 1991). This species is native to Palau and found growing on marshes that are areas of freshwater grasses, sedges, reeds, and other herbaceous plants (Hillmann Kitalong, DeMeo & Holm 2008).

Melastoma malabathricum L. var. *mariannum* (Naudin) Fosb. & Sach.: Southeastern Asia and the Seychelles through Malaysia into Australia and Polynesia (Smith 1985). Native to Palau and found growing on marshes that are areas of freshwater grasses, sedges, reeds, and other herbaceous plants (Hillmann Kitalong, DeMeo & Holm 2008).

Melicope denhamii (Seem.) T. G. Hartley: Indonesia and the Philippines to New Guinea and the Western Pacific. Native to Palau and found growing in volcanic lowland forests (Hillmann Kitalong, DeMeo & Holm 2008).

Phaleria nisidai Kaneh.: Malaysia, New Britain, New Guinea, and the Western Carolines (van Steenis & van Steenis-Kruseman 1972). In Palau it grows in volcanic lowland forest and in freshwater swamp forest (Hillmann Kitalong, DeMeo & Holm 2008).

Phyllanthus palauensis Hosok.: This is endemic to Palau (Hillmann Kitalong, DeMeo & Holm 2008).

Traditional Uses
Medicine for strengthening the heart.
Dianilla carolinensis (*kobesos*), *Phaleria nisidai* (*ongael*), *Limnophila aromatica* (*iaml*), *Cassytha filiformis* (*techelelachull*), *Melicope denhamii* (*kertub*), *Phyllanthus palauensis* (*dudurs*), and *Melastoma malabathricum* var. *mariannum* (*matakui*) are boiled together and consumed for the treatment of a weak heart. All plant parts are used except the roots. The plants are boiled together until the liquid is light yellow-green. The resulting decoction is bitter. It can be taken hot or cold, but tastes less bitter if taken warm. It can be kept at room temperature or cold. The treatment is usually taken in the morning, after food. The remaining liquid can be reheated without adding new leaves, with the addition of more water, until the liquid turns yellow-green again. The decoction is thrown away when the bitter flavor becomes weak. The treatment can be taken every day. The approximate dose if taken 1× daily is a 10 cc cough syrup dosage cap; a smaller dose can be used if administered 3× per day. The treatment is considered strong, and dose is taken appropriate to the weight of patient; taking too much causes dizziness [Dirraklang Merei Ngirametuker].

Pharmacological Properties
Cassytha filiformis L.: The crude ethanolic extract as well as alkaloids and flavonoids isolated from *C. filiformis* demonstrated vasorelaxing effects on precontracted rat aorta preparations (Tsai, Wang & Lin 2008). Compounds isolated from this plant showed inhibition of platelet aggregation induced by

arachidonic acid, collagen, ADP and platelet-activating factor (Chang *et al.*, 1998).

Dianella carolinensis Laut.: No pharmacological reports relevant to this use were identified.

Limnophila chinensis (Osb.) Merr. subsp. *aromatica* (Lam.) Yamazaki: An ethanol extract possessed anti-inflammatory properties, suppressing nitric oxide and tumor necrosis factor-alpha production by lipopolysaccharide-activated RAW 264.7 macrophages (Tuntipopipat, Muangnoi & Failla 2009).

Melastoma malabathricum L. var. *mariannum* (Naudin) Fosb. & Sach.: *Melastoma malabathricum* contains anti-inflammatory compounds such as flavonoids, quercetin, and pentacyclic triterpenes (Mazura, Susanti & Rasadah 2007).

Melicope denhamii (Seem.) T. G. Hartley: Several isolated compounds from related species (*Melicope semecarpifolia* and *M. confusa*) inhibited platelet aggregation *in vitro* (Chen, K.S. *et al.*, 2000; Chen, I.S. *et al.*, 2001; Chou *et al.*, 2005).

Phaleria nisidai Kaneh.: No pharmacological reports relevant to this use were identified.

Phyllanthus palauensis Hosok.: Various extracts of the related plants, *Phyllanthus polyphyllus*, *P. urinaria*, and *P. amarus*, showed anti-inflammatory effects on isolated gastric and hepatic cells, as well as systemically through a PAF receptor-mediated mechanism (Rao, Fang & Tzeng 2006; Lai *et al.*, 2008; Kiemer *et al.*, 2003; Fang, Rao & Tzeng 2008; Lin *et al.*, 2008; Kassuya *et al.*, 2006). A butanol extract of the leaves of another related plant, *Phyllanthus acidus*, decreased blood pressure in rats due to stimulation of nitric oxide release from the vascular endothelium (Leeya *et al.*, 2010).

Toxicology

Cassytha filiformis L.: A toxicological assessment of an aqueous extract of the stems and leaves revealed that a daily oral dose of 250-1,000 mg/kg for 28 days decreased levels of alkaline phosphatase and increased levels of serum cholesterol in rats. A decrease in relative weights of the heart and lung was also observed. The oral LD_{50} was determined to be greater than 500 mg/kg (Babayi *et al.*, 2007).

Dianella carolinensis Laut.: The related species, *Dianella revoluta,* is suspected in livestock poisoning and physiological disturbances in man when ingested. (Colegate, Dorling & Huxtable 1986, 1987). Isolation of the toxic compounds dianellidin, dianellinone, and stypandrol from *D. revoluta* indicates that possible caution should be exercised when ingesting this plant (Colegate, Dorling & Huxtable 1987, 1986). Stypandrol, isolated from *D. revoluta*, has been reported to induce toxicosis in goats and sheep, with acute intoxication causing weakness and paralysis of the hind limbs, sometimes leading to death (Dias, Silva & Urban 2009).

Limnophila chinensis (Osb.) Merr. subsp. *aromatica* (Lam.) Yamazaki: No reports of toxicity were identified.

Melastoma malabathricum L. var. *mariannum* (Naudin) Fosb. & Sach.: Oral doses up to 2,000 mg/kg of a cold water extract of *M. malabathricum* leaves showed no signs of toxicity in mice (Sunilson *et al.*, 2009).

Melicope denhamii (Seem.) T. G. Hartley: No reports of toxicity have been identified.

Phaleria nisidai Kaneh.: No reports of toxicity were identified.

Phyllanthus palauensis Hosok.: Aqueous extracts of the related species, *Phyllanthus amarus,* at 400 mg/kg was toxic to blood cells, promoted weight loss, and caused testicular degeneration in rats (Adedapo *et al.*, 2005; Adedapo, Adegbayibi & Emikpe 2005). Mice given 100 mg/kg of whole plant alcohol extracts of *P. amarus* were unable to get pregnant, possibly due to hormonal interference (Rao & Alice 2001). Chronic oral administration of the aqueous extract of the leaves of *P. amarus* caused hematological and histopathological changes indicative of potential toxicity in rats (Adedapo, Adegbayibi & Emikpe 2005).

a)

b)

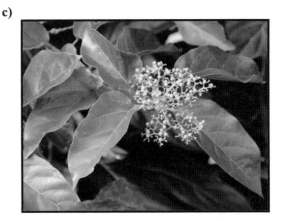

Figure 7. a) *Morinda citrifolia* leaves and fruit, with inset showing flower, flower buds, and fruit. [MB & AK]; **b)** *Piper betle* f. *densum* climbing vine. [MB]; **c)** *Premna serratifolia* leaves and flower buds. [MB]

Local and Scientific names:
ngel (Palauan); noni (English) - *Morinda citrifolia* L. (Rubiaceae)
kebui (Palauan); betel nut leaf (English) - *Piper betle* L. f. *densum* (Blume) Fosb. (Piperaceae)
chosm (Palauan) - *Premna serratifolia* L. (Lamiaceae)

Descriptions
Morinda citrifolia L.: A small tree 3 to 8 m in height, with a dbh of 10-30 cm and hairless, 4-angled stems. The simple, opposite, elliptic leaves are up to 45 cm long and 25 cm wide. The margins are entire, the surfaces are glossy, hairless and pliable, the stout petiole is up to 2 cm long. The flowers are borne in 75 to 90 flowered, oval to globe-like heads on a stalk about 3 cm long, with the calyx having a truncate rim with no lobes. The white corolla has 5 lobes that are slightly curled backward. The flower stalk is 1 to 3 cm long. The yellowish white, fleshy, soft and odiferous, irregular heads are about 5 cm long and 3 to 4 cm wide. The fruits have a wart-like appearance (Hillmann Kitalong, DeMeo & Holm 2008).

Piper betle L. f. *densum* (Blume) Fosb.: A woody climbing vine with dimorphic branching; leaf blades ovate, usually 12-20 × 6-12 cm, rachis of fruiting spike accrescent, at least 3 mm in diameter at maturity, the fruits congested or coalescent (Smith 1981).

Premna serratifolia L.: Low shrub or small tree, growing to 10 m in height, with compressed branchlets. The leaves are opposite, round to oval in shape, and 0.5-8 cm in length. The inflorescences are up to 2 cm in length, with small white cup-shaped calyces. The fruits are round, 2-4 mm in diameter, green ripening to black (Smith 1991).

Ranges

Morinda citrifolia L.: Indigenous to Indo-Malaysia, *Morinda citrifolia* ranges throughout the Pacific to Hawaiian Islands and other tropical regions around the world. In coastal forests, it is established as an understory plant often found near creeks, alongside the edge of mangrove swamps, and can be found growing up to 137 m above sea level (Smith 1988). In Palau, it is found along the volcanic forest edge and savanna (Hillmann Kitalong, DeMeo & Holm 2008).

Piper betle L. f. *densum* (Blume) Fosb.: A native of central and eastern Malaysia, but spreading in comparatively early times throughout tropical Asia and Malaysia, and later to Madagascar and eastern Africa. It is now cultivated in many other tropical areas, apparently being a recent introduction to places like Fiji (Smith 1981). Native in Palau, and grows in volcanic lowland forest and agroforest areas of cultivated forest and crop plants (Hillmann Kitalong, DeMeo & Holm 2008).

Premna serratifolia L.: A lowland species ranging from eastern Africa to Sri Lanka, southeastern Asia, the Ryuku Islands, Taiwan, Malaysia, and tropical Australia to the southern Pacific Islands. *Premna serratifolia* is found growing in beach thickets, dry lowland forest, along rocky shores, on the edges of mangrove swamps, and in agroforest areas (Balick *et al.*, 2009; Smith 1991). Native to Palau (Hillmann Kitalong, DeMeo & Holm 2008).

Traditional Uses

Medicine used for weight loss. Eight leaves of either *kebui* (*Piper betle*) or *kesebibui* (*P. hosokawae* Fosb.), *ngel* (*Morinda citrifolia*), *chosm* (*Premna serratafolia*), and 4 unripe fruits of *ngel* (*M. citrifolia*) are collected. The leaves of *Morinda* and *Premna* should not be the young new leaves but leaves right after the young stage (*omalk*). For the *Piper* leaf, the thickest leaves should be picked (*chedesaoch*) to make sure they are not yellow leaves. The ingredients are combined in a pot along with 1 gal of water and boiled. It needs to boil for 10 min and then cool it and drink. You can drink this instead of water, eat a normal diet but avoid sweets [Linda Omekat Belaio].

Pharmacological Properties

Morinda citrifolia L.: The fermented fruit juice (2 mL/kg) administered twice daily for 20 days to diabetic rats significantly reduced blood glucose levels (Nayak *et al.*, 2011). Damnacanthal, a compound isolated from the roots, increases antitumorigenic activity in human colorectal cancer cells (Nualsanit *et al.*, 2011), as well as epidermoid and cervical cancers (Thani *et al.*, 2010).

Piper betle L. f. *densum* (Blume) Fosb.: No pharmacological reports relevant to this use were identified.

Premna serratifolia L.: No pharmacological reports relevant to this use were identified.

Toxicology

Morinda citrifolia L.: Two publications reported three cases of liver toxicity linked to the ingestion of noni juice (Millonig, Stadelmann & Vogel 2005; Stadlbauer *et al.,* 2005). Some researchers believe that the risk of liver toxicity is unlikely due to very low concentrations of potentially hepatotoxic anthraquinones (Kamiya *et al.,* 2005; Pawlus *et al.,* 2005). *Morinda citrifolia* juice did not show any genotoxicity and the author concluded that pure *M. citrifolia* juice is safe for human consumption (Westendorf *et al.,* 2007).

Piper betle L. f. *densum* (Blume) Fosb.: No toxicological reports were identified for *Piper betle* or *P. hosokawae*.

Premna serratifolia L.: Isolated compounds from the chloroform extract of the leaves of the related species, *Premna tomentosa*, had carcinogenic effects on a healthy cell line (Chin *et al.*, 2006).

NOTES

CHAPTER THREE: BITES AND STINGS

Bites and stings are a common occurrence around the world, as many animals and other living creatures will bite when startled, scared, or provoked. Injuries sustained from bites can range from superficial scratches to deep, life-threatening wounds. If left untreated, bites can become infected by the bacteria passed from the mouth of the animal to the victim. Some animals and insects inject venom and others are poisonous when consumed or touched. These toxins have a wide range of noxious effects ranging from mild to life-threatening. Proper care requires wound inspection for injury to deeper structures, wound care, and decisions regarding closure of the wound, prophylactic antibiotics for wounds at high risk for infection, possible administration of antivenom and prophylaxis for tetanus and rabies as determined necessary by a qualified medical professional.

Anaphylactic Shock

Bites and stings may cause severe allergic reactions within minutes after exposure. Anaphylactic shock, the most severe allergic reaction, is a dramatic response by the body exposed to an allergen, an allergy-causing substance. When anaphylaxis occurs, blood vessels begin to leak fluid into the surrounding tissue causing blood pressure to drop quickly. During anaphylaxis, the flow and volume of blood decreases and less oxygen is delivered to the rest of the body, worsening functions of the brain and other vital organs (lungs, kidneys, etc). **This is a life-threatening situation that requires immediate treatment**. The body's response is to release antigens (substance capable of inducing a specific immune response). The antigens bind to mast cells that release many chemical mediators, notably histamine, which causes vasodilation that reduces blood pressure and causes local and systemic symptoms of anaphylaxis. Signs and symptoms of histamine release include: swelling in the skin, red rash and severe itching. **Anyone demonstrating sudden swelling and/or difficulty breathing should be brought to the hospital, clinic, public health outpost, or doctor's office for immediate treatment**.

Substances that can cause anaphylactic shock are:
- Bites and stings
- Certain foods and food additives
- Medicines such as penicillin or other antibiotics, or sulfur-containing drugs

Symptoms of anaphylactic shock are:
- Rapid pulse
- Difficulty breathing and/or shortness of breath
- Swelling of the lips, tongue or throat
- Hives (raised pink areas that arise quickly after exposure to a bite, sting or in allergic reactions)
- Pale, cool, damp skin
- Feeling faint (weak)
- Drowsiness, confusion, or loss of consciousness

Treatment of Anaphylactic Shock

Anaphylactic shock is an emergency situation and requires immediate treatment from a doctor. If you suspect shock (see symptoms listed above), take the person to an emergency room or medical facility immediately. If the person has stopped breathing call immediately for help and perform rescue breathing; additionally, if the person has no pulse, perform cardiopulmonary resuscitation (CPR).

Prevention of Anaphylactic Shock

Any person who has known allergies to bites/stings or food or has previously suffered from anaphylactic shock should carry a self-injecting form of epinephrine (Epipen) for use when a doctor is not available.

Simple First Aid for Bites and Stings

The goal in first aid is to immediately determine whether a life-threatening situation is developing (i.e. anaphylactic shock). After any immediate threats have been eliminated or treated, the next objective is to prevent the injury from worsening (i.e. enlargement of the wound) or further illness (infection or toxic reaction). All wounds should be cleaned with warm water and soap and any foreign material should be removed (stingers, insect parts) to prevent infection. Large openings (lacerations) in need of suturing should be closed (sutured) within 8-10 hours. After 24 hours, the risk of infection is too great to close a wound and the wound should be left open if it is superficial. Open wounds that require washing can be irrigated with boiled water (boiled for at least five minutes and allowed to cool) or sterile saline. A simple technique for irrigating wounds is pouring water over the wound for two minutes and letting the overflow carry out foreign debris (i.e. dirt). Most wounds can be dressed or covered after they have been cleaned, with sterile dry gauze or Band-Aid for small wounds. It is important to monitor wounds for signs of infection. An infected wound will appear red, swollen, hot, and painful (rubor, tumor, calor, and dolor). There may be pus or a foul smell. If the infection has spread to the rest of the body there will be fever, a red line may form above the wound, or the lymph nodes may become swollen and tender. Other clinical manifestations of bite and wound infections may include fever, erythema, swelling, tenderness, purulent drainage and lymphangitis. If any of these signs of infection are suspected, seek immediate medical attention (Werner, Thuman & Maxwell 1992).

Animal Bites

The most frequent animal bites are dog (*bilis*) and cat (*kato*) bites. Dogs account for the majority of bites and their bites tend to be ragged. Cat bites tend to be deeper and frequently become infected. Bites should be cleaned thoroughly and dressed immediately, and any severed parts should be closed (if a ligament or tendon is torn, it should be treated at the hospital). Facial wounds should be surgically closed. Hand wounds, if small, should be left open. Antibiotics should be prescribed. At this point, botanical medicines may be added; the wound dressings and medicines should be changed daily.

Human Bites

Human bites generally become bruises and rarely cause deep tears because human teeth are not sharp. If the bite breaks the skin, the person should take oral antibiotics to prevent infection. The wounds should be cleaned thoroughly. Topical applications of plant remedies (such as a poultice held together by a clean cotton gauze or cloth) could be used to prevent swelling, but should be changed daily, taking care to wash the area clean with sterile water each time.

Stingray Stings

Stingrays (*rrull*) have venomous barbs on the back of their tails. The majority of stings result from accidentally stepping on the stingray while walking in shallow water. Fragments can remain in the wound and should be removed to prevent infection. The venom is inactivated by heat, thus pain can be relieved by putting the limb in hot water for 30-90 minutes. After the wound is cleaned, traditional botanical medicines can be applied but should be changed daily to prevent infection.

Stonefish, Scorpionfish, Sea Urchin, and Crown of Thorn Stings

Stinging fish cause redness and swelling in the affected area. The fish usually have venom in the dorsal spine that is sensitive to heat. Soaking the limb in hot water for 30-90 minutes will reduce the pain of stonefish (*smuuch*), scorpionfish (*chesechid*), sea urchin (*cheualech*), and crown of thorn (*rrusech*) stings. Sea urchin spines can be dissolved in undiluted white vinegar. After the wound is cleaned, botanical medicines can be added but should be changed daily to prevent infection.

Coral, Sea Anemone, and Jellyfish Stings

Most corals (*marangd*), sea anemones (*etermall*), and jellyfish (*bidabd*, *butcherengel*, *chedead*), stings result in a painful rash. The rash can develop into blisters that fill with pus. The following is a general treatment suggested by the Merck Manual (Beers, Porter & Jones 2003):
- First, pour ocean water over the area (not freshwater)
- Soak the injured area in a solution of vinegar for 30-60 sec
- Remove the tentacles [by scraping them off using a hard-edged object (i.e. credit card or ruler). Do not use your hands as this might result in further stings]
- Pour flour or baking soda over the wound and carefully scrape the powder off with a sterilized knife
- Soak the area in vinegar again
- Apply an ointment or cream that has antihistamine (Benadryl) and/or anti-inflammatory properties (cortisone), and/or consider applying traditional botanical medicines as mentioned in this chapter

Stings and Rashes from Insects

Stings and certain parts of insects cause mild allergic reactions on the skin by creating hives or welts. This reaction is caused by the release of histamine. Treatment usually involves the application of a cream or salve to reduce the itching. An over-the-counter medication like Benadryl can be taken by mouth. The adult dose is 25-50 mg every six hours. The use of medications such as Benadryl (Diphenhydramine), which are from a class of medications called antihistamines, can cause sleepiness. It should be used as directed by a health care practitioner.

Chapter Three discusses six different plant species that have been reported to treat bites and stings of various animals, insects, and sea creatures.

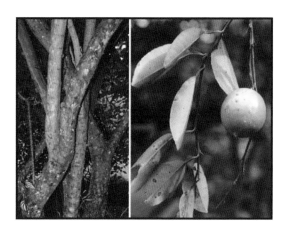

Figure 8. *Citrus aurantiifolia* branches and close-up of leaves and fruit. [WL]

Local names: *malchianged* (Palauan); bitter orange (English)
Scientific name: *Citrus aurantiifolia* (Christm.) Swingle
Family: Rutaceae (Citrus Family)

Description
A tree, 4-8 m tall, usually with many short spines; petioles narrowly winged, leaf blades ovate-elliptic, 4-12 × 2-7 cm. Flowers are small, 2-2.5 cm in diameter, have pale pink to white petals, and the fruits are ovoid, 3-6 cm in diameter and greenish yellow when ripe, with thin, adherent peel and greenish, very acid fruit (Smith 1985).

Range
Probably indigenous to Malaysia, and has spread throughout the tropics and subtropics (Smith 1985).

Traditional Uses
Medicine used for stings. Use juice from fruit and apply to sting [Rufino Alii].

Pharmacological Properties
The extract of the related species, *Citrus maxima,* exhibited strong antimicrobial action against *Escherichia coli, Staphylococcus aureus,* and *Bacillus subtilis,* with low minimum inhibitory concentrations (Tao *et al.*, 2010). A crude hexane extract of this fruit was found to inhibit the growth of *Bacillus cereus, Bacillus subtilis, Listeria monocytogenes,* and *Staphylococcus aureus* in another study (Suklampoo *et al.*, 2010).

Toxicology
There are many case reports of photosensitization due to topical exposure to compounds present in the leaves and fruits of *Citrus aurantiifolia* in combination with sunlight. Symptoms are similar to severe sunburn (Goskowicz, Friedlander &

Lawrence 1994; Pomeranz & Karen 2007; Thomson *et al.*, 2007).

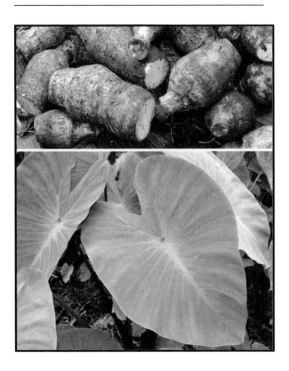

Figure 9. *Colocasia esculenta* harvested corms and leaves. [AL]

Local names: *dait* (Palauan); taro (English)
Scientific name: *Colocasia esculenta* L. Schott
Family: Araceae (Arum Family)

Description
Colocasia esculenta is an herb growing to 1 m in height with an underground corm. At the apex of this corm is a whorl of leaves. The leaves are 20-50 cm long, with an elongated oval shape. The lower lobes of the leaf may be rounded with dark red stems clasped at the base (Purseglove 1988).

Range
Colocasia esculenta originated from Southeast Asia. It is now widely cultivated for its edible corms, cormels, and leaves

throughout Africa, South and Southeast Asia, the Pacific and Caribbean Islands. Some varieties are also grown for their ornamental foliage (Lemmens & Bunyapraphatsara 2003; Purseglove 1988).

Traditional Uses
Medicine used to remove spine of urchin from foot. Wrap 5 leaves of *Colocasia esculenta* (*lel a dait*) with coconut oil around area where spine is [Clarence Kitalong].

Pharmacological Properties
The corm of *Colocasia esculenta* has been reported to have antiinflammatory properties (Cambie & Ferguson 2003).

Toxicology
There are reports of contact dermatitis associated with *Colocasia esculenta* (Lampe 1986). The leaves, stems and corms of uncooked *C. esculenta* contain calcium oxalate crystals and can cause injury to human mucous membranes (Nelson, Shih & Balick 2007).

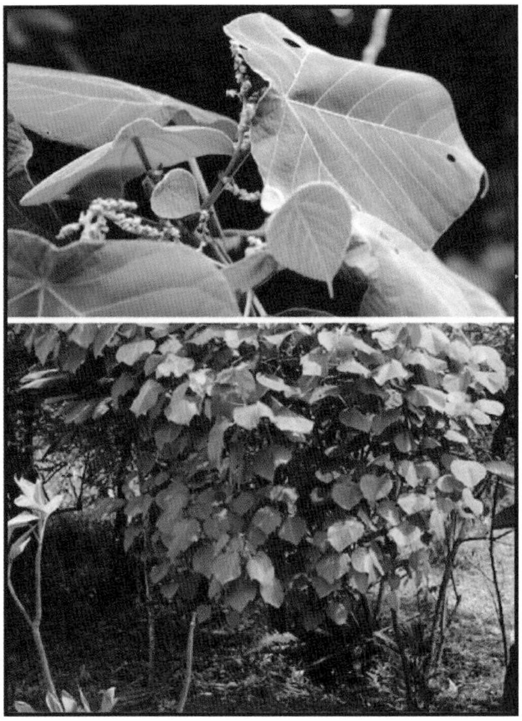

Figure 10. *Macaranga carolinensis* leaves and close-up of flowers (above); view of tree (below). [AK]

Local names: *bedel* (Palauan); macaranga (English)
Scientific name: *Macaranga carolinensis* Volk.
Family: Euphorbiaceae (Euphorbia Family)

Description
A small tree 3-10 m in height with a dbh of 3-40 cm. The simple, alternate, shield shaped leaves are 20-41 cm long, with hairy surfaces and veins radiating from one point. Male and female flowers both lack corollas and are found on separate plants (dioecious). The convex or flat-topped female cluster has the youngest flowers at the tip and is enclosed by a serrated triangular modified leaf and is borne on a stalk about 15 cm long. The male flowers are borne in a slender axillary compound cluster up to 25 cm long, with the youngest flowers at the tip. The solitary, globe-like, fuzzy capsules are about 5 mm

across (Hillmann Kitalong, DeMeo & Holm 2008).

Range

Macaranga carolinensis (*bedel*) is a fast-growing species common along forest edges, disturbed forests and secondary forests. It ranges from Indo-Malaya to Kosrae (Hillmann Kitalong, DeMeo & Holm 2008).

Traditional Uses

Styptic. Use any amount of leaves that fit in your mouth, chew and press the chewed leaves on the wound until the blood flow stops. There is no need to wrap the treatment onto the wound; wrapping is optional and for convenience [Dirraklang Merei Ngirametuker].

Pharmacological Properties

No pharmacological properties for *Macaranga carolinensis* were identified; however some related species in the genus *Macaranga* have shown antibacterial activity against *Escherichia coli* and *Micrococcus luteus* (Schutz *et al.*, 1995) and *Bacillus cereus, Micrococcus luteus*, and *Staphylococcus aureus* (Lim, Lim & Yule 2009).

Toxicology

No reports of toxicity were identified.

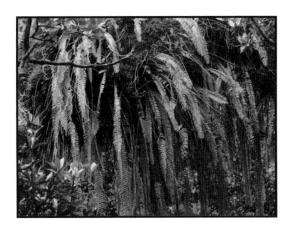

Figure 11. *Nephrolepis acutifolia.* [AK]

Local name: *delimes* (Palauan)
Scientific name: *Nephrolepis acutifolia* (Desv.) Christ
Family: Lomariopsidaceae (Sword Fern Family)

Description

A large epiphytic fern with short, erect, stoloniferous rhizomes and leathery fronds over 1 m long; the scaly rachises are red, with linear and marginal indusia; numerous pinnae (generally 20-50 pairs) (Hoshizaki & Moran 2001).

Range

Native to tropical Africa and from southeastern Asia to Polynesia (Hoshizaki & Moran 2001). Native to Palau and found growing in volcanic lowland forest and mangrove forest (Hillmann Kitalong, DeMeo & Holm 2008).

Traditional Uses

Antiseptic. Leaves are used as an antiseptic to clean wounds [Dirraklang Merei Ngirametuker, Gillian Johannes, Tsuneo Tesei, Kerngel Tesei].

Pharmacological Properties
No relevant pharmacological reports were identified.

Toxicology
Ferns of varying species, but not necessarily *Nephrolepis acutifolia*, have been shown to cause contact dermatitis in some patients (de Cock, Vorwerk & Bruynzeel 1998; Geller-Bernstein *et al.*, 1987; Stoof & Bruynzeel 1989).

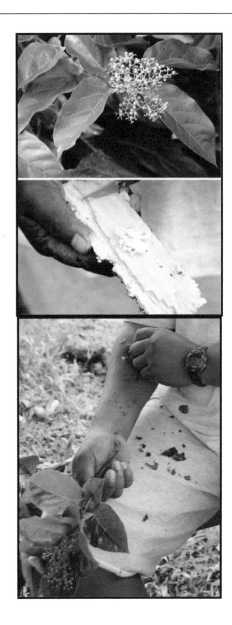

Figure 12. *Premna serratifolia* leaves, flowers, and inner bark. Also, crushed leaves rubbed on skin. [MB]

Local name: *chosm* (Palauan)
Scientific name: *Premna serratifolia* L.
Family: Lamiaceae (Mint Family)

Description
Premna serratifolia is a low shrub or small tree, growing to 10 m in height, with compressed branchlets. The leaves are opposite, round to oval in shape, and 0.5-8 cm in length. Inflorescences up to 2 cm in length, with small white cup-shaped calyces. The fruits are round, 2-4 mm in diameter, green ripening to black (Smith 1991).

Range
Premna serratifolia is a lowland species ranging from eastern Africa to Sri Lanka, southeastern Asia, the Ryuku Islands, Taiwan, Malaysia, and tropical Australia to the southern Pacific Islands. *Premna serratifolia* is found growing in beach thickets, dry lowland forest, along rocky shores, on the edges of mangrove swamps, and in agroforests (Balick 2009; Smith 1991). Native to Palau (Hillmann Kitalong, DeMeo & Holm 2008).

Traditional Uses
Medicine used for poison from fish spine. Remove the spine. Drip slime from inner bark of stem or branch of *chosm* (*Premna serratifolia*) onto a spoonful of coconut oil. Heat spoon from below and let the steam bathe the wound (*tabech*) [Tadashi Belchal, Risao Bausouch, Scott Yano]. Alternatively, you can heat the coconut oil and *chosm* slime mixture and apply directly to wound, and then bandage [Van-Ray Tadao].
Mosquito repellent. Crush 2-4 leaves and rub on arms and legs as mosquito repellent.

This can last for 2 hours, then reapply again [Henry Yuri].

Pharmacological Properties
The alcohol extract of the leaf of the related species, *Premna tomentosa,* possessed analgesic activity in rats (Devi *et al.,* 2003). Compounds isolated from the root nodule extract of another related species, *P. herbaceae* Roxb., enhanced antimicrobial activity against Gram-positive and Gram-negative bacteria (Murthy *et al.,* 2006). Compounds isolated from both of the related species, *P. schimperi* Engl. and *P. oligotricha* Baker showed *in vitro* antibacterial properties (Habtemariam *et al.,* 1990; Habtemariam, Gray & Waterman 1992).

Toxicology
Isolated compounds from the chloroform extract of the leaves of the related species, *Premna tomentosa,* had carcinogenic effects on a healthy cell line (Chin *et al.,* 2006).

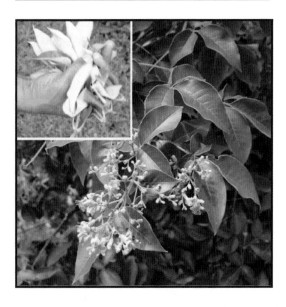

Figure 13. *Vitex trifolia* var. *trifolia* leaves and flowers, with inset showing four harvested branch tips [CT & AK]

Local names: *kelsechedui* (Palauan); simple-leaf chaste tree, Arabian lilac (English)
Scientific name: *Vitex trifolia* L. var. *trifolia*
Family: Lamiaceae (Mint Family)

Description
Small tree or shrub with leaves 3- or 5-foliolate, the central leaflets are petiolulate, the blades pubescent on both surfaces and oblong-elliptic to ovate-lanceolate. Flowers sessile; grayish to white, 2-4 mm long, 1.5-3 mm broad (Smith 1991).

Range
Southeastern Asia to southern Africa and Indian Ocean islands and eastward through Malaysia and northern Australia to Polynesia (Smith 1991). It was introduced to Palau and is now found growing in areas that typically have cultivated landscape with ornamental plants (Hillmann Kitalong, DeMeo & Holm 2008).

Traditional Uses
Mosquito repellent. Broken branches will emit odor which will keep mosquitoes away [Kerungil Augustin].

Pharmacological Properties
No pharmacological reports relevant to this use were identified.

Toxicology
No reports of toxicity were identified.

CHAPTER FOUR:
GASTROINTESTINAL DISORDERS

The condition of frequent, loose or liquid bowel movements is known as diarrhea. This occurs when stool, comprised of 60-90% water, is not effectively managed by the colon. In healthy individuals, the colon will reabsorb most of the water. When the colon does not absorb water, 90% of water is retained in the stool, resulting in diarrhea. This can range from mild to life-threatening. In most cases it is self-limiting, meaning that it resolves without medication, but requires that the patient drink enough fluids to prevent dehydration. **Caution: Seek immediate medical attention if diarrhea occurs for more than 72 hours, if there is blood in the stool, or if there is severe abdominal pain**.

Acute gastroenteritis or inflammation of the colon can result in diarrhea and ranks number four among the leading causes of hospital visits in Palau. Common symptoms that often accompany diarrhea include dehydration, nausea, bloating, cramping, increased mucus production, and gas. Children and the elderly are at greatest medical risk from diarrhea and often are the most susceptible. Diarrhea has many causes. Some of the most common causes of diarrhea include the following:

- Specific viral infections
- Bacterial infection or overgrowth (*Escherichia coli, Clostridium difficile*)
- Food poisoning
- Inability to digest dairy products
- Allergies to certain foods (especially seafood, crayfish, foods with sorbitol or a fat–free compound known as Olestra)

- Side effects of certain common medicines (antacids with magnesium and caffeine)
- Overuse of laxatives such as castor oil, bisacodyl, cascara, senna, sodium phosphate, lactulose, and docusate
- Blood in the stool which turns the stool black and increases gut movement or motility

Persistent diarrhea can also be caused by infectious organisms such as *Campylobacter*, *Yersinia* and parasites including *Giardia*, *Amoeba*, and *Cryptosporidium* that stimulate secretion. Chronic diarrhea can result from rare cancers of the gastrointestinal tract, overactive thyroid, inflammatory bowel disease, irritable bowel syndrome, tuberculosis, chronic HIV infection, and malaria. Diarrhea usually creates a condition of dehydration because the body is losing more water than it can take in.

The condition is worsened if vomiting occurs. Clinical signs of dehydration are:
- Increased thirst
- Dry/cracked lips
- Headaches
- A dark yellow color of the urine or little to no urination
- A dry mouth
- Sunken eyes
- Skin flushing
- A weak and rapid pulse
- Fatigue or weakness
- Changes in mental status

Treatment of Dehydration

Rehydrating the body is extremely important when you experience or treat symptoms of dehydration. Usually, in addition to loss of water (dehydration), sodium salts, potassium salts, and glucose (sugar) levels will be low in the body. Thus the primary objective of treatment is to restore water and electrolytes (specific mineral ions) back into the body lost through diarrhea. Powdered packets known as Oral Rehydration Salts (ORS) can be stirred into water or juice to rehydrate the body. Sports drinks, such as Gatorade® or Powerade®, can be used if available. In the tropics, coconut water is an effective alternative to ORS and other rehydration fluids.

A recipe for a homemade rehydration drink is:

- 1 liter of water
- ½ teaspoon of salt
- 8 level teaspoons of sugar
- Dilute this with half a cup of fruit juice, coconut water or mashed ripe banana (Werner, Thuman & Maxwell 1992)

If vomiting accompanies diarrhea, small sips of cool, not cold, water are advised. Intravenous fluids, if available, are helpful and occasionally even necessary to treat dehydration.

Chapter Four discusses 16 different plant remedies reported to treat diarrhea and gastric disorders on Palau.

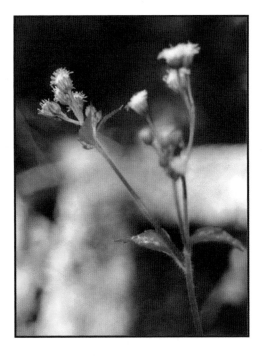

Figure 14. *Ageratum conyzoides* flowers. [RL]

Local names: *ngmak* (Palauan); goatweed, whiteweed (English)
Scientific name: *Ageratum conyzoides* L.
Family: Asteraceae (Daisy Family)

Description
Coarse herb 0.2-1 m high; opposite and simple leaves commonly subacute or obtuse to round at base; the corolla lobes and styles are white to pale lavender. Flowering heads usually 5-8 mm in diameter with 60-75 flowers. Flowering and fruiting observed throughout the year (Smith 1991).

Range
Mexico and the West Indies to South America, now often cultivated and established as an adventive in most warm countries. It was probably an early European introduction into the Pacific Islands as an ornamental (Smith 1991). Introduced to Palau and found growing in savanna grasslands and areas that typically have

cultivated landscape with ornamental plants (Hillmann Kitalong, DeMeo & Holm 2008).

Traditional Uses
Medicine used to treat dysentery and stomach trouble (gas). Decoction of boiled leaves is consumed (Del Rosario & Esguerra 2003).

Pharmacological Properties
A single oral dose of an *Ageratum conyzoides* ethanolic extract reduced gastric lesions in ibuprofen-, cold stress- and alcohol-induced ulcer models in rats (Shirwaikar *et al.*, 2003). The essential oil of the leaves of *A. conyzoides* was active against adult *Schistosoma mansoni* worms, the cause of schistosomiasis, and caused a reduction in number of eggs these worms produced (de Melo *et al.*, 2011).

Toxicology
No hepatotoxicity was observed with oral doses up to 500 mg/kg/day for 90 days in rats (Moura *et al.*, 2005).

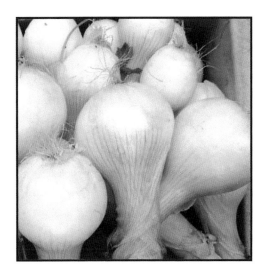

Figure 15. *Allium cepa* bulbs. [IA]

Local names: *sebulias* (Palauan); onion (English)
Scientific name: *Allium cepa* L.
Family: Liliaceae (Lily Family)

Description
Herb with bulbs broadly ovoid, usually solitary, rounded distally; peduncle conspicuously ventricose below middle; flowers in pedunculate umbels; perianth segments white or greenish (Smith 1979).

Range
Eurasia and cultivated elsewhere (Smith 1979). Introduced to Palau and found growing in agroforest and home gardens (Hillmann Kitalong, DeMeo & Holm 2008).

Traditional Uses
Medicine used for worms. Bulbs are used to expel intestinal worms (Del Rosario and Esguerra 2003).
Medicine used for GI issues. Bulbs are used to stimulate activity of the stomach, used as a tonic, and also used to treat diarrhea (Del Rosario and Esguerra 2003).

Pharmacological Properties
A polyethyleneglycol extract of onion bulb (*Allium cepa*) alone or mixed with coconut oil (*Cocos nucifera*) was active in both *in vitro* and *in vivo* against the *Trichuris muris* nematode (Klimpel *et al.*, 2011).

Toxicology
In a study on 16 subjects with heartburn, ingestion of one slice of raw onion in a meal significantly increased number of reflux episodes, heartburn episodes, belches and acidity in all subjects compared to the ingestion of the same meal excluding onion (Allen *et al.*, 1990). Two review articles (Stanghellini *et al.*, 2004; Saad & Chey 2006) state that subjects often complain of

dyspepsia, or indigestion, after meals including onion. High doses (500 mg/kg onion extract, i.p.) cause damage to the liver and lung tissues of rats, but low doses (50 mg/kg) were not harmful. Oral doses were much less toxic than intraperitoneal (Thomson *et al.*, 1998).

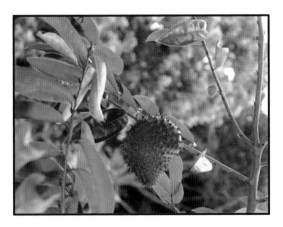

Figure 16. *Annona muricata* branches with leaves and fruit. [AK]

Local names: *sausab* (Palauan); soursop (English)
Scientific name: *Annona muricata* L.
Family: Annonaceae (Custard apple Family)

Description
A small evergreen tree about 7 m in height. The flowers are greenish and the fruits are characterized by numerous recurved spines on the rind, and are dark green with a white, fleshy pulp in the center (Smith 1981).

Range
Native from Central America to Peru, and is now widely cultivated in tropical regions including Palau (Smith 1981).

Traditional Uses
Medicine used for heartburn. Pick 2 or more young leaves and chew with water. The water should be warm or room temperature. This remedy should resolve the heartburn. If heartburn continues, take treatment again [Kerengel Tesei, Eriko Singeo, Raphaela Sumang].

Pharmacological Properties
No pharmacological reports relevant to this use were identified.

Toxicology
Dietary ingestion of *Annona muricata* fruits and fruit juice has been linked to cases of atypical Parkinson's disease. A case-control study of 87 patients showed that those with symptoms of atypical Parkinson's had diets higher in *A. muricata* (Caparros-Lefebvre & Elbaz 1999). Scientists believe that the acetogenins inhibit mitochondrial complex I, which produces dopaminergic neuronal death as effectively as rotenone by impairment of energy production (Lannuzel *et al.*, 2003). Neurodegenerative pathology manifests in an accumulation of tau proteins in neurons and brain imaging of patients found a correlation between tau protein lesions and *A. muricata* ingestion (Lannuzel, Ruberg & Michel 2008). A dose as low as 3.8 mg/kg in rats is sufficient to inhibit mitochondrial complex I (Champy *et al.*, 2004). This is estimated to be equivalent to eating one fruit or drinking one cup of tea per day. These toxins are not only present in the fruits as leaves of *A. muricata* extracted in water have 56 ± 22 mg/kg of annonacin (Ancuceanu & Istudor 2004). Annonacin and other acetogenins in *A. muricata* are thought to be topoisomerase poisons, which means that they can interfere with the cell's ability to replicate its DNA (Yuan *et al.*, 2003; Ancuceanu & Istudor 2004; Wang *et al.*, 2002; Lopez-Lazaro *et al.*, 2001).

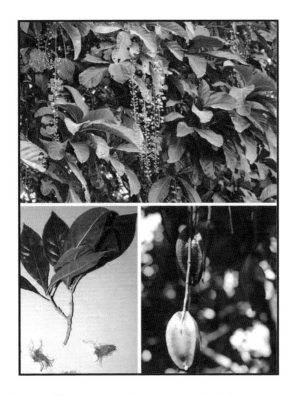

Figure 17. *Barringtonia racemosa* with close-ups of leaves, flowers, and fruits. [AK & CT]

Local names: *koranges* (Palauan); powder-puff tree (English)
Scientific name: *Barringtonia racemosa* (L.) Spreng.
Family: Lecythidaceae (Brazil Nut Family)

Description
Tree to 6 m in height or taller, with a medium sized trunk. The flowers have red buds opening into reddish purple or green calyces. The petals are white with creamy, yellow anthers and a pinkish-white style. The fruits are green and ripen to brown or red (Smith 1981).

Range
This species is found in eastern and southern Africa to India and throughout Micronesia, Malaysia, and the Pacific Islands. It grows in forests, along rivers and the edges of mangrove swamps (Smith 1981). Native to Palau and found growing in lowland volcanic forest and freshwater swamp forests (Hillmann Kitalong, DeMeo & Holm 2008).

Traditional Uses
Medicine used for heartburn. The stem and/or fruits are grated (*mengseus*) and squeezed through a coconut fiber sieve (*techir*); the juice is consumed. Alternatively, the leaves are boiled in water and consumed [Clarence Kitalong, Walter Ringang Metes].

Pharmacological Properties
No pharmacological reports relevant to the treatment of heartburn were identified.

Toxicology
Daily doses of a 50% methanolic seed extract of *Barringtonia racemosa*, up to 12 mg/kg i.p., for 14 days did not produce any acute or short-term toxicity in mice, but a 24 mg/kg daily i.p. dose was accompanied by an elevation in serum urea levels, indicating potential kidney or metabolic malfunctioning. LD_{50} of a single i.p. dose was found to be 36 mg/kg (Thomas *et al.*, 2002).

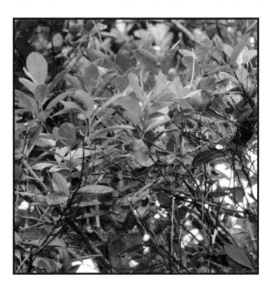

Figure 18. *Citrus mitis* leaves and fruit. [AK]

Local names: *kingkang* (Palauan); acid orange, calamondin orange (English)
Scientific name: *Citrus mitis* Blanco
Family: Rutaceae (Citrus Family)

Description
Tree 2-7.5 m high, erect, slender, often quite cylindrical, densely branched beginning close to the ground, slightly thorny. Leaves alternate, aromatic 4-7.5 cm long, faintly toothed at the apex, with short, narrowly-winged petioles. Flowers fragrant, with white petals, borne singly or in 2's or 3's. Fruits are round or oblate, 4.5 cm wide, with very aromatic, orange-red peel, glossy (Morton 1987).

Range
Believed to be native to China and thought to have been taken in early times to Indonesia and the Philippines. It is widely grown in India and throughout southern Asia and Malaysia. It is a common ornamental dooryard tree in Hawaii, the Bahamas, some islands of the West Indies, and parts of Central America (Morton 1987). Introduced to Palau and growing in agricultural and agroforest areas (Hillmann Kitalong, DeMeo & Holm 2008).

Traditional Uses
Medicine used for worms. Leaves are used in an unspecified way

Pharmacological Properties
No pharmacological reports relevant to this use were identified.

Toxicology
There were no reports of toxicity, adverse effects or drug interactions for *Citrus mitis*. Other species in the genus *Citrus* have been shown to interfere with the metabolism of drugs by cytochrome P450 3A4 (CYP3A4).

CYP3A4 is an enzyme involved in the intestinal absorption and metabolism of many drugs in use today. Chemicals that inhibit CYP3A4 can increase the bioavailability of the drug *in vivo*. Flavonoids found in grapefruit (*C. paradisi*), pomelo (*C. maxima*), and bitter orange (*C. aurantiifolia*) have all been shown to inhibit CYP3A4 (Adepoju & Adeyemi 2010; Egashira *et al.*, 2004; Grenier *et al.*, 2006; Hanley *et al.*, 2011; Xu, Go & Lim 2003).

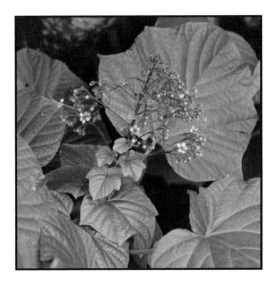

Figure 19. *Clerodendrum paniculatum* leaves and flowers. [MB]

Local names: *butcherchar* (Palauan); pagoda, orange tower (English)
Scientific name: *Clerodendrum paniculatum* L.
Family: Lamiaceae (Mint Family)

Description
Shrub 1-2 m high; branchlets medullose to hollow, bluntly quadrangular, the node with a broad band of hairs; leaves opposite, petioles 20 cm long, the blades 4-15 × 7-20 cm; inflorescences axillary or terminal. Panicles large, multi-flowered, to 45 cm long and

broad, the pedicels reddish, filiform 4-15 mm long, the flowers slightly fragrant; calyx red or orange-red to scarlet or rarely white, puberulent, the tube slender to 2 cm long. Fruit drupaceous, greenish-blue to black at maturity (Smith 1991).

Range
India, China, and Taiwan south to the Andaman and Nicobar Islands and into Malaysia, cultivated elsewhere (Smith 1991). Introduced to Palau and found growing in areas that typically have cultivated landscape with ornamental plants (Hillmann Kitalong, DeMeo & Holm 2008).

Traditional Uses
Medicine used for diarrhea. Boil dried leaves with water and drink [Flora Wasisang].
Medicine used for stomachache. Boil five mature leaves and drink [Gloria Emesiochel]. Crush leaves, place inside a glass of water, and drink (5 leaves for adults, 3 leaves for children) [Bedebii Chiokai].

Pharmacological Properties
No pharmacological reports relevant to this use were identified.

Toxicology
No toxicological reports were identified.

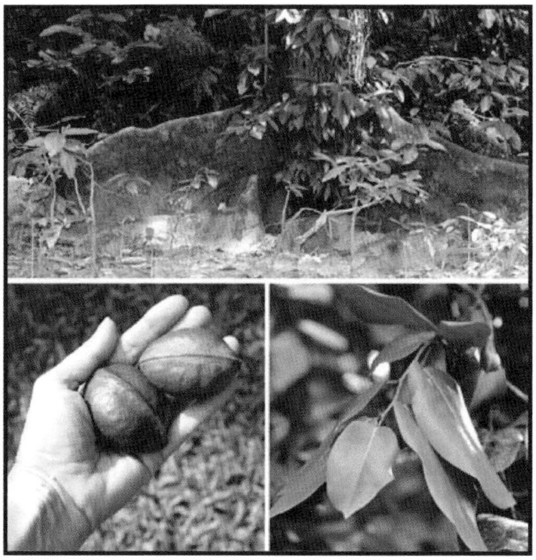

Figure 20. *Heritiera littoralis* with close-ups of buttressed roots, fruits, and leaves. [AK]

Local names: *chebibech* (Palauan); looking glass tree, salt water chestnut (English)
Scientific name: *Heritiera littoralis* Dryander
Family: Malvaceae (Hibiscus Family)

Description
A medium size tree up to 15 m in height, dbh 50-200 cm, often buttressed. The bark is whitish gray and cracked. The simple, alternate leaves are 8-35 cm long and 3-12 cm wide. The dark-green upper surface is usually covered with lichens and bryophytes and the lower surface is silvery white. The small, white flowers are on axillary panicles (compound flower cluster with the younger flowers at the apex or center) measuring 4-6 mm long. The brown fruit has a keeled hard elliptical woody nut that is 5-7 cm long and 3-5 cm wide (Hillmann Kitalong, DeMeo & Holm 2008).

Range
Heritiera littoralis is found at the landward edge of mangroves, along channels or rivers through the upper part of the mangroves and

occasionally at the mangrove coastal strand interface and lowland forests. It ranges throughout Southeast Asia and the Pacific (Hillmann Kitalong, DeMeo & Holm 2008).

Traditional Uses
Medicine used as an emetic (induce vomiting) and to treat diarrhea and/or dysentery. Use water extract of leaves and/or fruits (Hillmann Kitalong, DeMeo & Holm 2008).

Pharmacological Properties
No pharmacological reports relevant to this use were identified.

Toxicology
No relevant toxicological reports were identified.

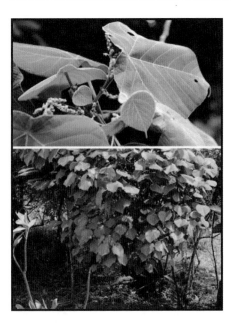

Figure 21. *Macaranga carolinensis* leaves and close-up of flowers (above); view of tree (below). [AK]

Local names: ***bedel*** (Palauan); macaranga (English)
Scientific name: *Macaranga carolinensis* Volk.
Family: Euphorbiaceae (Euphorbia Family)

Description
A small tree 3-10 m in height with a dbh of 3-40 cm. The simple, alternate leaves are 20-41 cm long, with hairy surfaces. Male and female flowers both lack corollas and are found on separate plants (dioecious). The convex or flat-topped female cluster is enclosed by a serrated triangular modified leaf and is borne on a stalk about 15 cm long. The male flowers are borne in a slender axillary compound cluster with the youngest flowers at the tip. The solitary, globe-like, fuzzy capsules are about 5 mm across (Hillmann Kitalong, DeMeo & Holm 2008).

Range
Macaranga carolinensis (*bedel*) is a fast-growing species common along forest edges, disturbed forests and secondary forests. It ranges from Indo-Malaya to Kosrae (Hillmann Kitalong, DeMeo & Holm 2008).

Traditional Uses
Medicine used for stomachache and diarrhea. Young leaves are boiled and consumed [David Ngirakesau].
Medicine for relieving stomachache pain. Chew small handful of very young leaves, and swallow. Repeat 1-2 times until stomach pain goes away [Henry Yuri].
Medicine used for mild diarrhea. The young leaves are chewed and have a bitter taste, and then swallowed. This dose is taken with 1 cup of water. The treatment is taken once daily, but if the diarrhea does not cease, it can be retaken. Treatment must be stopped when diarrhea ceases, otherwise the effect will be constipating. Use young leaves due to

the soft texture of the underside of the leaf. Used for mild cases of diarrhea due to bad food or water, not in more severe cases such as amoebic dysentery [Dirraklang Merei Ngirametuker].

Pharmacological Properties
No pharmacological reports relevant to this use were identified.

Toxicology
No toxicological reports were identified.

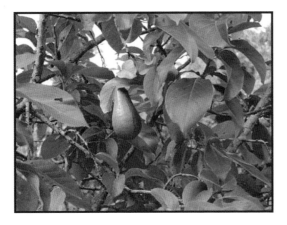

Figure 22. *Persea americana* leaves and fruit. [MB]

Local names: *bata* (Palauan); avocado (English)
Scientific name: *Persea americana* Mill.
Family: Lauraceae (Cinnamon Family)

Description
Tree 7-10 m high (but can grow 20 m or more). Fragrant flowers have a perianth 10-15 mm in diameter, the segments being yellow or yellowish-white; the conspicuous staminoids are orange to brown. The fruit, green to purplish when edible, is globose to pyriform and attains a size of 20 × 10 cm; the large seed is up to 5 cm in diameter (Smith 1981).

Range
Native to Central America, spreading early in cultivation into South America and somewhat later into the West Indies; the species is now cultivated in most tropical and subtropical areas (Smith 1981). Introduced to Palau and found growing in agricultural and agroforest areas (Hillmann Kitalong, DeMeo & Holm 2008).

Traditional Uses
Medicine used for diarrhea. Leaves are boiled in water and taken only once to treat diarrhea (3 leaves for young child and 5 leaves for adults) [Gloria Emesiochel].

Pharmacological Properties
The aqueous extract of the leaves produced dose-dependent, anti-inflammatory effects in mice and rats *in vivo* (Adeyemi, Okpo & Ogunti 2002).

Toxicology
Oral consumption of leaves is severely toxic and may cause death to some animals, such as goats, horses, and rabbits (Grant *et al.*, 1991; McKenzie & Brown 1991; Singh, W.R. *et al.*, 2010). The methanolic extracts of leaves and fruit were genotoxic to human peripheral lymphocytes *in vitro* (Kulkarni, Paul & Ganesh 2010).

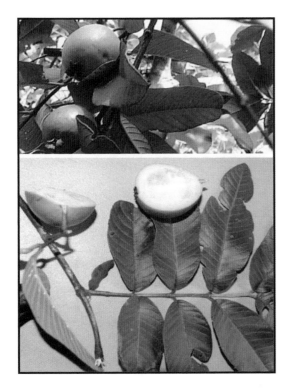

Figure 23. *Psidium guajava* leaves and fruit. [AK & WL]

Local names: *kuabang* (Palauan); guava (English)
Scientific name: *Psidium guajava* L.
Family: Myrtaceae (Myrtle Family)

Description
Psidium guajava is an evergreen shrub or small tree to 10 m in height. The leaves are 4-10 cm long and oval. The flowers are white and fragrant and 5 cm long. The fruits are small, round and yellow, with sweet, pink-seeded flesh when ripe (Merlin *et al.*, 1992; Smith 1979).

Range
Native to tropical Central America ranging from Mexico to northern South America, *Psidium guajava* is now pantropical. It is found growing at all elevations, often forming thickets along roadsides and clearings (Smith 1979). It has been cultivated throughout the world for its fruit (Morton 1987).

Traditional Uses
Medicine used for diarrhea. Boil young leaves and drink [Ngemelas Kitalong, Clarence Kitalong, Ann Hillmann Kitalong, Patrick Tellei]. Chew 2 leaf tips (*eberdil*) and drink with 4 oz of water. Alternatively, get 10 leaves from the second stage of growth (*omalk*) and boil with 1 gal of water for 15-25 min.

Pharmacological Properties
An alcohol extract of the young leaf exhibited microbicidal properties, particularly against pathogens that cause diarrhea (Vieira *et al.*, 2001). The leaves and stem bark showed antiamoebic activities (Tona *et al.*, 1998). This species also demonstrated antimicrobial properties (Chah *et al.*, 2006).

Toxicology
No reports of toxicity were identified.

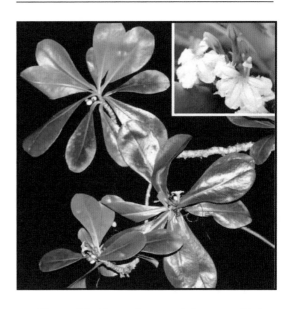

Figure 24. *Scaevola taccada* leaves, with inset showing flowers. [MB & AK]

Local names: *kirrai*, *korrai* (Palauan); beach naupaka (English)
Scientific name: *Scaevola taccada* (Gaertn.) Roxb.
Family: Goodeniaceae (Naupaka Family)

Description
Freely branching, spreading shrub 0.5-5 m high. The vegetative parts and inflorescences soft-white-sericeous to glabrous (but with hair tufts in leaf axils); petioles winged to base; leaf blades obovate to spathulate, variable in size 8-26 cm long, 4-12 cm broad. Inflorescences axilary, few-flowered, 2-5 cm long, corolla 12-22 mm long, the tube white to greenish or purplish; fruit white, globose to ovoid, 10-18 mm in diameter when fresh (Smith 1991).

Range
Widespread in the Indo-Pacific, usually restricted to open sandy beaches or rocky coasts on most islands and continental shores from East Africa northward to Ceylon, India, and southern Japan, and eastward through Malaysia to tropical Australia and into eastern Polynesia and Hawaii (Smith 1991). In Palau, found growing in freshwater swamp forests and in limestone forests, atolls, and strand vegetation along the coasts (Hillmann Kitalong, DeMeo & Holm 2008).

Traditional Uses
Medicine used for stomachache. Pick leaves in the morning, and boil as many leaves as can fit in a pot and drink [Clarence Kitalong].

Pharmacological Properties
No pharmacological reports relevant to this use were identified.

Toxicology
Oral and interperitoneal administration of a *Scaveola taccada* methanolic extract (2,000 mg/kg) showed evidence of toxicity in rats (Umadevi, Mohanta & Manavalan 2006).

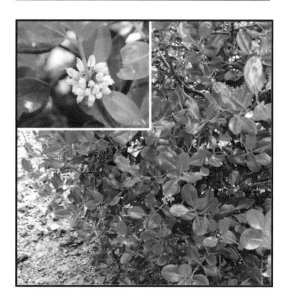

Figure 25. *Scyphiphora hydrophyllacea* leaves, with inset showing flowers. [AK]

Local name: *kuat* (Palauan)
Scientific name: *Scyphiphora hydrophyllacea* C. F. Gaertn.
Family: Rubiaceae (Coffee Family)

Description
A small shrub 1.5-5 m in height. The branchlets are reddish, smooth and flexible. The simple, opposite leaves are 4-8 cm long and 3-5 cm wide. The white-pinkish clusters of fragrant flowers are borne between the leaf and stem. The flowers are 1-1.2 cm long, with white petals tinged with pink. The light green fleshy fruit is 1-seeded, with 8 longitudal ridges measuring 5 to 11 mm long (Hillmann Kitalong, DeMeo & Holm 2008).

Range
Found in Palau along channels and in the middle to landward edge of the mangrove forest. It ranges from Southern India and Malaysia to New Caledonia. In Palau it often grows in association with *Lumnitzera littorea* (Jack) Voigt. This is an uncommon tree found near the docks of Ulimang, Ngaraard and the inner mangrove edge in Airai and Aimeliik (Hillmann Kitalong, DeMeo & Holm 2008).

Traditional Uses
Medicine for stomachache. Use warm water extract of leaves and drink to alleviate stomach pain (Hillmann Kitalong, DeMeo & Holm 2008).

Pharmacological Properties
No pharmacological reports relevant to this use were identified.

Toxicology
No toxicological reports were identified.

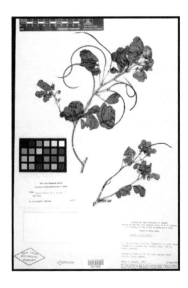

Figure 26. NYBG voucher specimen of *Senna obtusifolia*. [W.R.A.]

Local name: *kuroterariang* (Palauan)
Scientific name: *Senna obtusifolia* (L.) H.S. Irwin & Barneby
Family: Fabaceae (Legume Family)

Description
A coarse herb or shrub up to 1.2 m tall; having leaflets in three pairs. Leaf blades are obovate and broadly rounded at apex. The short, 2-flowered racemes have pedicels 4-15 mm long, sepals 6 mm long, and petals are yellow up to 10 mm long. Pod is often curved, slender, 4-6 mm in diameter (Smith 1985).

Range
Paleotropical, from India and Ceylon eastward into Polynesia (Smith 1985).

Traditional Uses
Medicine used to kill intestinal worms. Young parts of leaves are eaten raw. Just take once with water [Elin Rebluud].

Pharmacological Properties
Leaves of the related plant, *Senna alata* (L.) Roxb., have been demonstrated to have purgative and laxative effects in humans and rats due to the presence of anthraquinone derivatives (Hennebelle *et al.*, 2009).

Toxicology
The alcohol extract and compounds isolated from the leaves of the related species *Senna alata* (L.) Roxb., may cause subtle hepato-renal (liver and kidney) toxicity in rats (Yagi, Tigani & Adam 1998).

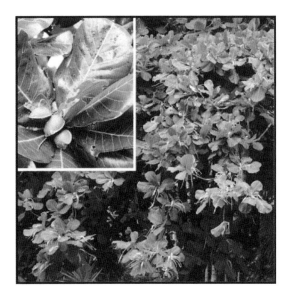

Figure 27. *Terminalia catappa* with inset showing fruits. [AK & MB]

Local names: *miich* (Palauan); Indian almond (English)
Scientific name: *Terminalia catappa* L.
Family: Combretaceae (Combretum Family)

Description
A large tree, normally up to 30 m tall. Leaves in whorls at ends of branches, broad and inversely oval, generally dark green and glossy. Older leaves turn brilliant shades of red and orange before dropping. Flowers small in whitish-yellow clusters with racemes (or spikes) 5-15 cm long. Fruits are flattened and egg-shaped, green when young but turn reddish-yellow when ripe. Edible cylindrical seeds are encased in a tough fibrous husk with a fleshy outer layer (Hillmann Kitalong, DeMeo & Holm 2008).

Range
Usually found in atoll forests, inland from ocean beaches near river mouths and around coastal areas in general. Native to coastal areas of Eastern India, Indochina, Malaysia, Indonesia, Northern Australia, Oceania, the Philippines and Taiwan. Widely planted and naturalized in the lowland tropical regions of the rest of the world (Hillmann Kitalong, DeMeo & Holm 2008).

Traditional Uses
Medicine used for diarrhea. Boil fruit skin in water and drink [Tadashi Belchal].

Pharmacological Properties
The alcohol extract of the leaf has strong antibacterial properties against a wide range of pathogens (Goun *et al.*, 2003; Kloucek *et al.*, 2005).

Toxicology
No reports of toxicity were identified.

COMBINATION THERAPIES

a)

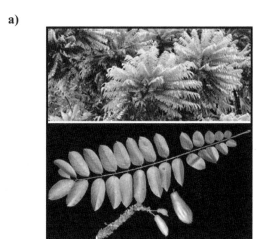

b)

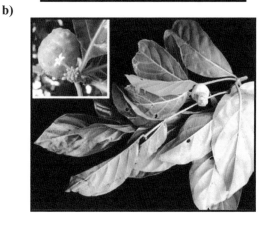

c)

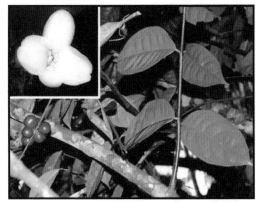

d)

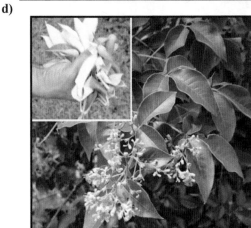

Figure 28. **a)** *Averrhoa bilimbi* showing close-up of leaves and fruits. [AK & MB]; **b)** *Morinda citrifolia* leaves and fruit, with inset showing flower, flower buds, and fruit. [MB & AK]; **c)** *Phaleria nisidai* fruits and leaves, with inset showing flower. [AK & CT]; **d)** *Vitex trifolia* var. *trifolia* leaves and flowers, with inset showing four harvested branch tips. [CT & AK]

Local and Scientific names:

imekurs (Palauan); bilimbi (English) - *Averrhoa bilimbi* L. (Oxalidaceae)
ngel (Palauan); noni (English) - *Morinda citrifolia* L. (Rubiaceae)
ongael, delalakar (Palauan); mother of medicine (English) - *Phaleria nisidai* Kaneh. (Thymelaeaceae)
kelsechedui (Palauan); simple-leaf chastetree, Arabian lilac (English) - *Vitex trifolia* L. var. *trifolia* (Lamiaceae)

Descriptions

Averrhoa bilimbi L.: Shrub or small tree 4-15 m high, with yellowish red to purple sepals and red petals. It is usually cauliflorous and ramiflorous, the leaves having 15-41 leaflets with predominant oblong blades usually 3-7 × 1.5-2.5 cm, acute at apex, a few proximal ones smaller than the distal ones. Fruits are green, terete to obtusely angled, ellipsoid to obovoid, up to 10 × 5 cm, with seeds 6-8 × 4-6 mm and lacking arils (Smith 1985).

Morinda citrifolia L.: A small tree 3-8 m in height, with a dbh of 10-30 cm and hairless, 4-angled stems. The simple, opposite, elliptic leaves are up to 45 cm long and 25 cm wide. The margins are entire, the surfaces are glossy, hairless and pliable; the stout petiole is up to 2 cm long. The flowers are borne in 75 to 90-flowered, oval to globe-like heads on a stalk about 3 cm long, with the calyx having a truncate rim with no lobes. The white corolla has 5 lobes that are slightly curled backward. The flower stalk is 1-3 cm long. The yellowish-white, fleshy, soft and odiferous, irregular heads are about 5 cm long and 3-4 cm wide. The fruits have a wart-like appearance (Hillmann Kitalong, DeMeo & Holm 2008).

Phaleria nisidai Kaneh.: A ca. 15 m tall tree with opposite leaves, 15-20 cm long, 7-8 cm wide; the corolla tube is white, 15 mm long (Kanehira 1933). The drupe is red at maturity. It is native to Palau (Hillmann Kitalong, DeMeo & Holm 2008).

Vitex trifolia L. var. *trifolia*: Small tree or shrub with leaves 3- or 5-foliolate, the central leaflets are petiolulate, the blades hairy on both surfaces and oblong-elliptic to ovate-lanceolate. Flowers sessile; grayish to white, 2-4 mm long, 1.5-3 mm broad (Smith 1991).

Ranges

Averrhoa bilimbi L.: Exact origin unknown, but often seen as a relict of former cultivation in eastern Melanesia (Smith 1985). Introduced to Palau, it is found growing in agricultural and agroforest areas, as well as in urban areas that typically have cultivated landscape and ornamental plants (Hillmann Kitalong, DeMeo & Holm 2008).

Morinda citrifolia L.: Indigenous to Indo-Malaysia, *Morinda citrifolia* ranges throughout the Pacific to Hawaiian Islands and other tropical regions around the world. In coastal forests, it is established as an understory plant often found near creeks, alongside the edge of mangrove swamps, and can be found growing up to 137 m above sea level (Smith 1988). In Palau, it is found along the volcanic forest edge and savanna (Hillmann Kitalong, DeMeo & Holm 2008).

Phaleria nisidai Kaneh.: Southeastern Asia and Ceylon through Malaysia to Micronesia, Australia, and eastward in the Pacific to Samoa and Tonga (Smith 1981). In Palau, it grows in volcanic lowland forest and in freshwater swamp forest (Hillmann Kitalong, DeMeo & Holm 2008).

Vitex trifolia L. var. *trifolia*: Southeastern Asia to southern Africa and Indian Ocean islands and eastward through Malaysia and northern Australia to Polynesia (Smith 1991). Introduced to Palau and found growing in areas that have cultivated landscape with ornamental plants (Hillmann Kitalong, DeMeo & Holm 2008).

Traditional Uses

Medicine used to keep body hydrated (preserve water). Get 1 handful of leaves of *Vitex trifolia* var. *trifolia* (*kelsechedui*), and combine with 4 leaves from second growth stages (*omalk*) of *Morinda citrifolia* (*ngel*), *Phaleria nisidai* (*ongael*), and *Averrhoa bilimbi* (*imekurs*). Boil with 2 gal of water for 15-25 min, and then drink 8 oz in the morning through evening after every meal. This remedy is for a person who needs hydration. Women who have gone through their menstrual period, or are pregnant are not allowed to use this remedy; it will cause abortion or too much menstrual flow [Ingas Spesungel].

Pharmacological Properties

Averrhoa bilimbi L.: No pharmacological reports relevant to this use were identified.

Morinda citrifolia L.: No pharmacological reports relevant to this use were identified.

Phaleria nisidai Kaneh.: No pharmacological reports relevant to this use were identified.

Vitex trifolia L. var. *trifolia*: No pharmacological reports relevant to this use were identified.

Toxicology

Averrhoa bilimbi L.: Feeding of the fruit at daily oral doses of 250-1,000 mg/kg for 15 days did not result in any obvious toxicity in rats (Ambili, Subramoniam & Nagarajan 2009).

Morinda citrifolia L.: Two publications reported cases of liver toxicity linked to the ingestion of noni juice (Millonig, Stadelmann & Vogel 2005; Stadlbauer *et al.,* 2005). Some researchers believe that the risk of liver toxicity is unlikely due to very low concentrations of potentially hepatotoxic anthraquinones (Kamiya *et al.*, 2005; Pawlus *et al.*, 2005). *Morinda citrifolia* juice did not show any genotoxicity and the author concludes that pure *M. citrifolia* juice is safe for human consumption (Westendorf *et al.,* 2007).

Phaleria nisidai Kaneh.: No reports of toxicity were identified.

Vitex trifolia L. var. *trifolia*: No reports of toxicity were identified.

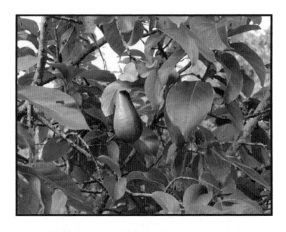

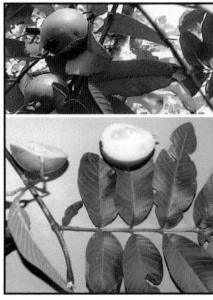

Figure 29. *Persea americana* leaves and fruit. [MB] (top); *Psidium guajava* leaves and fruit. [AK & WL] (bottom)

Local and Scientific names:
bata (Palauan); avocado (English) - *Persea americana* Mill. (Lauraceae)
kuabang (Palauan); guava (English) - *Psidium guajava* L. (Mrytaceae)

Descriptions
Persea americana Mill.: See earlier in this chapter.
Psidium guajava L.: See earlier in this chapter.

Ranges
Persea americana Mill.: See earlier in this chapter.
Psidium guajava L.: See earlier in this chapter.

Traditional Uses
Medicine used for diarrhea. Leaves of avocado and guava are boiled and consumed (3 each for a young child and 5 each for an adult). This is taken once daily to treat diarrhea [Gloria Emesiochel].

Pharmacological Properties
Persea americana Mill.: No pharmacological reports relevant to this use were identified.
Psidium guajava L.: The alcohol extract of the leaf sprout exhibited microbicidal properties, particularly against pathogens that cause diarrhea (Vieira *et al.*, 2001). The leaves and stem bark showed antiamoebic activities (Tona *et al.*, 1998) and demonstrated antimicrobial properties (Chah *et al.*, 2006).

Toxicology
Persea americana Mill.: Oral consumption of leaves is severely toxic and may cause death to some animals, such as goats, horses, and rabbits (Grant *et al.*, 1991; McKenzie & Brown 1991; Singh, W.R. *et al.*, 2010). The methanolic extracts of leaves and fruit were genotoxic to human peripheral lymphocytes *in vitro* (Kulkarni, Paul & Ganesh 2010).
Psidium guajava L.: No reports of toxicity were identified.

CHAPTER FIVE: SKIN DISORDERS

The skin is the largest organ in the body and can be affected by a variety of disorders that require treatment. In this chapter we discuss skin disorders such as fungi, boils, skin rashes and burns. In most cases, diseases of the skin are limited to the skin alone, but there can be particular situations when a skin condition can reflect a serious internal medical conditions requiring more intensive medical care.

Boils and Abscesses

Boils and abscesses are infections of the skin that are pus-filled sacs, red, warm to the touch, and usually painful. These can also be accompanied by swollen lymph nodes and fever. Signs of a spreading infection include widening of the inflamed area and increased pain. Generally, boils that enlarge 1-2 inches in diameter become classified as abscesses and need to be drained. This can be done by a health care practitioner who can open the abscess, drain the pus, and wash the pocket with a sterile solution. Occasionally, the boil or abscess will open by itself; in this case, the drainage can be assisted by applying hot compresses over the area. The boil or abscess should then be properly cleaned with soap and water.

Fungal Infections

Fungal infections usually occur in moist areas of the body; typically on the scalp, between the toes or fingers, between the legs (especially in the groin area), in the axilla (armpit), under the breasts, in beards, or in skin folds that are repeatedly moist.

Commonly, the rash of a fungal infection will present in the form of a ring and will create itchiness, redness and scale formation (i.e. ringworm) whereas thrush, an oral infection from *Candida albicans* is usually more diffuse. If it occurs in an area where hair grows, loss of hair may occur. If the fungal infection occurs under the nail, the nail will usually darken and its appearance will change from smooth to rough and irregular in texture. A very common mild fungal infection *Tinea versicolor* caused by the yeast *Malassezia furfur* occurs in the tropics and causes white spots on the face and body, and is often distributed on the neck, chest and back. Generally there is no itching or scale. This can be treated with a commonly available shampoo that contains selenium sulfide at 2.5% concentration or ketoconazole. This should be applied for ten minutes daily, and then washed off, for a duration of ten days in a row. Leprosy also causes pale spots but is never completely white and is associated with reduced feeling over the white area. The decreased sensation can be tested by lightly pricking the area with a pin. If leprosy is suspected a health care practitioner should be contacted immediately.

Treatment of Fungal Infections

Treatment for fungal infections can include cleaning the infected area with soap and water daily and keeping the area dry, especially in moist environments. Over-the-counter creams and powders which often eliminate the fungal infection include the active ingredients clotrimazole, econazole, oxiconazole, ciclopirox, ketoconazole, terbinafine, and butenafine, to name a few. These preparations should be used daily until the rash clears and continued to be used for at least one week after symptoms abate.

Occasionally, a fungal infection will become so severe that it could lead to a bacterial infection. Any area of the skin with oozing pus should be evaluated for this potential problem, and might require antibiotics. Oral antifungal medications can be prescribed for persistent fungal infections.

Skin Allergies

Allergic rashes are noninfectious irritations caused by touching, eating, injecting, or breathing in something that triggers an allergic response. This response in the skin is most commonly presented as hives or as a rash that is red and itchy. In certain cases, touching plants or other allergens creates a "contact" rash or contact dermatitis that causes blistering and redness associated with itching. The best treatment focuses on reduction of the redness and itching as well as identification of the allergic trigger. Redness can be reduced by bathing in cool water or use of cool compresses (cloth soaked in cold water). An over-the-counter antihistamine such as chlorpheniramine can be used, however, before use a health care professional should be consulted. Light steroid creams can be useful in reducing the allergic response. Shingles (*Herpes zoster*) can also present with blisters, but unlike contact dermatitis, shingles are very painful. It presents on only one side of the body (unilateral) on the chest, neck, or face. A doctor should be consulted, especially if the shingles rash is on the face.

Burns

Burns are an injury to the skin that results from heat (thermal), radiation, chemicals, or electricity. When the skin is burned, tissues are damaged, causing general swelling and pain. The specific classification of burns is defined by the depth and extent of damage to the skin. First degree burns or minor burns are superficial, affecting only the top most layer of the skin known as the epidermis. Minor burns usually present with redness and swelling in the burned areas. Second degree burns or moderate burns go into the middle layers of the skin known as the dermis. This results in blistering that may burst and ooze. Third degree burns or severe burns damage all three layers of the skin, the epidermis, dermis and fat layer (adipose tissue) beneath the dermis. Usually in third degree burns, nerves, hair follicles and sweat glands are injured. These burns appear charred with exposed raw areas. Since many of the nerves are damaged, pain is less severe with a third degree burn; however, fluid can be lost and infections can occur causing serious problems due to the depth of the burn, dehydration, and sepsis (profound infection). Burns involving the face, hands, joints, groin region, buttocks, and feet should be considered serious burns and should receive professional medical treatment.

Treatment of Burns

For first-degree burns, oral treatment with aspirin or a non-steroidal anti-inflammatory (NSAID) and cold water compresses are sufficient (placing the burn under cold running water for 15 minutes). It is crucial to protect second degree burns from rupturing as this greatly reduces the risk of infection. Vaseline or Neosporin ointment is applied to the blister, and gauze to protect it with daily dressing changes are the preferred treatment strategy. Honey is a natural agent that can prevent and control infection by acting as a natural barrier for wound care. Third degree burns can cause extensive damage to the skin. Therefore, infection and fluid loss are a primary concern in wound care. **If a third degree burn occurs, this is a medical emergency and medical attention should be sought immediately**. The burns can be covered lightly with room to breathe; however, no ointments or ice water should be applied. **Do not put ice on any burn as this will cause further damage**.

Chapter Five discusses 21 different plant remedies reported to treat abscesses, boils, and other skin related conditions.

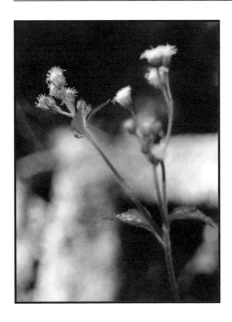

Figure 30. *Ageratum conyzoides* flowers. [RL]

Local names: ***ngmak*** (Palauan); goatweed, whiteweed (English)
Scientific name: *Ageratum conyzoides* L.
Family: Asteraceae (Daisy Family)

Description
Coarse herb 0.2-1 m high; opposite and simple leaves commonly subacute or obtuse to round at base; the corolla lobes and styles are white to pale lavender. Flowering heads usually 5-8 mm in diameter with 60-75 flowers. Flowering and fruiting seen throughout the year (Smith 1991).

Range
Mexico and the West Indies to South America, and now often cultivated and established as an adventive in most warm countries. It was probably an early European introduction into the Pacific Islands as an ornamental (Smith 1991). Introduced to Palau and found growing in savanna grasslands and in urban areas that typically have cultivated landscape and ornamental plants (Hillmann Kitalong, DeMeo & Holm 2008).

Traditional Uses
Medicine used for boils. Poultices of the leaves are used for boils and other skin diseases, particularly leprosy (Del Rosario & Esguerra 2003). Rub leaves together, apply coconut oil to the boil and place leaves on top of boil [Elin Rebluud, Rideph Emesiochel].

Pharmacological Properties
Oral administration of an ethanolic leaf extract of *Ageratum conyzoides* for 90 days reduced subchronic and chronic inflammation in rats (Moura *et al.*, 2005). A methanolic extract of this plant improved wound healing parameters in a rat model (Oladejo *et al.*, 2003).

Toxicology
No hepatotoxicity was observed with oral doses up to 500 mg/kg/day for 90 days in rats (Moura *et al.*, 2005).

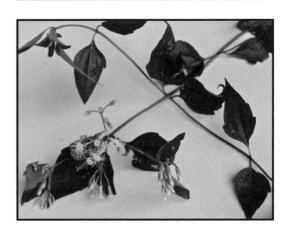

Figure 31. *Chromolaena odorata.* [MB]

Local names: *ngesngesil* (Palauan); Siam weed (English)
Scientific name: *Chromolaena odorata* (L.) R. M. King & H. Rob.
Family: Asteraceae (Daisy Family)

Description
Shrub or herb 1-2 m high, with many branches. Leaves strongly aromatic. Flowers in flat topped clusters of 20-35 florets, involucre green, corolla lilac to off-white, seeds black [M.J. Balick 3447, 4383] (Arvigo & Balick 1998).

Range
Native to the American continent, and introduced to tropical Asia, West Africa, and parts of Australia. It was introduced to Palau and now is considered an invasive (Hillmann Kitalong, DeMeo & Holm 2008).

Traditional Uses
Medicine used for cuts, boils, infections. The top 4 youngest leaves of *lius* are pounded with the top 4 youngest leaves of *Chromolaena odorata*. This creates a sticky substance that is used to draw out blood from cuts, remove pus and blood from boils, draw out splinters, and draw out snake fangs [Dirraklang Merei Ngirametuker, Gillian Johanes, Tsuneo Tesei, Kerngel Tesei].

Pharmacological Properties
Aqueous leaf extracts of *Chromolaena odorata* showed anti-inflammatory actions in rats (25-200 mg/kg) supporting use for wounds and inflammation (Owoyele, Adediji & Soladoye 2005) and flavonoids isolated from this plant demonstrated anti-inflammatory and analgesic activity *in vitro* (Owoyele *et al.*, 2008). An ethanol extract of *C. odorata* enhanced proliferation of fibroblasts, endothelial cells and keratinocytes *in vitro* (Thang *et al.*, 2001).

Growth enhancement of human keratinocytes (human skin cells) and the migration of keratinocytes into damaged tissue were stimulated by *C. odorata* extracts at low concentrations *in vitro* (Phan, Hughes & Cherry 2001). Collagen lattice contraction was irreversibly inhibited at 200 µg/ml and 400 µg/ml (Phan *et al.*, 1996). Improved wound healing due to *C. odorata* extract is enhanced by the upregulation of adhesion complex proteins and fibronectin produced by human keratinocytes (Phan *et al.*, 2000). *Chromolaena odorata* extract also has antimicrobial and antifungal properties, inhibiting the growth of *Pseudomonas aeruginosa* and *Streptococcus faecalis* (Irobi 1992). Ethanolic extracts of the leaves of *C. odorata* showed antibacterial activity against both Gram-positive and Gram-negative bacteria (Irobi 1992; 1997). Aqueous ethanol extracts of leaves showed antifungal activity (Ngono Ngane *et al.*, 2006). Administration of *C. odorata* extract inhibited carrageenan-induced paw edema in rats (Owoyele, Adediji & Soladoye 2005; Oludare *et al.*, 2000).

Toxicology
Administration of aqueous extract of *Chromolaena odorata* leaves caused a reduction in the size of testicles and reduced the number of spermatozoa in rats. Thus, *C. odorata* possesses antiandrogenic properties at the testicular level interfering with fertility (Yakubu, Akanji & Oladiji 2007). Oral administration of *C. odorata* extract produced a significant reduction in testicular body weight ratio, acid phosphatase activities, and protein, cholesterol, glycogen, sialic acid, and testosterone concentrations further indicating that this plant may possess anti-androgenic effects (Yakubu, Akanji & Oladiji 2007). At high concentrations the *C. odorata* extract was toxic to keratinocytes (Phan, Hughes & Cherry 2001).

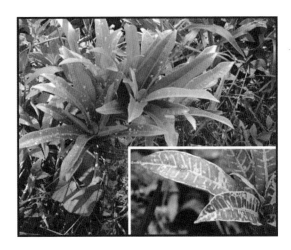

Figure 32. *Codiaeum variegatum* leaves and flowers, with inset showing close-up variegated leaves. [WL & AK]

Local names: *kesuk* (Palauan); variegated croton (English)
Scientific name: *Codiaeum variegatum* (L.) Blume
Family: Euphorbiaceae (Euphorbia Family)

Description

Shrub or small tree. Leaves variously colored, alternate (spirally arranged), the blades simple; inflorescences axillary, racemose, solitary or paired; male flowers with 5-6 minute petals; female flowers lack petals; fruit a subglobose, 3-lobed, schizocarp, dehiscent (Smith 1981).

Range

Malaysia, northern Australia, and eastward into the Pacific (Smith 1981). Introduced to Palau and found growing in areas that have cultivated landscape with ornamental plants (Hillmann Kitalong, DeMeo & Holm 2008).

Traditional Uses

Medicine used for skin rash. Break the leaf base (petiole); the sap coming out of it is used on skin rashes. Young leaves are not used; lower, older leaves carry more sap.

Pharmacological Properties

Extracts of *Codiaeum variegatum* have demonstrated antimolluscicidal activity (Yadav & Singh 2001).

Toxicology

Some species in the family Euphorbiaceae have sesquiterpene lactones which might be responsible for the contact dermatitis sometimes associated with *Codiaeum variegatum* (Hausen & Schulz 1977; Tafelkruyer & van Ketel 1976; van Ketel 1979; Warshaw & Zug 1996). An extract of *C. variegatum* leaves showed Epstein-Barr virus-inducing activity at low concentrations in human lymphoblastoid cell lines harboring EBV, indicating potential tumor promotion (Norhanom & Yadav 1995).

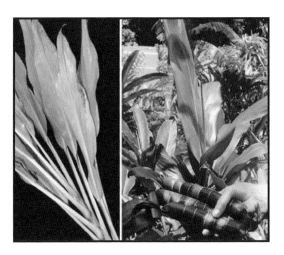

Figure 33. *Cordyline fruticosa* leaves (left); leaves used to wrap food (right). [MB & WL]

Local names: *sis* (Palauan); ti plant, good luck plant (English)
Scientific name: *Cordyline fruticosa* L. Chev.
Family: Laxmanniaceae (Laxmannia Family)

Description
Cordyline fruticosa is a shrub growing 2-4 m in height. The leaves are oppositely arranged, leathery and shaped like a knife blade. They range from 30-50 cm in length and may be red or green in color. The flower is a raceme of small white, purple or red flowers. The fruits are red, fleshy berries (Burkill 1935; Lee Ling 1998).

Range
Cordyline fruticosa is indigenous to the Himalayas, Southeast Asia, Malaysia and northern Australia and has become naturalized in the Pacific Islands (Smith 1991). Throughout its range, *C. fruticosa* has been widely cultivated as an ornamental for its colorful leaves (Burkill 1935).

Traditional Uses
Medicine used for rashes. Leaves are crushed and applied to rash [Gloria Emesiochel].

Pharmacological Properties
No pharmacological reports relevant to this use were identified.

Toxicology
No reports of toxicity were identified.

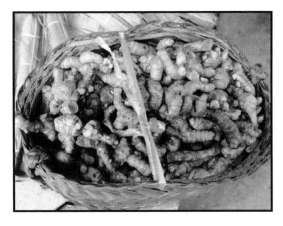

Figure 34. *Curcuma longa* showing harvested tubers. [AK]

Local names: *kesol* (Palauan); turmeric (English)
Scientific name: *Curcuma longa* L.
Family: Zingiberaceae (Ginger Family)

Description
An herb 1 m high with a spike of pale yellow flowers surrounded by white bracts. The tuber is orange brown on the outside and bright yellow orange on the inside (Smith 1979).

Range
Cultivated throughout the tropical regions of China, India, and Indo-Malaysia. The origin is thought to be South Asia, however, the species is so widely naturalized throughout the Pacific Islands that it appears indigenous (Smith 1979). Introduced to Palau, it is found growing in agricultural and agroforest areas (Hillmann Kitalong, DeMeo & Holm 2008).

Traditional Uses
Medicine used for skin rash and black spots (melasma). Use a clean, peeled root— crush it, and boil with coconut oil. The oil will take on a yellow color. Cool and apply to affected area, at least 2× daily, in the morning after bathing and in the evening.

Also used for hotbath for mothers after birth of a child. Helps remove stretch marks [Eriko Singeo].

Pharmacological Properties
Curcumin, isolated from the roots of *Curcuma longa* counteracted inflammation and irritation associated with experimental models of skin conditions in rats (Mukhopadhyay, Basu & Ghatak 1982). A methanol extract of *C. longa* root showed dose-dependent inhibition of porcine pancreatic- and human leukocyte elastase *in vitro*. Inhibitors of elastase, the enzyme responsible for the breakdown of elastic protein fibers of connective tissue in human skin, are being investigated for anti-aging properties and for beneficial effects on dry and damaged skin (Lee *et al.*, 1999).

Toxicology
No reports of toxicity were identified.

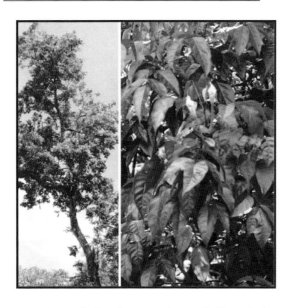

Figure 35. *Dolichandrone spathacea* (left); and close-up of leaves and flowers (right). [AK]

Local names: *rriu* (Palauan); trumpet mangrove (English)
Scientific name: *Dolichandrone spathacea* (L. f.) K. Schum.
Family: Bignoniaceae (Catalpa Family)

Description
Tree 30 m high, dbh 1 m, bark gray to dark brown, twigs lenticellate, leaves compound and opposite. Solitary large white flowers. Fruit a follicle, 35 cm long and dark brown, (Prosperi *et al.*, 2005; M.J. Balick 4433).

Range
Distributed in tropical Southeast Asia, southern India throughout Malaysia, Papua New Guinea, Micronesia, and New Caledonia (Prosperi *et al.*, 2005). Native to Palau and found growing in the mangrove forests (Hillmann Kitalong, DeMeo & Holm 2008).

Traditional Uses
Medicine used for treatment of the skin disease called yaws (*kerdik*), which is caused by the bacterium *Treponema pertenue* (Hillmann Kitalong, DeMeo & Holm 2008).

Pharmacological Properties
No pharmacological reports relevant to this use were identified.

Toxicology
No reports of toxicity were identified.

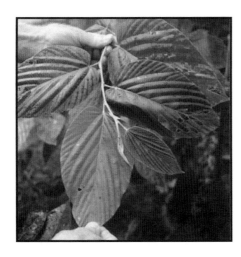

Figure 36. *Flemingia strobilifera* showing young and mature leaves. [AK]

Local names: *besungelaiei* (Palauan); wild hops (English)
Scientific names: *Flemingia strobilifera* (L.) R. Br.
Family: Fabaceae (Legume Family)

Description
Shrub up to 2 m tall, the stipules striate, leaves trifoliolate, the leaflet blades covered with small glands especially on the lower surface, and prominently nerved beneath. Inflorescences axillary or terminal, usually multi-flowered, flowers white with pink veins, calyx 5-lobed, lobes longer than the tube; fruits oblong-ovoid, inflated, dehiscent (Smith 1985).

Range
Paleotropical, Himalayas to India and Ceylon to China and into Malaysia (Smith 1985). It was introduced to Palau and it is found growing in the savanna grasslands, as well as in urban areas that typically have cultivated landscape and ornamental plants (Hillmann Kitalong, DeMeo & Holm 2008).

Traditional Uses
Medicine used for pain and itch.
Pick a couple of leaves and add it to about 12 oz of boiling coconut oil. When cooled, rub it on affected area to stop pain and itchiness caused by the Palau poison tree (*Semecarpus venenosus*: *tonget*). Can also be used for other types of pain and itchiness [Alfonsa Bintorio, Maria Kim, Nona Luii, Eriko Singeo, Hinako Takeo].

Pharmacological Properties
Chemicals isolated from the roots showed moderate antioxidant and antimicrobial activities *in vitro* (Madan *et al.*, 2009).

Toxicology
No reports of toxicity were identified.

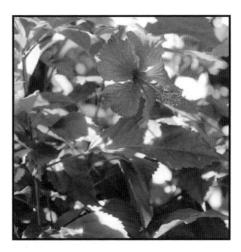

Figure 37. *Hibiscus rosa-sinensis* var. *rosa-sinensis* leaves and flowers. [AK]

Local names: *bussonge* (Palauan); hibiscus (English)
Scientific name: *Hibiscus rosa-sinensis* L. var. *rosa-sinensis*
Family: Malvaceae (Hibiscus Family)

Description
Hibiscus rosa-sinensis is a shrub 1-3 m tall with a narrow trunk. The leaves are alternate and ovate with serrated margins. The conspicuous flowers range in color from yellow to pink, orange, red and crimson with long stamens and have yellow seeds (Smith 1981).

Range
Hibiscus rosa-sinensis is probably native to eastern Africa, although its exact origin is unknown. It has been widely cultivated throughout the tropics and subtropics as an ornamental, often used as hedgerows (Smith 1981).

Traditional Uses
Medicine used for boils. Boil leaves in water and put this on boil; pound flower buds or petals until becoming slimy and soft, then rub on the center of the boil until it is very clean and open, after 2-3 min of cleaning the area, put 1 petal to cover the boil, it helps to suck out the pus from the boil, then it will heal fast [Siabal L. Kitalong].

Pharmacological Properties
No pharmacological reports relevant to this use were identified.

Toxicology
No reports of toxicity were identified.

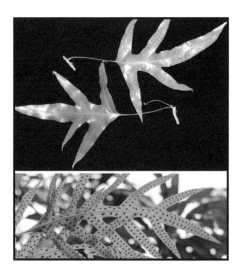

Figure 38. *Microsorum scolopendria* fronds and rhizomes (above); and close-up of sori (below). [MB & AK]

Local name: *chebechab* (Palauan)
Scientific name: *Microsorum scolopendria* (Burm. f.) Copel.
Synonym: *Phymatosorus scolopendria* (Burm. f.) Pic. Serm.
Family: Polypodiaceae (Fern Family)

Description
Herb, epiphytic or terrestrial; creeping rhizome up to 10 mm in diameter. The deeply pinnatifid, leathery fronds, up to 0.9 m long, are widely spaced along the rhizome. The stipe (leaf stalk) is up to 4 cm long. The leaf blade is divided into narrowly oblong lobes. The somewhat sunken sori are round to oval, 2-3 mm in diameter and occur in 1 or 2 rows on either side of the costa (Roux 2005).

Range
Widespread in the Old World, occurring from Australia, throughout Polynesia and Asia and extending to Madagascar and Africa (Roux 2005). Native to Palau and found growing on volcanic lowland forests, as well as in cultivated landscapes as ornamental plants (Hillmann Kitalong, DeMeo & Holm 2008).

It can grow beside saltwater beaches and shady moist forest (Roux 2005).

Traditional Uses
Medicine used to remove and heal skin scars and black marks (melasma). The green juices pressed from the frond heals and removes scars or black marks on the skin [Dirraklang Merei Ngirametuker].

Pharmacological Properties
No pharmacological reports relative to this use were identified.

Toxicology
Ferns of varying species, but not necessarily *Microsorum scolopendria*, have been shown to cause contact dermatitis in some patients (de Cock, Vorwerk & Bruynzeel 1998; Geller-Bernstein *et al.*, 1987; Stoof & Bruynzeel 1989).

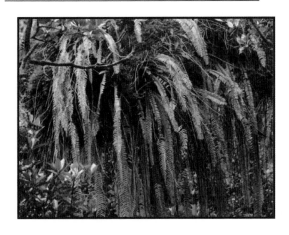

Figure 39. *Nephrolepis acutifolia.* [AK]

Local name: *delimes* (Palauan)
Scientific name: *Nephrolepis acutifolia* (Desv.) Christ
Family: Lomariopsidaceae (Sword Fern Family)

Description
A large epiphytic fern with short, erect, stoloniferous rhizomes and leathery fronds over 1 m long; the scaly rachises are red, with linear and marginal indusia; numerous pinnae (generally 20-50 pairs) (Hoshizaki & Moran 2001).

Range
It is native to tropical Africa and from southeastern Asia to Polynesia (Hoshizaki & Moran 2001). Native to Palau and found growing in the volcanic lowland forests and mangrove forests (Hillmann Kitalong, DeMeo & Holm 2008).

Traditional Uses
Antiseptic. The fronds are used as an antiseptic, to clean wounds [Dirraklang Merei Ngirametuker, Gillian Johannes, Tsuneo Tesei, Kerngel Tesei].

Pharmacological Properties
No pharmacological reports relevant to this use were identified.

Toxicology
Ferns of varying species, but not necessarily *Nephrolepis acutifolia*, have been shown to cause contact dermatitis in some patients (de Cock, Vorwerk & Bruynzeel 1998; Geller-Bernstein *et al.*, 1987; Stoof & Bruynzeel 1989).

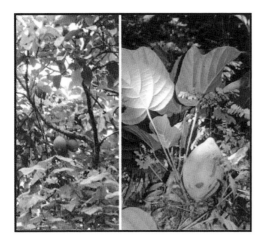

Figure 40. *Pangium edule* branch showing leaves and fruits (left); fallen fruit and leaves (right). [AK & MB]

Local names: *riamel* (Palauan); false durian (English)
Scientific name: *Pangium edule* Reinw. ex Blume
Family: Achariaceae (Acharia Family)

Description
Tree 12-20 m tall, dbh 30 cm. Leaves with shiny dark green above, paler beneath. Flowers with yellow stamens, anthers orange, perianth green; flowers with strong, sweet odor. The fruit is 15 cm long, ovoid shape with brown, warty skin [D.H. Lorence 9646; M.J. Balick 3805].

Range
Native to Southeast Asia. Likewise, it was introduced and now naturalized in Palau and found growing on volcanic lowland forests (Hillmann Kitalong, DeMeo & Holm 2008).

Traditional Uses
Medicine used for hemorrhoids. Warm oil is placed on the leaves and this is placed on the affected area. It soothes the area and makes the problem go away [Dorothy Yukie Yano, Oderai Beouch].

Pharmacological Properties
No pharmacological activities relevant to this use were identified.

Toxicology
No toxicological reports relevant to the topical use of this plant were identified.

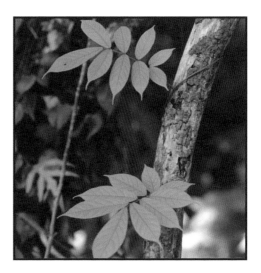

Figure 41. *Paraderris eliptica* liana showing leaves. [MB]

Local names: *dub* (Palauan); derris root, poison vine (English)
Scientific name: *Paraderris elliptica* (Wall.) Adema
Family: Fabaceae (Legume Family)

Description
Paraderris elliptica is a liana or scrambling shrub. The leaves are entire and oblong in shape, 15 cm long 2.5 cm wide. The stalks have a purple hue and the flower petals are pink. The fruits have a brownish color and are usually 2 cm long 5 cm wide, and have a wing 1-5 mm broad along both sutures (Smith 1985).

Range

Paraderris elliptica is a cultivated species growing near sea level to an elevation of about 400 m and has naturalized along roadsides and creek banks from India throughout Malaysia (Smith 1985). Introduced to Palau and found growing in agricultural and agroforest areas, as well as in areas that typically have cultivated landscapes and ornamental plants (Hillmann Kitalong, DeMeo & Holm 2008).

Traditional Uses

Medicine used for skin irritation. Leaves are pounded and mixed with coconut oil; it can be used to treat skin irritation [Kerungil Augustin].

Pharmacological Properties

The organic and alcohol extracts from various plant parts of *Paraderris elliptica* and the related species, *P. indica*, and *P. trifoliata*, have demonstrated a wide range of antibacterial activity. The strongest activities were found from alcohol and organic solvent extracts of the root bark, leaves and root heart-wood of *P. indica* and *P. trifoliata* (Khan, Omoloso & Barewai 2006).

Toxicology

Case reports in humans on the effect of rotenone present in the root of *Paraderris elliptica* indicated that direct contact caused conjunctivitis, dermatitis, pharyngitis, and rhinitis. Additionally, oral ingestion of rotenone produced gastrointestinal irritation, nausea, and vomiting. Inhalation of rotenone dust can cause respiratory stimulation followed by depression and convulsions (Hardman, Limbird & Gilman 2001). Rotenone is a highly potent mitochondrial poison, blocking NADH oxidation (Hayes & Laws 1991).

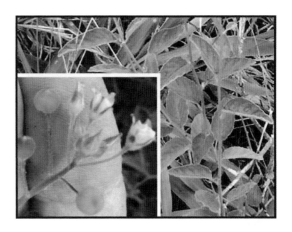

Figure 42. *Piriqueta racemosa* with inset showing close-up of flowers. [DL]

Local name: rigid stripeseed (English)
Scientific name: *Piriqueta racemosa* (Jacq.) Sweet
Family: Turneraceae (Turnera Family)

Description

Herbaceous, erect to 40 cm tall; flowers yellow (USDA 2011).

Range

Native to South America (USDA 2011). Introduced to Palau and found growing in the savanna grasslands and urban areas that have cultivated and ornamental plants (Hillmann Kitalong, DeMeo & Holm 2008).

Traditional Uses

Medicine used for skin itch. Leaves are used with coconut oil and applied to itchy area [Elin Rebluud].

Pharmacological Properties

No relevant pharmacological reports were identified.

Toxicology

No relevant toxicological reports were identified.

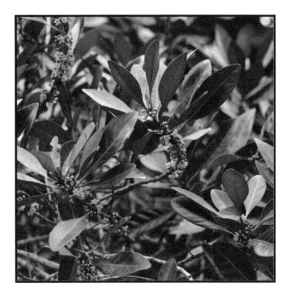

Figure 43. *Pouteria obovata* leaves and flowers. [AK]

Local names: *chelangel* (Palauan); northern yellow boxwood (English)
Scientific name: *Pouteria obovata* (R. Br.) Baehni
Family: Sapotaceae (Sapodilla Family)

Description A shrubby to tall tree about 18 m in height, with a dbh of 30-60 cm. The simple, alternate elliptic-oblong leaves are 8-12 cm long and 3.5-5 cm wide, with a distinct coppery underside. Greenish-white flowers grow in axilliary clusters of 1-5. The young fruits are green for over a month and turn black as they ripen. The black, flattened, kidney-shaped, fleshy fruits are 3-5 cm long, and contain one large seed (Hillmann Kitalong, DeMeo & Holm 2008).

Range
Commonly found in both volcanic and limestone forests of Palau. It is broadly distributed in the tropics from India and Malaysia to Australia and the Pacific Islands (Hillmann Kitalong, DeMeo & Holm 2008).

Traditional Uses
Medicine used for rashes. Boil leaves, fruits, stems and flowers in water and use as a bath when cooled [Linda Omekat Belaiok].
Medicine used for acne. Boil leaves in pot and use the water to wash your face. Do not use soap or any other face wash when you are using this. Use for a couple of days to a week and start to see acne disappear and the face become smooth [Linda Omekat Belaiok]

Pharmacological Properties
No pharmacological properties relevant to these uses were identified.

Toxicology
No relevant toxicological reports were identified.

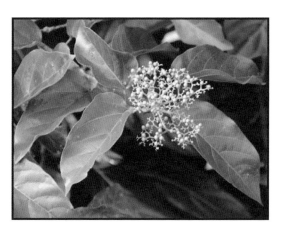

Figure 44. *Premna serratifolia* leaves, flowers, and inner bark. [MB]

Local name: *chosm* (Palauan)
Scientific name: *Premna serratifolia* L.
Family: Lamiaceae (Mint Family)

Description
Premna serratifolia is a low shrub or small tree, growing to 10 m in height, with compressed branchlets. The leaves are opposite, round to oval in shape, and 0.5-8

cm in length. The inflorescences are up to 2 cm in length, with small white cup-shaped calyces. The fruits are round, 2-4 mm in diameter, green ripening to black (Smith 1991).

Range
Premna serratifolia is a lowland species ranging from eastern Africa to Sri Lanka, southeastern Asia, the Ryuku Islands, Taiwan, Malaysia, and tropical Australia to the southern Pacific Islands. *Premna serratifolia* is found growing in beach thickets, dry lowland forest, along rocky shores, on the edges of mangrove swamps, and in agroforest areas (Balick 2009; Smith 1991). It is native to Palau (Hillmann Kitalong, DeMeo & Holm 2008).

Traditional Uses
Medicine used for ringworm. Leaves are rubbed together and put on infected area for ringworm (*besokel*) and then it will dry and just peel off [Tadashi Belchal, Risao Bausouch, Scott Yano].

Pharmacological Properties
Compounds isolated from the extract of root nodules from the related species, *Premna herbaceae* Roxb., enhanced antimicrobial activity against Gram-positive and Gram-negative bacteria and fungi (Murthy *et al.*, 2006).

Toxicology
Isolated compounds from the chloroform extract of the leaves of the related species, *Premna tomentosa*, had carcinogenic effects on a healthy cell line (Chin *et al.*, 2006).

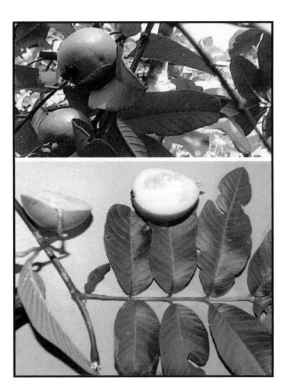

Figure 45. *Psidium guajava* leaves and fruit. [AK & WL]

Local names: *kuabang* (Palauan); guava (English)
Scientific name: *Psidium guajava* L.
Family: Myrtaceae (Myrtle Family)

Description
Psidium guajava is an evergreen shrub or small tree to 10 m in height. The leaves are 4-10 cm long and oval. The flowers are white and fragrant and 5 cm long. The fruits are small, round and yellow, with sweet, pink-seeded flesh when ripe (Merlin *et al.*, 1992; Smith 1979).

Range
Native to tropical Central America ranging from Mexico to northern South America, *Psidium guajava* is now pantropical. It is found growing at all elevations, often forming thickets along roadsides and clearings (Smith 1979). It has been cultivated

throughout the world for its fruit (Morton 1987).

Traditional Uses
Medicine used for rash. One bundle of leaves is boiled and the person bathes with this water. Bathe repeatedly to cure rash [Gloria Emesiochel].

Pharmacological Properties
The alcohol extract of the leaf sprout exhibited antimicrobial activity against strains of *Escherichia coli* and *Staphylococcus aureus* (Vieira *et al.*, 2001). Another study demonstrated the methanolic extract of the leaves of *P. guajava* showed inhibitory activity against strains of *E. coli*, *S. aureus*, *Pseudomonas aeruginosa*, *Proteus* spp., and *Shigella* spp. multidrug-resistant wound isolates from hospital patients in Nigeria. This same extract also improved wound healing parameters in rats (Chah *et al.*, 2006).

Toxicology
No reports of toxicity were identified.

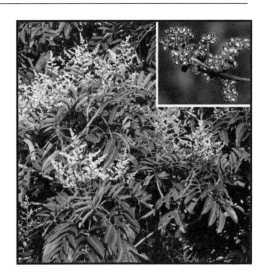

Figure 46. *Rhus taitensis* leaves and flowers, with inset showing fruits. [AK]

Local names: *cheues* (Palauan); sumac (English)
Scientific name: *Rhus taitensis* Guill.
Family: Anacardiaceae (Cashew Family)

Description
A medium size tree 10-15 m tall, dbh 25-70 cm. The branchlets are smooth and hairy with a reddish color. Leaves are compound, 5-10 cm long and 2-3 cm wide. Yellowish-white flower clusters grow at the end of the branchlets. The black fruit is 4-5 mm wide and covered with fine hairs (Hillmann Kitalong, DeMeo & Holm 2008).

Range
A common tree growing in the volcanic forests of Babeldaob Island. Small trees are found along the forest edge and larger trees within the interior. It is distributed in Palau, Yap, the Philippines, and Tahiti (Hillmann Kitalong, DeMeo & Holm 2008).

Traditional Uses
Medicine used for skin fungus. Roll some leaves, cut and dispose of the base. Use the leaves and pound it so its juices can come out. Then you spread it on the affected area of the skin. A few leaves rolled together are good for fungal skin problems (*Tinea versicolor*) [Kerungil Tesei].

Pharmacological Properties
Methanolic extracts of the related species, *Rhus glabra,* showed strong antibiotic activity and moderate, though diverse, antifungal activity (McCutcheon *et al.*, 1994).

Toxicology
Poison sumac, ivy, and oak are all former members of the *Rhus* or sumac genus. They were moved to the genus *Toxicodendron* to isolate the plants containing high quantities

of urushiol, which causes dermatitis and other allergic responses (Gladman 2006). The urushiol content of *Rhus taitensis* is not known (Kuo *et al.*, 1991).

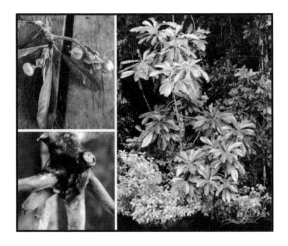

Figure 47. *Semecarpus venenosus* fruits and leaves (top left); point of leaf attachment (bottom left); and branches (right). [WL & MB]

Local names: *tonget* (Palauan); Palau poison tree (English)
Scientific name: *Semecarpus venenosus* Volk.
Family: Anacardiaceae (Cashew Family)

Description

A medium sized tree about 10 m tall, dbh to 80 cm. Simple alternate leaves 25-35 cm long and 10-12 cm wide and cluster at the branch tips. White flower clusters grow at the branch tips with the younger flowers at the center. Male and female flowers occur on separate plants. Male flower clusters are 6-8 cm long without a flower stalk. The petals are thick, leathery and pointed and 3-4 mm long. The red freshly one-seeded fruit is compressed and globe-like in shape (Hillmann Kitalong, DeMeo & Holm 2008).

Range

Semecarpus venenosus (*tonget*) or poison tree grows in the limestone and volcanic forests of Babeldaob and Koror. It is also common in riparian areas. The distribution of *S. venenosus* is restricted to Palau and Yap (Hillmann Kitalong, DeMeo & Holm 2008).

Traditional Uses

Medicine used for ringworm. If placed on area infected by ringworm (*besokel*) it becomes inflamed and slowly heals [Dr. Victor Yano].

Pharmacological Properties

No pharmacological reports relevant to this use were identified.

Toxicology

The related species, *Semecarpus anacardium* L. as well as other species of the genus *Semecarpus*, contain urushiol and related substances which can induce contact dermatitis (Bruneton 1999).

COMBINATION THERAPIES

a)

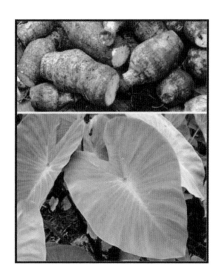

b)

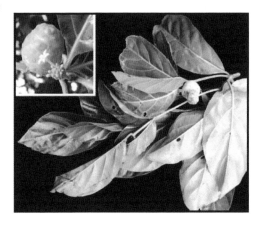

Figure 48. **a)** *Colocasia esculenta* harvested corms and leaves. [AK]; **b)** *Morinda citrifolia* leaves and fruit, with inset showing flower, flower buds, and fruit. [MB & AK]

Local and Scientific names:

dait (Palauan); taro (English) - *Colocasia esculenta* L. Schott (Araceae)

ngel (Palauan); noni (English) - *Morinda citrifolia* L. (Rubiaceae)

Descriptions

Colocasia esculenta L. Schott: *Colocasia esculenta* is an herb growing to 1 m in height with an underground corm. At the apex of this corm is a whorl of leaves. The leaves are 20-50 cm long, with an elongated oval shape. The lower lobes of the leaf may be rounded with dark red stems clasped at the base (Purseglove 1988).

Morinda citrifolia L.: A small tree 3-8 m in height, with a dbh of 10-30 cm and hairless, 4-angled stems. The simple, opposite, elliptic leaves are up to 45 cm long and 25 cm wide. The margins are entire, the surfaces are glossy, hairless and pliable, the stout petiole is up to 2 cm long. The flowers are borne in 75-90 flowered, oval to globe-like heads on a stalk about 3 cm long, with the calyx having a truncate rim with no lobes. The white corolla has 5 lobes that are slightly curled backward. The flower stalk is 1-3 cm long.

The yellowish-white, fleshy, soft and odiferous, irregular heads are about 5 cm long and 3-4 cm wide. The fruits have a wart-like appearance (Hillmann Kitalong, DeMeo & Holm 2008).

Ranges

Colocasia esculenta L. Schott: *Colocasia esculenta* originated from Southeast Asia. It is now widely cultivated for its edible corms, cormels, and leaves throughout Africa, South and Southeast Asia, the Pacific and Caribbean Islands. Some varieties are also grown for their ornamental foliage (Lemmens & Bunyapraphatsara 2003; Purseglove 1988). *Morinda citrifolia* L.: Indigenous to Indo-Malaysia, *Morinda citrifolia* ranges throughout the Pacific to Hawaiian Islands and other tropical regions around the world. In coastal forests, it is established as an understory plant often found near creeks, alongside the edge of mangrove swamps, and can be found growing up to 137 m above sea level (Smith 1988). In Palau, it is found along the volcanic forest edge and savanna (Hillmann Kitalong, DeMeo & Holm 2008).

Traditional Uses

Medicine used for boils. Cover 5 leaves each of *Colocasia esculenta* (*dait*) and *Morinda citrifolia* (*ngel*), with coconut oil, and stick to the boil to draw out pus and liquids [Clarence Kitalong].

Pharmacological Properties

Colocasia esculenta L. Schott: The corm of *Colocasia esculenta* has been reported to have anti-inflammatory properties (Cambie and Ferguson 2003).

Morinda citrifolia L.: The fruit extract has potent antibacterial properties (Zaidan *et al.*, 2005). The fruit extract of the related species, *Morinda pubescens* Sm., accelerated wound healing in rats (Mathivanan *et al.*, 2006).

Toxicology

Colocasia esculenta L. Schott: There are reports of contact dermatitis associated with *Colocasia esculenta* (Lampe 1986). The leaves, stems and tubers of *C. esculenta* contain calcium oxalate crystals and can cause injury to the mucous membranes of the mouth when eaten raw. Cooking the tuber inactivates these crystals (Nelson, Shih & Balick 2007).

Morinda citrifolia L.: Two publications reported cases of liver toxicity linked to the ingestion of noni juice (Millonig, Stadelmann & Vogel 2005; Stadlbauer *et al.,* 2005). Some researchers believe that the risk of liver toxicity is unlikely due to very low concentrations of potentially hepatotoxic anthraquinones (Kamiya *et al.,* 2005; Pawlus *et al.,* 2005). *Morinda citrifolia* juice did not show any genotoxicity and the author concluded that pure *M. citrifolia* juice is safe for human consumption (Westendorf *et al.*, 2007).

b)

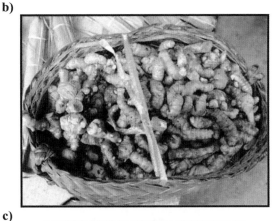

c)

a)

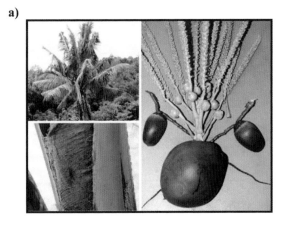

Figure 49. a) *Cocos nucifera* leaves, husk, and fruits. [DL & WL]; **b)** *Curcuma longa* tubers. [AK]; **c)** *Musa × paradisiaca* with fruits. [AK].

Local and Scientific names:

lius (Palauan); coconut (English) - *Cocos nucifera* L. (Arecaceae)
kesol (Palauan); turmeric (English) - *Curcuma longa* L. (Zingiberaceae)
tuu (Palauan); banana (English) - *Musa × paradisiaca* L. (Musaceae)

Descriptions

Cocos nucifera L.: *Cocos nucifera* is a tall palm, reaching heights of 20-30 m. It bears a terminal crown of leaves. The trunk is grayish-brown in color and is 20-40 cm in diameter. The fruits are green, yellow or red depending on the variety. This species may live up to 80-100 years (Purseglove 1988; Smith 1979).

Curcuma longa L.: An herb 1 m high with a spike of pale yellow flowers surrounded by white bracts. The tuber is orange-brown on the outside and bright yellow-orange on the inside (Smith 1979).

Musa × paradisiaca L.: *Musa × paradisiaca* is a tall perennial herb, 2-10 m in height, resembling a tree in habit. The large flower is reddish brown with clustering fruits varying in size, color and shape, though the cultivated variety usually has larger fruits. The skin can vary from thin and tender to thick and tough. The flesh of the fruit can be starchy, sweet, yellowish, green, or red, and is often seedless. A cross between *Musa acuminate* Colla. and *M. balbisiana* Colla., *Musa × paradisiaca* has hundreds of cultivars (Smith 1979).

Ranges

Cocos nucifera L.: A pantropical species, *Cocos nucifera* is native to the Old World tropics, most likely the Pacific Islands (*Cocos nucifera*, TRAMIL 2008). It has been cultivated extensively throughout the tropics as an important economic crop. Due to its wide distribution, commonness, and unwieldy size, few voucher collections are made of this species (Smith 1979).

Curcuma longa L.: Cultivated throughout the tropical regions of China, India, and Indo-Malaysia. The origin is thought to be South Asia, however, the species is so widely naturalized throughout the Pacific Islands that it appears indigenous (Smith 1979). Introduced to Palau, it is found growing in agricultural and agroforest areas (Hillmann Kitalong, DeMeo & Holm 2008).

Musa × paradisiaca L.: The center of origin for this crop is thought to be in Southeast Asia. *Musa* species are now pantropical and widely cultivated for food (Purseglove 1988). Introduced to Palau and found growing in agricultural and agroforest areas, as well as in areas that have cultivated and ornamental plants (Hillmann Kitalong, DeMeo & Holm 2008).

Traditional Uses

Medicine used for skin fungus. Root of *kesol* is used to treat skin fungus (*tebkabk*) that is believed to be caused by "black magic." Grind the roots of *Curcuma longa* (*kesol*) and combine with ground *Cocos nucifera* (*kles el lius*) and place inside *C. nucifera* fiber, then wrap it in banana (*tuu*) leaves and burn for about 30 min. Then pick out the extremely burned portions of the poultice and wrap it in a white cloth and that is then pressed onto the fungus on the skin for 1 min, then remove the poultice at least 30 sec, then reapply again, and again about 5 min [Ingas Spesungel].

Pharmacological Properties

Cocos nucifera L.: The oil from the nut is valued as an emollient and the extract from the husk fiber is used in remedies to treat skin infections due to its antibacterial and antiviral properties (Aburjai & Natcheh 2003; Mendonça-Filho *et al.*, 2004).

Curcuma longa L.: No pharmacological reports relevant to this use were identified.

Musa × paradisiaca L.: No pharmacological reports relevant to this use were identified.

Toxicology

Cocos nucifera L.: No reports of toxicity were identified.

Curcuma longa L.: No reports of toxicity relevant to the topical use of *Curcuma longa* were identified.

Musa × paradisiaca L.: Pulp extracts of *Musa × paradisiaca* enhanced the growth of pathogenic Gram-negative bacterial strains of *Escherichia coli*, *Shigella flexneri*, *Enterobacter cloacae*, and *Salmonella typhimurium* (Lyte 1997). The fruit is involved in a rare but potentially fatal clinical entity of type I allergy to fruits without concomitant allergy to other common airborne/contact allergens (Saraswat & Kumar 2005). Similarly, individuals with sensitivity to bananas should be cautious of foods such as avocado, orange and chestnut that are known to cross-react with banana antigens (Moreno-Ancillo *et al.*, 2004).

c)

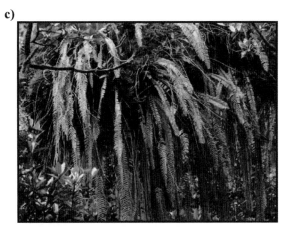

a)

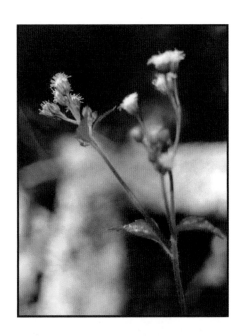

b)

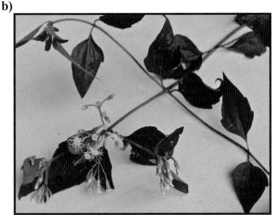

Figure 50. a) *Ageratum conyzoides* flowers. [RL]; **b)** *Chromolaena odorata*. [MB]; **c)** *Nephrolepis acutifolia*. [AK]

Local and Scientific names:
ngmak (Palauan); goatweed, whiteweed (English) - *Ageratum conyzoides* L. (Asteraceae)
ngesngesil (Palauan); Siam weed (English) - *Chromolaena odorata* (L.) R. M. King & H. Rob. (Asteraceae)
delimes (Palauan) - *Nephrolepis acutifolia* (Desv.) Christ (Lomariopsidaceae)

Descriptions
Ageratum conyzoides L.: Coarse herb 0.2-1 m high; opposite and simple leaves commonly subacute or obtuse to round at base; the corolla lobes and styles are white to pale lavender. Flowering heads usually 5-8 mm in diameter with 60-75 flowers. Flowering and fruiting seen throughout the year (Smith 1991).
Chromolaena odorata (L.) R. M. King & H. Rob.: Shrub or herb 1-2 m high, with many branches. Leaves strongly aromatic. Flowers in flat topped clusters of 20-35 florets, involucre green, corolla lilac to off-white, seeds black [M.J. Balick 3447, 4383] (Arvigo & Balick 1998).
Nephrolepis acutifolia (Desv.) Christ: A large epiphytic fern with short, erect, stoloniferous rhizomes and leathery fronds over 1 m long; the scaly rachises are red, with linear and marginal indusia; numerous

pinnae (generally 20-50 pairs) (Hoshizaki & Moran 2001).

Ranges

Ageratum conyzoides L.: Mexico and the West Indies to South America, now often cultivated and established as an adventive in most warm countries. It was probably an early European introduction into the Pacific Islands as an ornamental (Smith 1991). Introduced to Palau and found growing in savanna grasslands and in urban areas that typically have cultivated landscape and ornamental plants (Hillmann Kitalong, DeMeo & Holm 2008).

Chromolaena odorata (L.) R. M. King & H. Rob.: Native to the American continent, and introduced to tropical Asia, West Africa, and parts of Australia. It was introduced to Palau and now is considered an invasive (Hillmann Kitalong, DeMeo & Holm 2008).

Nephrolepis acutifolia (Desv.) Christ: Native to tropical Africa and from southeastern Asia to Polynesia (Hoshizaki & Moran 2001). Native to Palau and found growing in volcanic lowland forest and mangrove forest (Hillmann Kitalong, DeMeo & Holm 2008).

Traditional Uses

Medicine used for boils. The top 4 leaves of *lius* (*Cocos nucifera*) are pounded with the top 4 leaves of *ngesngesill* (*Chromolaena odorata*). [It is possible that another species is used, *ngmak*, *Ageratum conyzoides*—in the non-flowering stage the plants can easily be confused]. This creates a sticky substance that is used to suck out blood from cuts, take out pus and blood from boils, draw out splinters, and draw out snake fangs. Young leaves are pounded and put on cuts to soak up blood [Dirraklang Merei Ngirametuker, Gillian Johannes, Tsuneo Tesei, Kerngel Tesei].

Pharmacological Properties

Ageratum conyzoides L.: Oral administration of an ethanolic leaf extract of *Ageratum conyzoides* for 90 days reduced subchronic and chronic inflammation in rats (Moura *et al.*, 2005). A methanolic extract of this plant improved wound healing parameters in a rat model (Oladejo *et al.*, 2003).

Chromolaena odorata (L.) R. M. King & H. Rob.: Aqueous leaf extracts of *Chromolaena odorata* showed anti-inflammatory actions in rats (25-200 mg/kg) supporting use for wounds and inflammation (Owoyele, Adediji & Soladoye 2005) and flavonoids isolated from this plant demonstrated anti-inflammatory and analgesic activity *in vitro* (Owoyele *et al.*, 2008). An ethanol extract of *C. odorata* enhanced proliferation of fibroblasts, endothelial cells and keratinocytes *in vitro* (Thang *et al.*, 2001). Growth enhancement of human keratinocytes (human skin cells) and the migration of keratinocytes into damaged tissue were stimulated by *C. odorata* extracts at low concentrations *in vitro* (Phan, Hughes & Cherry 2001). Collagen lattice contraction was irreversibly inhibited at 200 μg/ml and 400 μg/ml (Phan *et al.*, 1996). Improved wound healing due to *C. odorata* extract is enhanced by the upregulation of adhesion complex proteins and fibronectin produced by human keratinocytes (Phan *et al.*, 2000). *Chromolaena odorata* extract also has antimicrobial and antifungal properties, inhibiting the growth of *Pseudomonas aeruginosa* and *Streptococcus faecalis* (Irobi 1992). Ethanolic extracts of the leaves of *C. odorata* showed antibacterial activity against both Gram-positive and Gram-negative bacteria (Irobi 1992; 1997). Aqueous ethanol extracts of leaves showed antifungal activity (Ngono Ngane *et al.*, 2006). Administration of *C. odorata* extract inhibited carrageenan-induced paw edema in rats (Owoyele,

Adediji, & Soladoye 2005; Oludare *et al.*, 2000).

Nephrolepis acutifolia (Desv.) Christ: No pharmacological reports relevant to this use were identified.

Toxicology

Ageratum conyzoides L.: No hepatotoxicity was observed with oral doses up to 500 mg/kg/day for 90 days in rats (Moura *et al.*, 2005).

Chromolaena odorata (L.) R. M. King & H. Rob.: Administration of aqueous extract of *C. odorata* leaves to rats caused a reduction in the size of testicles and reduced the number of spermatozoa. Thus, *Chromolaena odorata* possesses antiandrogenic properties at the testicular level interfering with fertility (Yakubu, Akanji & Oladiji 2007). Oral administration of *C. odorata* extract produced a significant reduction in testicular body weight ratio, acid phosphatase activities, and protein, cholesterol, glycogen, sialic acid, and testosterone concentrations further indicating that this plant may possess anti-androgenic effects (Yakubu, Akanji & Oladiji 2007). At high concentrations the *C. odorata* extract was toxic to keratinocytes (Phan, Hughes & Cherry 2001).

Nephrolepis acutifolia (Desv.) Christ: Ferns of varying species, but not necessarily *Nephrolepis acutifolia*, have been shown to cause contact dermatitis in some patients (de Cock, Vorwerk & Bruynzeel 1998; Geller-Bernstein *et al.*, 1987; Stoof & Bruynzeel 1989).

NOTES

CHAPTER SIX: CUTS, WOUNDS, AND BROKEN BONES

Cuts or tears in tissue (lacerations), scrapes (abrasions), and puncture wounds are common health concerns and can be caused by bites, sharp or pointed objects, blades, or numerous other types of injuries. Depending on the severity, a majority of wounds heal rapidly without complications. More severe wounds can cause extensive blood loss and have a greater chance of becoming infected. Deeper wounds can become complicated by infection or injury to other structures, such as nerves, tendons, or blood vessels.

Wounds can be painful at first, but usually the pain lessens after the first day. If a cut affects a nerve or tendon, the injured person may lose partial or full range of motion and/or experience numbness. If a foreign object remains inside a punctured wound, the part of the wound near the object can be painful to the touch. Pain that worsens one day or more after the injury is often the first sign of infection. The symptoms of infection include fever, redness and swelling of the area, and abscess (localized collection of pus) or oozing pus. These are signs that a wound may require oral antibiotic treatment.

Infection can develop when a wound is contaminated with dirt and bacteria. Although any wound can become infected, infection is particularly likely in deep scrapes, which grind dirt into the skin, and in puncture wounds, which introduce contamination deep under the skin layer. Additionally, wounds that contain foreign material (such as splinters, glass, or clothing fragments) are likely to be contaminated with dirt and/or bacteria and therefore are much more likely to become infected.

First-Aid Treatment

While bleeding helps clean a wound, the first step in treating a cut or open wound is to stop the bleeding. Shallow cuts to most areas of the skin rarely bleed much and often stop bleeding on their own. In the vast majority of cases, bleeding can be stopped by firmly compressing a clean cloth or gauze to the bleeding area with a finger or hand for at least five minutes. If bleeding does not stop after 15 minutes of continous pressure, seek professional medical care. Cuts to the hand and face/head/scalp as well as cuts to arteries and larger veins tend to bleed vigorously and often require more extensive and invasive treatments. Whenever possible, the bleeding part should be elevated above the level of the heart (i.e. by raising a limb above the head). Tourniquets shut off all blood flow to a body part depriving it of oxygen and therefore should be used rarely, or if necessary, only for a short duration of time (≤10 min).

After the bleeding has been controlled, the wound must be cleaned to prevent infection. The longer a wound remains contaminated, the more likely infection will develop. Large particles should be carefully removed first. Smaller dirt and particles that cannot be seen are removed by washing with clean/sterile running water. The wound can be held under running water, or a tub can be filled with water and a cup used to pour the water over the wound. A mild soap can be added to the water. Dirt and particles that remain after washing often can be removed with a more highly pressured stream. Deep scrapes should be scrubbed gently to remove all debris. After gently cleaning, antibiotic ointment and a bandage should be applied. After the wound is cleaned, traditional botanical medicines can be applied but should be changed daily to prevent infection. If a wound is very small, it can be kept closed with commercially available tapes or super glue. Most of these small wounds heal within a few days. Stitches may be needed for deep or large cuts. Harsher agents, such as alcohol, iodine, and peroxide, are not recommended for cleaning deep wounds. These solutions can cause tissue damage and make it harder for the wound to heal properly.

Professional medical assistance is urgently needed under the following circumstances:

- **If the cut is jagged**
- **If a cut becomes tender or inflamed**
- **If a cut is longer than about $^1/_3$ in, is on the face, appears deep, or has edges that separate**
- **If the cut bleeds in spurts**
- **If bleeding does not stop within several (approximately fifteen) minutes or after pressure is applied**
- **If there are symptoms of a nerve or tendon injury**
- **If a scrape is deep or has dirt and particles that are difficult to remove**
- **If there is a puncture wound, particularly if it is suspected that a foreign object is imbedded in the wound**
- **If the person has not had a tetanus vaccination within the past 10 years**

All wounds, whether treated at home or by medical professionals, should be observed for symptoms of infection during the first several days after treatment. If any symptoms of infection develop, medical assistance should be sought within several hours and the appropriate antibiotic initiated at that time.

Chapter Six discusses 20 different plant remedies reported to treat cuts and wounds.

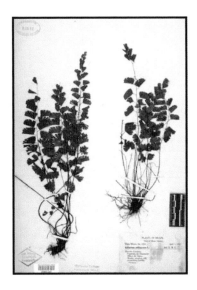

Figure 51. NYBG voucher specimen of *Adiantum philippense*. [Y.E.J.M]

Local names: *oecherela kesebekuu* (Palauan); maiden hair (English)
Scientific name: *Adiantum philippense* L.
Family: Pteridaceae (Pteris Fern Family)

Description

Rhizome short, suberect or creeping with tufted fronds, dark-brown subulate rhizome-scales about 3 mm long. Stipe castaneous, up to 15 cm long, glabrous. Frond arching, herbaceous, often proliferous at the apex. Lamina up to 42 × 9.5 cm, lanceolate in outline, pinnate; pinnae up to 2 × 4.6 cm, mostly very broadly oblong to rhombic, more reduced and obcuneate towards the apex of the frond. Sori borne on the apices of the pinna lobes; indusial flaps up to 2 cm long, linear to shallowly lunate, glabrous (Schelpe 1970).

Range

Pantropical. Native to Palau and found growing in the volcanic lowland forests (Hillmann Kitalong, DeMeo & Holm 2008).

Traditional Uses

Styptic. Leaves are crushed and applied to a wound to stop bleeding (DeFilipps, Maina & Pray 1988).

Pharmacological Properties

Intraperitoneal and oral administration of a methanolic extract of the related species, *Adiantum latifolium* Lam., produced dose-dependent analgesic and anti-inflammatory activity in mice (Nonato *et al.*, 2010). Methanolic extracts of the related species, *A. capillus-veneris* and *A. venustum,* demonstrated antimicrobial activity against *Escherichica coli* and *Aspergillus terreus*, respectively (Singh *et al.*, 2008).

Toxicology

A single oral dose of 1,000 mg/kg did not produce any toxicity in mice (Nonato *et al.*, 2010).

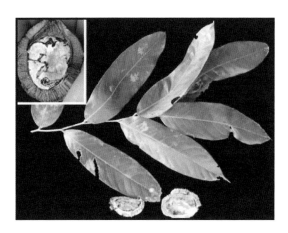

Figure 52. *Atuna racemosa* subsp. *racemosa* with inset showing cross section of fruit.
[MB & WL]

Local names: *cheritem* (Palauan); parinarium nut (English)
Scientific name: *Atuna racemosa* Raf. subsp. *racemosa*
Family: Chrysobalanaceae (Coco-plum Family)

Description

A medium tree 10-15 m tall with a dbh from 20-35 cm. The branchlets are smooth, slender and dark. The simple, alternate leaves are 10-15 cm long and 3-6 cm wide. The lavender flower clusters grow on a main axis (raceme) with the youngest flowers at the tip. The funnel-shaped flowers are up to 1.5 cm in diameter. The calyx has 5 hairy sepals. The fleshy, brown one-seeded fruit is 5-10 cm in diameter with a brown exocarp that is hard and rough, with a fleshy mesocarp (Hillmann Kitalong, DeMeo & Holm 2008).

Range

Atuna racemosa subsp. *racemosa* is found in the volcanic and urban forests of Babeldaob Island, typically along rivers and stream banks. It is distributed in the Philippines, Borneo, Malasia and the Micronesian Islands of Yap, Pohnpei, and Chuuk (Hillmann Kitalong, DeMeo & Holm 2008).

Traditional Uses

Medicine used for wounds. Peel bark and grind wood and squeeze on the wound until juice comes out. This will stop the bleeding. Leave on wound for 1 day and change it the next day. Stop putting it on when the wound is dry and healing [Johnson Emesiochel].

Pharmacological Properties

An ethanolic extract of *Atuna racemosa* was active against methicillin-resistant *Staphylococcus aurea* (MRSA) *in vitro* (Buenz *et al.*, 2007).

Toxicology
In a phase I clinical trial the maximum tolerated topical dose of an *Atuna racemosa* ethanolic extract was determined to be between 500 and 1,000 µg/ml. No adverse effects were reported in any of the test subjects (Buenz *et al.*, 2007).

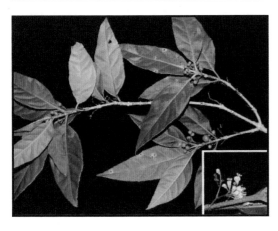

Figure 53. *Callicarpa elegans* leaves and fruits with inset showing flowers. [SP]

Local name: ***keruiau*** (Palauan)
Scientific name: *Callicarpa elegans* Hayek
Family: Lamiaceae (Mint Family)

Description
Shrub to 2.5 m tall; dbh 2 cm; leaves simple, opposite; flowers white [M.J. Balick 4549, 4492].

Range
Native to Palau and growing on the volcanic lowland forests (Hillmann Kitalong, DeMeo & Holm 2008).

Traditional Uses
Medicine used for treating wounds. Boil 1 handful of leaves with 1 gal of water for 15-25 min, and pour into basin. Mix with cool water, so that it will not burn the skin, and clean the infected area or wound before medication or dressing the infected skin or wound [Ingas Spesungel].

Pharmacological Properties
No pharmacological reports relevant to the treatment of cuts, wounds, or broken bones were identified.

Toxicology
No reports of toxicity were identified.

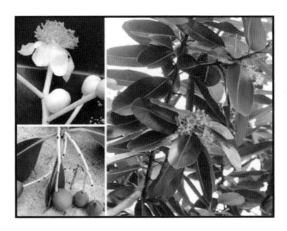

Figure 54. *Calophyllum inophyllum* branches, flowers, and fruits. [AK & CK]

Local names: ***btaches*** (Palauan); galip nut, beach mahogany (English)
Scientific name: *Calophyllum inophyllum* L.
Family: Clusiaceae (Clusia Family)

Description
Large and spreading tree 6-25 m high, with white latex and a massive trunk to 1.5 m in diameter. The fragrant flowers have white perianth segments and yellow anthers; the fruit is green to yellow, eventually becoming purplish or blackish (Smith 1981).

Range
Eastern Africa and India throughout Malaysia and eastward into the Tuamotus; it was presumably an aboriginal introduction into Hawaii (Smith 1981). Likewise, it is native to

Palau and found growing in volcanic lowland forests, savanna grasslands, and limestone forests, atolls and strand vegetation along the coast (Hillmann Kitalong, DeMeo & Holm 2008).

Traditional Uses
Medicine used for wounds. Oil is extracted from the fruit. Used to heal wounds and prevent infection due to its antibacterial properties (Kitalong, DeMeo & Holm 2008).

Pharmacological Properties
A coumarin isolated from *Calophyllum inophyllum* exhibits anticoagulant properties and might also work as an anti-inflammatory agent (Arora, Mathur & Seth 1962; Bhalla *et al.*, 1980) perhaps due to a PAF-related mechanism as demonstrated on rabbit platelets (bin Jantan, Jalil & Warif 2001). An oral dose of a methanolic stem bark extract protected mice from thermally-induced pain in the hot plate test (Mishra *et al.*, 2010). A methanol extract of the stem bark of *C. inophyllum* inhibited Gram-positive and Gram-negative bacteria *in vitro* (Mishra *et al.*, 2010).

Toxicology
Oil extracted from the seed of *Calophyllum inophyllum* has been reported to cause contact dermatitis (Le Coz 2004). Rats fed *C. inophyllum* seed oil (5% of diet) for 8 weeks showed signs of liver, kidney and heart damage and demonstrated evidence of atherosclerosis (Ajayi *et al.*, 2008). After an oral dose of a stem bark methanolic extract at 2,000 mg/kg, no acute toxicity was observed in mice (Mishra *et al.*, 2010). There are cases of contact dermatitis from the seed oil (Le Coz 2004). Anticoagulant properties of coumarins isolated from this plant may interfere with the intrinsic wound-healing

capacity of blood (Arora, Mathur & Seth 1962).

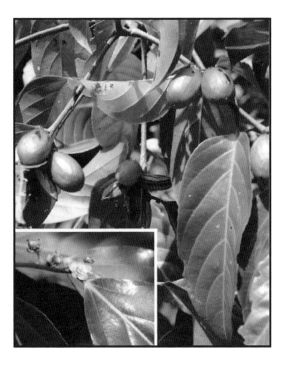

Figure 55. *Casearia hirtella* leaves and fruits with inset showing flowers. [AK]

Local names: *ngiwoden*, *kesengelengolm* (Palauan)
Scientific name: *Casearia hirtella* Hosok.
Family: Salicaceae (Willow Family)

Description
Tree or shrub ranging 3-5 m tall; dbh 2 cm; leaves green; immature fruit green, turning yellow with reddish seed [M.J. Balick 4364, 4408].

Range
It is endemic to Palau and grows on volcanic lowland forests and limestone forests, atolls, and strand vegetation along the coasts (Hillmann Kitalong, DeMeo & Holm 2008).

Traditional Uses
Styptic. New young leaves are chewed and placed on small cuts to stop bleeding [Tadashi Belchal, Risao Bausouch, Scott Yano].

Pharmacological Properties
An aqueous extract of the leaves of the related species, *Casearia sylvestris,* showed protection against bee and snake venom through partial inhibition of phospholipase A2 present in these venoms (Borges *et al.*, 2000). The extract was able to inhibit several isolated phospholipase A2s, which are involved in pain and inflammation at wound sites (de Mattos *et al.*, 2007). Essential oil from *C. sylvestris* leaves has demonstrated anti-inflammatory activity (Esteves *et al.*, 2005). An ethanolic extract of *C. sylvestris* demonstrated analgesic activity in ovalbumin- and acetic acid-induced pain models in mice (de Mattos *et al.*, 2007). The essential oil of the *C. sylvestris* leaves showed inhibition of carageenan-induced rat paw inflammation when administered orally to mice (Esteves *et al.*, 2005).

Toxicology
The crude leaf extract of the related species, *Casearia tomentosa*, induced chromosomal changes in bone marrow cells and primary spermatocytes in mice (Awasthy *et al.*, 2000). The oral LD_{50} of the leaf crude ethanolic extract of the related species, *C. sylvestris*, was determined to be 1,840 mg/kg in rats, indicating low acute internal toxicity (Basile *et al.*, 1990).

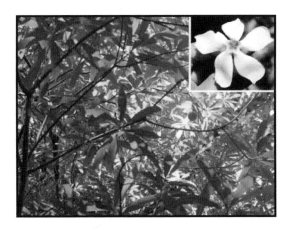

Figure 56. *Cerbera manghas* branches with fruit and inset showing close-up of flower. [AK]

Local names: *chemeridech* (Palauan); milkwood, sea mango (English)
Scientific name: *Cerbera manghas* L.
Family: Apocynaceae (Dogbane Family)

Description
Small tree 7-10 m tall. Leaves simple, alternate, narrowly obovate, 16-35 cm long × 3-8 cm wide. Flowers white, fragrant, in terminal cluster of 10-30 flowers, fruits large, 6-8 cm long × 4-6 cm wide, dark red in color (Hillmann Kitalong, DeMeo & Holm 2008).

Range
A small tree normally found in riparian areas in the volcanic forests of Babeldaob. It is native to Palau and is also found in tropical north Australia, Papua New Guinea and eastern Indonesia (Hillmann Kitalong, DeMeo & Holm 2008).

Traditional Uses
Medicine used for cuts. Milky latex is placed over cuts as a liquid bandage (Hillmann Kitalong, DeMeo & Holm 2008).

Pharmacological Properties
Ethanolic leaf extracts of the related species, *Cerbera odollam*, caused an increase in

reaction time to thermal pain in mice (Hiên, Navarro-Delmasure & Vy 1991).

Toxicology

There are no reports of toxicity concerning the topical use of this plant; however ingestion of the seeds of *Cerbera manghas* is extremely toxic. Self-poisoning with the seeds of this plant led to seven deaths observed at a teaching hospital in Sri Lanka between 2001 and 2002. Symptoms typical of cardiac glycoside poisoning including cardiac disarrhythmias and hyperkalemia were evident (Eddleston & Haggalla 2008). Another instance of self-poisoning with this plant comes from a 50-year-old man in China who experienced numbness of the face and upper extremities, and presented digoxin-like poisoning, including hyperkalemia, in general after eating three seeds of this plant in a suicide attempt (Tsai Y.C. *et al.,* 2008). While the seeds are the typical route of poisoning, plants in the Apocynaceae family have been known to have cardiac glycosides in all parts of the plant (Cheenpracha *et al.*, 2004; Radford *et al.*, 1986).

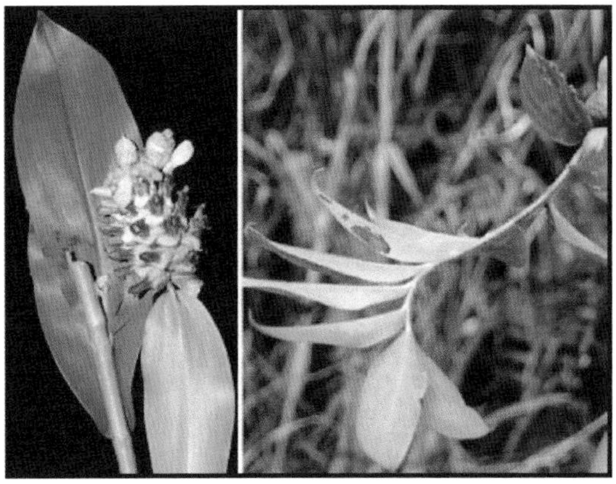

Figure 57. *Cheilocostus speciosus* leaves and flowers.
[MB & KS]

Local names: *isebsab* (Palauan); Malay ginger, spiral flag (English)
Scientific name: *Cheilocostus speciosus* (J. Koenig) C. Specht
Family: Costaceae (Costus Family)

Description

Coarse herb 1-4 m high. Ovoid inflorescence is 5-10 cm long, with bracts green to red or red-purple; the outer perianth segments are purplish, the inner ones white; the labellum is white with a yellow center and 5 cm long or more; the filament is white. The fruit is bright red (Smith 1979).

Range

Indo-Malaysia from the Himalayas to New Guinea, but widely cultivated and sometimes naturalized elsewhere (Smith 1979). It was introduced to Palau and it is now naturalized; found growing in the volcanic lowland forests (Hillmann Kitalong, DeMeo & Holm 2008).

Traditional Uses

Antiseptic. Use leaves to clean wounds.

Pharmacological Properties

No pharmacological reports relevant to the treatment of cuts, wounds or broken bones were identified.

Toxicology

No reports of toxicity were identified.

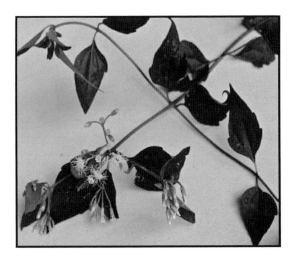

Figure 58. *Chromolaena odorata.* [MB]

Local name: *ngesngesil* (Palauan); Siam weed (English)
Scientific name: *Chromolaena odorata* (L.) R.M. King & H. Rob.
Family: Asteraceae (Daisy Family)

Description
Shrub or herb 1-2 m high, with many branches. Leaves strongly aromatic. Flowers in flat topped clusters of 20-35 florets, involucre green, corolla lilac to off-white, seeds black [M.J. Balick 3447, 4383] (Arvigo & Balick 1998).

Range
Native to the American continent, and introduced to tropical Asia, West Africa, and parts of Australia. It was introduced to Palau and now is considered an invasive (Hillmann Kitalong, DeMeo & Holm 2008).

Traditional Uses
Medicine used for cuts, boils, infections. The top 4 youngest leaves of *lius* (*Cocos nucifera*) are pounded with the top 4 youngest leaves of *ngesngesil* (*Chromolaena odorata*). This creates a sticky substance that is used on cuts to draw out blood from cuts, remove pus and blood from boils, draw out splinters, and draw out snake fangs [Dirraklang Merei Ngirametuker, Gillian Johanes, Tsuneo Tesei, Kerngel Tesei].

Pharmacological Properties
Aqueous leaf extracts of *Chromolaena odorata* showed anti-inflammatory actions in rats (25-200 mg/kg) supporting use for wounds and inflammation (Owoyele, Adediji & Soladoye 2005) and flavonoids isolated from this plant demonstrated anti-inflammatory and analgesic activity *in vitro* (Owoyele *et al.*, 2008). An ethanol extract of *C. odorata* enhanced proliferation of fibroblasts, endothelial cells and keratinocytes *in vitro* (Thang *et al.*, 2001). Growth enhancement of human keratinocytes (human skin cells) and the migration of keratinocytes into damaged tissue was stimulated by *C. odorata* extracts at low concentrations *in vitro* (Phan, Hughes & Cherry 2001; Phan *et al.*, 2001). Collagen lattice contraction was irreversibly inhibited at 200 µg/ml and 400 µg/ml (Phan *et al.*, 1996). Improved wound healing due to *C. odorata* extract is enhanced by the upregulation of adhesion complex proteins and fibronectin produced by human keratinocytes (Phan *et al.*, 2000). *Chromolaena odorata* extract also has antimicrobial and antifungal properties. Extract inhibited the growth of *Pseudomonas aeruginosa* and *Streptococcus faecalis* (Irobi 1992). Ethanolic extracts of the leaves of *C. odorata* showed antibacterial activity against both Gram-positive and Gram-negative bacteria (Irobi 1992; 1997). Aqueous ethanol extracts of leaves showed antifungal activity (Ngono Ngane *et al.*, 2006). Oral administration of *C. odorata* extract inhibited carrageenan-induced paw edema in rats (Owoyele, Adediji & Soladoye 2005; Oludare *et al.*, 2000).

Toxicology

Pyrrolizidine alkaloids are hepatotoxic and possibly tumorigenic. However it appears that the leaves and stems of *Chromolaena odorata* do not contain the alkaloids (Biller *et al.*, 1994). Compounds from the flowers of *C. odorata* show moderate cytotoxicity against human small cell lung cancer cells MIC 19.2 µM and weak toxicity against HBC (MIC 38.4 µM) (Suksamrarn *et al.*, 2004). Administration of aqueous extract of leaves of *C. odorata* in rats showed a reduction in the size of testicles and reduced number of spermatozoa. Thus, *C. odorata* possesses antiandrogenic properties at the testicular level interfering with fertility (Yakubu, Akanji & Oladiji 2007). Concentrations of 350 µg/ml were found to be toxic to keratinocytes (Phan, Hughes & Cherry 2001). Oral administration of *C. odorata* extract produced a significant reduction in testicular body weight ratio, acid phosphatase activities, and protein, cholesterol, glycogen, sialic acid, and testosterone concentrations and had anti-androgenic effects (Yakubu, Akanji & Oladiji 2007).

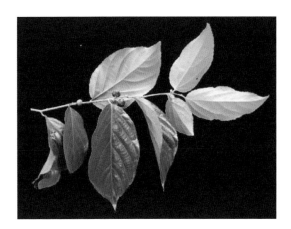

Figure 59. *Flacourtia rukam* var. *micronesica* leaves and fruits [MB]

Local name: *chemechong* (Palauan)
Scientific name: *Flacourtia rukam* Zoll. & Mor. var. *micronesica* Fosb. & Sach.
Family: Salicaceae (Willow Family)

Description

Chemechong is a medium size tree about 12 m in height with easily breakable stems with a dbh of 35 cm. The simple, alternate, elliptic to oval leaves are 1-20 cm long × 6-10 cm wide. Male and female flowers grow on different trees. The female flowers have a light green, rounded and glabrous calyx. The male flowers have 30-45 yellow stamens sticking out 2-4 mm long and no corolla. The red to purple berry-like fruit is about 1.3 cm long × 1 cm wide (Hillmann Kitalong, DeMeo & Holm 2008).

Range

Flacourtia rukam var. *micronesica* grows in limestone forests as well as old and young volcanic forests of Babeldaob. It is distributed throughout Micronesia and is found in Palau, Chuuk, and Pohnpei (Hillmann Kitalong, DeMeo & Holm 2008).

Traditional Uses

Medicine used for cuts. Use leaves to treat smaller cuts such as from a knife. Take some of the youngest leaves, chew them and put on cut. This will stop bleeding when used once (depending on the size of the cut) and change the leaves as needed, until the cut is healed [Clarence Kitalong, Ingas Spesungel].

Pharmacological Properties

No pharmacological reports relevant to the treatment of cuts, wounds or broken bones were identified.

Toxicology

No studies were found investigating the toxicity of *Flacourtia rukam*. A methanol extract of the related species, *F. jangomas,* showed no toxicity when orally administered to rats at a dose of 2,000 mg/kg (Singh, A.K., *et al.,* 2010).

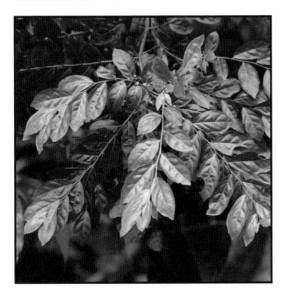

Figure 60. *Glochidion ramiflorum* leaves and fruits. [MB]

Local name: *ngolm* (Palauan)
Scientific name: *Glochidion ramiflorum* J.R. Forst. & G. Forst.
Family: Phyllanthaceae (Phyllanthus Family)

Description

A small tree about 10 m in height, dbh 6-32 cm. The simple, alternate leaves are 3-18 cm long, often unequally sided. The long-stalked yellow female flower is 4 mm wide and grows singly at the base of the male raceme. The male flowers grow on the axis of a long simple flower cluster up to 15 cm long. The green, flattened capsule is 5-15 mm in diameter, with unequal lobes. Fruits look like miniature pumpkins (Hillmann Kitalong, DeMeo & Holm 2008).

Range

Glochidion ramiflorum (*ngolm*) is found in both limestone and volcanic primary and secondary forests of Palau. *Ngolm* is native in Palau and is distributed throughout Micronesia and Polynesia (Hillmann Kitalong, DeMeo & Holm 2008).

Traditional Uses

Medicine used for cuts. Use leaves to treat smaller cuts such as from a knife. Take some of the youngest leaves, chew them and put on cut. This will stop bleeding when used once (depending on the size of the cut) and change the leaves as needed, until the cut is healed. These leaves are thicker than other species and thus preferred [Clarence Kitalong].

Pharmacological Properties

No pharmacological reports relevant to the treatment of cuts, wounds or broken bones were identified.

Toxicology

No reports of toxicity were identified.

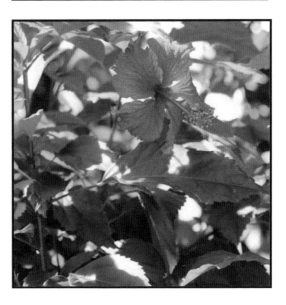

Figure 61. *Hibiscus rosa-sinensis* var. *rosa-sinensis* leaves and flowers. [AK]

Local names: *bussonge* (Palauan); hibiscus (English)
Scientific name: *Hibiscus rosa-sinensis* L. var. *rosa-sinensis*
Family: Malvaceae (Hibiscus Family)

Description
Hibiscus rosa-sinensis is a shrub 1-3 m tall with a narrow trunk. The leaves are alternate and ovate with serrated margins. The conspicuous flowers range in color from yellow to pink, orange, red and crimson with long stamens and have yellow seeds (Smith 1981).

Range
Hibiscus rosa-sinensis is probably native to eastern Africa, although its exact origin is unknown. It has been widely cultivated throughout the tropics and subtropics as an ornamental, often used as hedgerows (Smith 1981).

Traditional Uses
Medicine used for wounds. Use leaves and flowers to clean wounds, boils, and inflammations. Take the leaves and flowers and mash in cool water and wash affected area (face, hands, body, etc.) 3-4 times daily [Subediang Ubedei].

Pharmacological Properties
No pharmacological reports relevant to the treatment of cuts, wounds or broken bones were identified.

Toxicology
No reports of toxicity were identified.

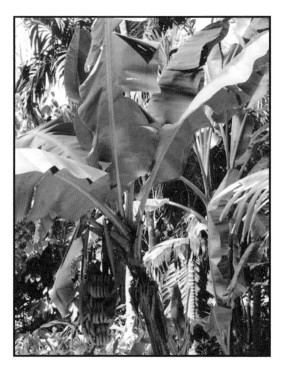

Figure 62. *Musa × paradisiaca* with fruits. [AK]

Local name: *miskebesang* (Palauan)
Scientific name: *Musa × paradisiaca*
Family: Musaceae (Banana Family)

Description
Herbaceous plant with thick, fleshy stems to 24 feet tall, arising from a corm. Leaves spirally arranged, growing to 2-3 m long × 60 cm wide. Inflorescence arising from the base of the crown, producing fruits that ripen to a yellow color (Banana, Wikipedia 2011).

Range
Bananas are found throughout the tropics and subtropics, particularly at lower elevations.

Traditional Uses
Medicine used for deep cuts. Take fibers of old stem and squeeze juice on cut and use banana fibers to wrap like gauze and leave for 2 days and do not get it wet. Another leaf

is pounded and put onto the gauze with coconut oil [Martha Nabeyama].

Pharmacological Properties
No relevant pharmacological properties were identified.

Toxicology
Pulp and peel extracts of *Musa* × *paradisiaca* enhanced the growth of pathogenic Gram-negative bacterial strains *Escherichia coli*, *Shigella flexneri*, *Enterobacter cloacae*, and *Salmonella typhimurium* (Lyte 1997). The fruit is involved in a rare but potentially fatal clinical entity of type I allergy to fruits without concomitant allergy to other common airborne/contact allergens (Saraswat & Kumar 2005). Similarly, individuals with sensitivity to bananas should be cautious of foods such as avocado, orange and chestnut that are known to cross-react with banana antigens (Moreno-Ancillo *et al.*, 2004).

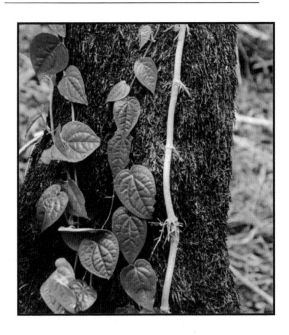

Figure 63. *Piper betle* f. *densum* climbing vine. [MB]

Local name: *kebui* (Palauan)
Scientific name: *Piper betle* L. f. *densum* (Blume) Fosb.
Family: Piperaceae (Pepper Family)

Description
Woody climbing vine with dimorphic branching; leaf blades ovate, usually 12-20 × 6-12 cm, rachis of fruiting spike accrescent, at least 3 mm in diameter at maturity, the fruits congested or coalescent (Smith 1981).

Range
A native of central and eastern Malaysia, but spreading in comparatively early times throughout tropical Asia and Malaysia, and later to Madagascar and eastern Africa. It is now cultivated in many other tropical areas, apparently being a recent introduction to places like Fiji (Smith 1981). Native in Palau, and grows in volcanic lowland forest and agroforest areas (Hillmann Kitalong, DeMeo & Holm 2008).

Traditional Uses
Styptic. Chew leaf and put mass on wound [Bedebii Chiokai, Tadashi Belchal, Ellabed Rebluud].

Pharmacological Properties
The crude ethanol extract of *Piper betle* leaves and a compound isolated from this extract show anti-inflammatory activity in an animal model by suppression of iNOS and COX-2 (Sarkar *et al.*, 2008). In another study, an ethanolic extract of the leaves was able to downregulate T-helper 1 cell pro-inflammatory responses in a model of arthritis in rats (Ganguly *et al.*, 2007). Ethyl acetate and ethanol leaf stalk extracts of *P. betle* have shown activity against human pathogenic bacteria (Shitut, Pandit & Mehta 1999). Hydroxychavicol, isolated from the aqueous leaf extract of *P. betle* has

demonstrated *in vitro* antifungal activity against *Candida* and *Aspergillus* species related to topical infections (Ali *et al.*, 2010).

Toxicology

No toxicity related to the topical use of *Piper betle* has been reported. Several studies demonstrated an antifertility effect in rats and mice with internal administration of *P. betle* (Adhikary *et al.*, 1989; Sarkar *et al.*, 2000; Tewari, Chaturvedi & Dixit 1970). Oral administration of the leaf extracts caused no toxicity in mice in other studies (Sen, Talukder & Sharma 1989; Sengupta *et al.*, 2000; Choudhary & Kale 2002).

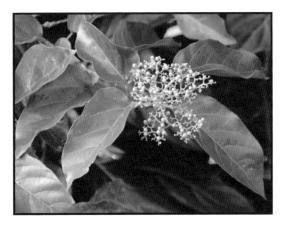

Figure 64. *Premna serratifolia* leaves and immature fruits. [MB]

Local name: *chosm* (Palauan)
Scientific name: *Premna serratifolia* L.
Family: Lamiaceae (Mint Family)

Description

Premna serratifolia is a low shrub or small tree, growing to 10 m in height, with compressed branchlets. The leaves are opposite, round to oval in shape, and 0.5-8 cm in length. The inflorescences are up to 2 cm in length, with small white cup-shaped calyces. The fruits are round, 2-4 mm in diameter, green ripening to black (Smith 1991).

Range

Premna serratifolia is a lowland species ranging from eastern Africa to Sri Lanka, southeastern Asia, the Ryuku Islands, Taiwan, Malaysia, and tropical Australia to the southern Pacific Islands. *Premna serratifolia* is found growing in beach thickets, dry lowland forest, along rocky shores, on the edges of mangrove swamps, and in agroforest areas (Balick 2009; Smith 1991). It is native to Palau (Hillmann Kitalong, DeMeo & Holm 2008).

Traditional Uses

Medicine used for cuts. Chew or crush leaves and apply directly on wound [Flora Wasisang, Martha Nabeyama, Subediang Ubedei, Gloria Emesiochel, Victor Yano, Clarence Kitalong].

Medicine used for deep cuts. The outer skin of the young stems is taken off and the white interior is scraped into a cotton-like fiber. The fiber with its juice is placed on the cut. The amount of scraped *chosm* depends on the size of the cut. Put on wound and cover with cloth and apply pressure. Keep on cut until bleeding stops. When bathing, change dressing or change once daily. Use for 3-4 days. [Flora Wasisang, Subediang Ubedei]. Instead of scraping the fiber, place slimy inner bark on wound with white cloth, changing twice a day for 3 to 4 days or until bleeding stops—use only once [Flora Wasisang, Subediang Ubedei, Van-Ray Tadao].

Medicine for head injury. Scrape *chosm* branch and squeeze out mucous material and apply to injury [Rufino Alii].

Pharmacological Properties

Compounds isolated from the extract of root nodules from related species, *Premna herbaceae* Roxb. enhanced antimicrobial activity against Gram-positive and Gram-negative bacteria and fungi (Murthy *et al.,* 2006). Compounds isolated from other related species, *P. schimperi* Engl. and *P. oligotricha* Baker showed *in vitro* antibacterial activity against *Staphylococcus aureus* and *Bacillus subtilis* (Habtemariam *et al.,* 1990; Habtemariam, Gray & Waterman 1992).

Toxicology

Isolated compounds from the chloroform extract of the leaves of the related species, *Premna tomentosa,* exhibited cytotoxic activity against three human cancer cell lines but showed possible cancerous effects to one normal cell line (Chin *et al.*, 2006).

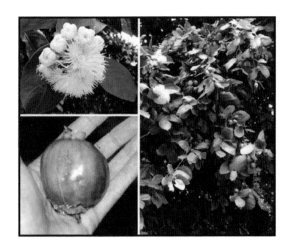

Figure 65. *Syzygium samarangense* flowers, matured fruit, and branches. [CT & AK]

Local name: *rebotel* (Palauan)
Scientific name: *Syzygium samarangense* (Blume) Merr. & Perry
Family: Myrtaceae (Mrytle Family)

Description

Shrub or tree 1-15 m high. Leaves are often subsessile, the petioles 1-7 mm long, the blades 10-25 × 5-12 cm, cordate to rounded at base; inflorescences terminal, axillary, or in axils of fallen leaves; flowers 3-5 cm across expanded stamens, petals and filaments are white; the fruits are borne on branches and when mature are red and as large as 15 × 8 cm (Smith 1985).

Range

Indigenous to the Indo-Malaysia region, but has long been cultivated and naturalized so its precise origin is unknown (Smith 1985). It was introduced to Palau and now found growing on agricultural and agroforest areas, as well as areas that typically have cultivated landscapes and ornamental plants (Hillmann Kitalong, DeMeo & Holm 2008).

Traditional Uses

Medicine used for deep cuts. Take some of the youngest leaves, chew them and put on cut. This will stop bleeding when used once (depending on the size of the cut) and change the leaves as needed, until the cut is healed. This species has more of a 'lime' flavor and it will help 'freeze' the cut as compared to other plants used for this purpose [Clarence Kitalong].

Pharmacological Properties

Stercurensin, an active compound isolated from the leaves, exhibited anti-inflammatory activity through an NF-κB mechanism *in vitro* and *in vivo* (mice model) (Kim *et al.*, 2011).

Toxicology

No relevant toxicological reports were identified.

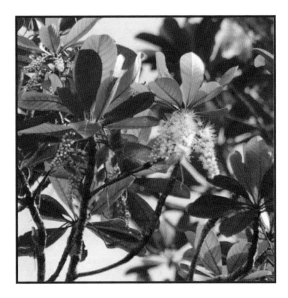

Figure 66. *Terminalia crassipes* branches with leaves and flowers. [AK]

Local name: ***chesemiich*** (Palauan)
Scientific name: *Terminalia crassipes* Kaneh. & Hatus.
Family: Combretaceae (Combretum Family)

Description
Tree 6 m tall, trunk 12 cm dbh, branches whorled, new leaves bronze-color, dark, shiny green when mature. Flowers are greenish-white, fragrant. Young fruits green with brownish pubescence [D.H. Lorence 8226].

Range
Endemic to Palau and found growing in the volcanic lowland forests (Hillmann Kitalong, DeMeo & Holm 2008).

Traditional Uses
Medicine used for cuts. Leaves are crushed and applied to wound [Van-Ray Tadao].

Pharmacological Properties
The alcohol extract of the leaf of related species, *Terminalia catappa*, has strong inhibition against *Bacillus* spp., *Enterococcus faecalis, Staphylococcus* spp., *Bacteroides fragilis, Escherichia coli,* and *Pseudomonas aeruginosa* as well as antifungal properties against various fungal species (Goun *et al.*, 2003; Kloucek *et al.*, 2005).

Toxicology
No toxicological reports were identified.

COMBINATION THERAPIES

a)

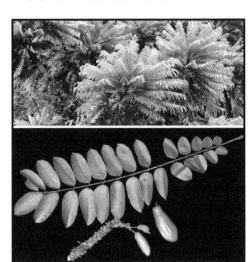

b)

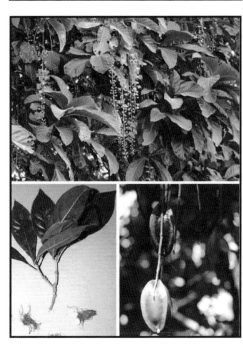

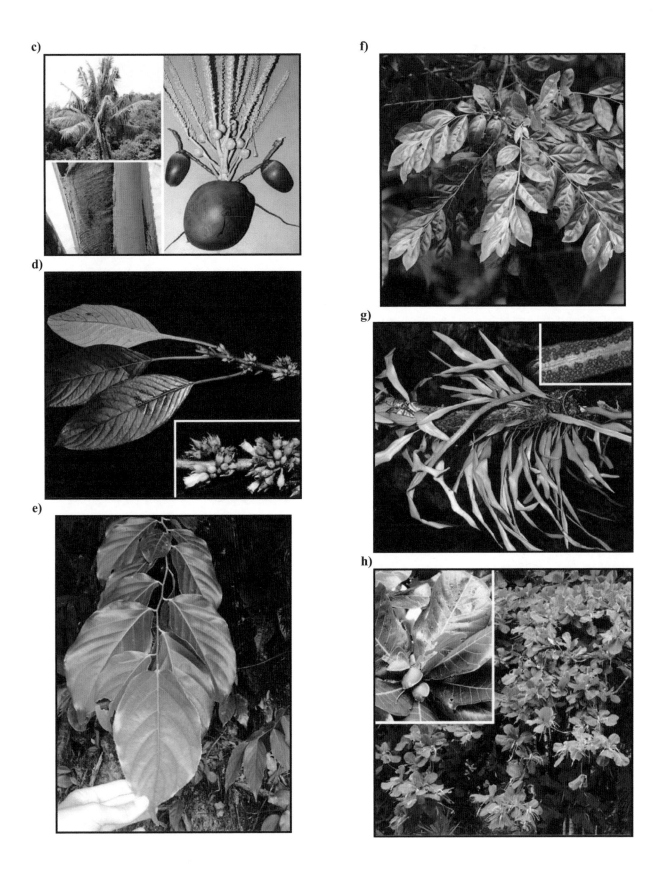

Figure 67. a) *Averrhoa bilimbi* showing close-up of leaves and fruits. [AK & MB]; **b)** *Barringtonia racemosa* with close-ups of leaves, flowers, and fruits. [AK & CT]; **c)** *Cocos nucifera* leaves, husk, and fruits. [DL & WL]; **d)** *Cyrtandra palawensis* with inset showing close-up of flowers. [SP]; **e)** *Flacourtia inermis* leaves. [AK]; **f)** *Glochidion ramiflorum* leaves and fruits. [MB]; **g)** *Pyrrosia lanceolata* with inset showing close-up of sori. [CT]; **h)** *Terminalia catappa* with inset showing fruits. [AK & MB]

Local and Scientific names:

imekurs (Palauan); bilimbi (English) - *Averrhoa bilimbi* L. (Oxalidaceae)

koranges (Palauan); powder-puff tree (English) - *Barringtonia racemosa* (L.) Spreng. (Lecythidaceae)

lius (Palauan); coconut (English) - *Cocos nucifera* L. (Arecaceae)

melkii (Palauan) - *Cyrtandra palawensis* Schltr. (Gesneriaceae)

chemechong (Palauan); batoko plum (English) - *Flacourtia inermis* Roxb. (Salicaceae)

ngolm (Palauan) - *Glochidion ramiflorum* J.R. Forst. & G. Forst. (Phyllanthaceae)

ar ra beluu (Palauan) - *Pyrrosia lanceolata* (L.) Farw. (Polypodiaceae)

miich (Palauan); Indian almond (English) - *Terminalia catappa* L. (Combretaceae)

Descriptions

Averrhoa bilimbi L.: Shrub or small tree 4-15 m high, with yellowish red to purple sepals and red petals. It is usually cauliflorous and ramiflorous, the leaves having 15-41 leaflets with predominant oblong blades usually 3-7 × 1.5-2.5 cm, acute at apex, a few proximal ones smaller than the distal ones. Fruits are green, terete to obtusely angled, ellipsoid to obovoid, up to 10 × 5 cm, with seeds 6-8 × 4-6 mm and lacking arils (Smith 1985).

Barringtonia racemosa (L.) Spreng.: Tree to 6 m in height or taller, with a medium sized trunk. The flowers have red buds opening into reddish purple or green calyces. The petals are white, with creamy, yellow anthers and a pinkish white style. The fruits are green and ripen to brown or red (Smith 1981).

Cocos nucifera L.: *Cocos nucifera* is a tall palm, reaching heights of 20-30 m. It bears a terminal crown of leaves. The trunk is grayish brown in color and is 20-40 cm in diameter. The fruits are green, yellow or red depending on the variety. This species may live up to 80-100 years (Purseglove 1988; Smith 1979).

Cyrtandra palawensis Schltr.: Shrub 1-2 m tall; flowers white [S. Perlman 20834].

Flacourtia inermis Roxb.: Tree about 5 m tall; leaves are dark green, glossy, alternate, simple leaves; flowers are small, green petals, with yellow stamens and pistils; immature fruits are green and bright red when mature, 2 cm diameter [D.E. Atha 823].

Glochidion ramiflorum J.R. Forst. & G. Forst.: A small tree about 10 m in height, dbh 6-32 cm. The simple, alternate, elliptic to spear-shaped leaves are 3-18 cm long, often unequally sided. The long-stalked yellow female flower is 4 mm wide and grows singly at the base of the male raceme. The male flowers grow on the axis of a long simple flower cluster up to 15 cm long. The green, flattened capsule is 5-15 mm in diameter, with unequal lobes, and grows on a stalk about 1 cm long. Fruits look like miniature pumpkins (Hillmann Kitalong, DeMeo & Holm 2008).

Pyrrosia lanceolata (L.) Farw.: Epiphytic and rarely terrestrial. Rhizome about 1.3 mm in diameter, widely creeping, with widely spaced fronds. Frond stipitate, thinly coriaceous. Lamina up to 16 × 1.5 cm, simple, linear to lanceolate to narrowly elliptic, narrowly acute to obtuse, entire but usually with a narrowly reflexed margin. Sori emergent through the tomentum (Schelpe 1970).

Terminalia catappa L.: A large tree, normally up to 30 m tall. Leaves in whorls at ends of branches, broad and inversely oval, generally dark green and glossy. Older leaves turn brilliant shades of red and orange before dropping. Flowers small in whitish-yellow clusters with racemes (or spikes) 5-15 cm long. Fruits are flattened and egg-shaped, green when young but turn reddish yellow when ripe. Edible cylindrical seeds are encased in a tough fibrous husk with a fleshy outer layer (Hillmann Kitalong, DeMeo & Holm 2008).

Ranges

Averrhoa bilimbi L.: Exact origin unknown, but often seen as a relict of former cultivation in eastern Melanesia (Smith 1985). Introduced to Palau, it is found growing in agricultural and agroforest areas, as well as in urban areas that typically have cultivated landscape and ornamental plants (Hillmann Kitalong, DeMeo & Holm 2008).

Barringtonia racemosa (L.) Spreng.: This species is found in eastern and southern Africa to India and throughout Micronesia, Malaysia, and the Pacific Islands. It grows in forests, along rivers and the edges of mangrove swamps (Smith 1981). Native to Palau and found growing on volcanic lowland forests and freshwater swamp forests (Hillmann Kitalong, DeMeo & Holm 2008).

Cocos nucifera L.: A pantropical species, *Cocos nucifera* is native to the Old World tropics, most likely the Pacific Islands (*Cocos nucifera*, TRAMIL 2008). It has been cultivated extensively throughout the tropics as an important economic crop. Due to its wide distribution, commonness, and unwieldy size, few voucher collections are made of this species (Smith 1979).

Cyrtandra palawensis Schltr.: Endemic to Palau and found growing in volcanic lowland forests (Hillmann Kitalong, DeMeo & Holm 2008).

Flacourtia inermis Roxb.: Native to the Philippines, and has naturalized in tropical Asia and Africa. Similarly, it is native to Palau and found growing in volcanic lowland forests (Hillmann Kitalong, DeMeo & Holm 2008).

Glochidion ramiflorum J.R. Forst. & G. Forst.: *Glochidion ramiflorum* (*ngolm*) is found in both limestone and volcanic primary and secondary forests of Palau. *Ngolm* is native in Palau and is distributed throughout Micronesia and Polynesia (Hillmann Kitalong, DeMeo & Holm 2008).

Pyrrosia lanceolata (L.) Farw.: Distributed in Cameroon, Gabon, Congo, Mozambique, Madagascar, India to China, Indo-China, Malaysia, Australia and the Pacific (Schelpe 1970). Native to Palau and found growing in volcanic lowland forests, and in freshwater swamp forests (Hillmann Kitalong, DeMeo & Holm 2008).

Terminalia catappa L.: Usually found in atoll forests, inland from ocean beaches near river mouths and around coastal areas in general. Native to coastal areas of Eastern India, Indochina, Malaysia, Indonesia, Northern Australia, Oceania, the Philippines and Taiwan. Widely planted and naturalized in the lowland tropical regions of the rest of the world (Hillmann Kitalong, DeMeo & Holm 2008).

Traditional Uses
Medicine used to treat wounds. Get 2 tips with young leaves (*eberdil*) from *Barringtonia racemosa* (*koranges*), *Flacourtia inermis* (*chemchong*), *Pyrrosia lanceolata* (*arbeluu*), *Glochidion ramiflorum* (*ngolm*), *Averrhoa bilimbi* (*imekurs*), *Cyrtandra palawensis* (*melkii*), and *Terminalia catappa* (*miich*). Pound them together to make a poultice and leave some

of it aside. Grind the white meat of the fallen coconut *(lius, Cocos nucifera)* that has turned brown and combine with some of the pounded plants. Squeeze the poultice through a white cloth or coconut fiber onto the wound or cut. Next, take the remaining pounded plants that were not combined with the ground coconut and apply to wound. This remedy stops bleeding and helps control swelling. After 1 week the wound should be healed [Ingas Spesungel; Kerengel Tesei].

Pharmacological Properties

Averrhoa bilimbi L.: No pharmacological reports relevant to this use were identified.

Barringtonia racemosa (L.) Spreng.: A root extract of *Barringtonia racemosa* demonstrated *in vivo* antibacterial activity (Khan *et al.*, 2001). The bark showed a wide spectrum of antifungal activity *in vitro* (Wijesundera, Deraniyagala & Amarasekara 1996; Gowri *et al.*, 2009).

Cocos nucifera L.: The oil from the nut is valued as an emollient and the extract from the husk fiber is used in remedies to treat skin infections due to its antibacterial and antiviral properties (Aburjai & Natcheh 2003; Mendonça-Filho *et al.*, 2004). The crude water extract and low molecular weight fractions of *Cocos nucifera* inhibited histamine- and serotonin-induced rat paw edema (Rinaldi *et al.*, 2009).

Cyrtandra palawensis Schltr.: No pharmacological reports relevant to this use were identified.

Flacourtia inermis Roxb.: An acetone extract (50 mg/ml) from the fruit of *Flacourtia inermis* inhibited the growth of *Apergillus fumigatus, Aspergillus niger, Aspergillus flavus, Mucor ramosissimus,* and *Chrysosporum* fungal species (Shibumon & Benny 2010).

Glochidion ramiflorum J.R. Forst. & G. Forst.: No pharmacological reports relevant to this use were identified.

Pyrrosia lanceolata (L.) Farw.: No pharmacological reports relevant to this use were identified.

Terminalia catappa L.: The alcohol extract of the leaf of *Terminalia catappa,* has strong inhibition against *Bacillus* spp., *Enterococcus faecalis, Staphylococcus* spp., *Bacteroides fragilis, Escherichia coli,* and *Pseudomonas aeruginosa* as well as antifungal properties against various fungal species (Goun *et al.*, 2003; Kloucek *et al.*, 2005).

Toxicology

Averrhoa bilimbi L.: Feeding of the fruit at daily oral doses of 250-1,000 mg/kg for 14 days did not result in any obvious toxicity (Ambili, Subramoniam & Nagarajan 2009).

Barringtonia racemosa (L.) Spreng.: Daily doses up to 12 mg/kg i.p. for 14 days did not produce any acute or short-term toxicity, but a 24 mg/kg daily i.p. dose was accompanied by an elevation in serum urea levels, indicating potential kidney or metabolic malfunctioning when used internally (Thomas *et al.*, 2002).

Cocos nucifera L.: No reports of toxicity were identified.

Cyrtandra palawensis Schltr.: No reports of toxicity were identified.

Glochidion ramiflorum J.R. Forst. & G. Forst.: No reports of toxicity were identified.

Flacourtia inermis Roxb.: No reports of toxicity were identified.

Pyrrosia lanceolata (L.) Farw.: No reports of toxicity were identified.

Terminalia catappa L.: No reports of toxicity were identified.

a)

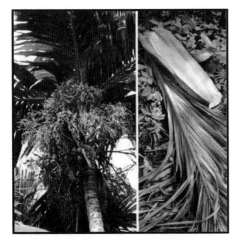

b)

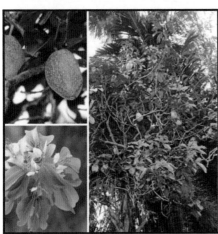

c)

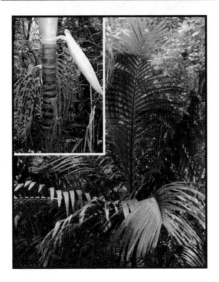

Figure 68. a) *Areca catechu* flowers, fruits, and a dried, fallen leaf. [AK]; **b)** *Crateva religiosa* with close-ups of fruits and flowers. [AK]; **c)** *Pinanga insignis* leaves, with inset showing red fruits and flower. [CT]

Local and Scientific names:
buuch (Palauan); betel nut (English) - *Areca catechu* L. (Arecaceae)
chedebsungel (Palauan) - *Crateva religiosa* G. Forst. (Capparidaceae)
chebouch (Palauan); Pinang palm, black fiber palm (English) - *Pinanga insignis* Becc. (Arecaceae)

Descriptions
Areca catechu L.: Small palm tree with solitary, green, and prominently ringed stem, about 10-30 m high, dbh 15-20 cm. Leaves about 2 m long with 12 pinnae on each side, and usually 2-3 ribbed. Inflorescence with staminate and pistillate flowers with small sepals. The fruit is oblong to ovoid in shape 4-5 cm long, dull orange to red (Smith 1979).
Crateva religiosa G. Forst.: Tree, usually 5-15 m high. Sepals are green, the petals white, becoming cream-colored or yellowish, the filaments distally pink or purple, and the fruit pale green, up to 20 × 9.5 cm but usually smaller, drying grayish (Smith 1981).
Pinanga insignis Becc.: Small palm tree 5-8 m in height, dbh 7-31 cm. The compound, pinnate leaves 1-3 m long are stiffly ascending and arch downward. The simply branched inflorescences are up to 1 m long. The asymmetrical male flowers have a short, 3-lobed calyx and acute tipped petals with many stamens. The female flowers have partly overlapping or fused sepals and overlapping petals. The red, acute tipped, ellipsoid fruits are 1.7-2.2 cm long and 0.9-1.3 cm wide (Hillmann Kitalong, DeMeo & Holm 2008).

Ranges

Areca catechu L.: The origin of *Areca catechu* is uncertain. It is distributed across India and Sri Lanka to southeastern Asia, Indonesia, and the Philippines. It is widely cultivated in the Asiatic tropics, including Pohnpei Island (Smith 1979).

Crateva religiosa G. Forst.: Himalayan India and Burma eastward through Micronesia and Malaysia to the Gambier Islands in the Tuamotus (Smith 1981). Native to Palau and found growing in the savanna grassland (Hillmann Kitalong, DeMeo & Holm 2008).

Pinanga insignis Becc.: A common understory species in volcanic forests of Babeldaob. *Chebouch* is distributed in Palau and the Philippines (Hillmann Kitalong, DeMeo & Holm 2008).

Traditional Uses

Medicine used for broken bones. Pound 7-10 leaves of *chedebsungel* (*Crateva religiosa*). Place pounded leaves around the appendage and wrap leaf sheath (*keai*) of either *chebouch* (*Pinanga insignis*) or *buuch* (*Areca catechu*) around and tie. Leaves act as a muscle relaxant and the *keai* stabilizes the bone while it heals. Leave *keai* in place and do not get wet. Replace if necessary [Clarence Kitalong].

Pharmacological Properties

Areca catechu L.: No pharmacological reports relevant to this use have been reported.

Crateva religiosa G. Forst.: Lupeol is the active compound in *Crateva religiosa* (Bani *et al.*, 2006). Lupeol has been shown to have some antinociceptive activity by binding to glutamate (Martini *et al.*, 2007). Lupeol has been shown to have anti-inflammatory activity, acting on a wide range of molecular pathways (Saleem 2009) and exerted a significant dose dependent effect on acute and chronic inflammation in rat models of arthritis (Geetha & Varalakshmi 1999). Extracts of *C. religiosa* have demonstrated antibacterial activity against *Staphylococcus aureus* and *Escherichia coli* strains (Grosvenor, Supriono & Gray 1995).

Pinanga insignis Becc.: No pharmacological reports relevant to this use were identified.

Toxicology

Areca catechu L.: No reports on the toxicity of topical use of *Areca catechu* have been identified.

Crateva religiosa G. Forst.: The LD_{50} of lupeol exceeds 2 g/kg (Bani *et al.*, 2006). In mice and rats, no toxicity or mortality was reported following topical or oral administration (Saleem 2009).

Pinanga insignis Becc.: No reports on the toxicity of topical use of *Pinanga insignis* were identified.

a)

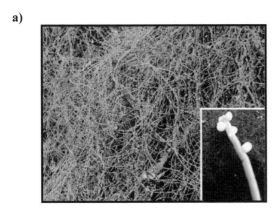

b)

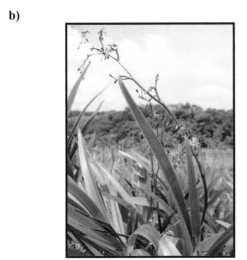

c)

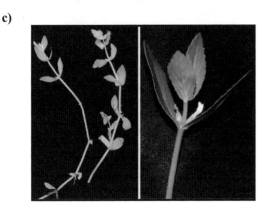

d)

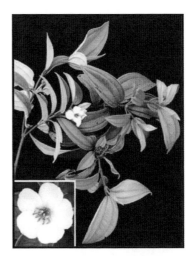

e)

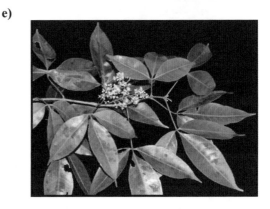

Figure 69. a) *Cassytha filiformis* with inset showing flowers. [MB]; **b)** *Dianella carolinensis* leaves and flowers. [CT]; **c)** *Limnophila chinensis* subsp. *aromatica* leaves and close-up of flowers. [MB & WL]; **d)** *Melastoma malabathricum* L. var. *mariannum* leaves, flower, and fruit, with inset showing close-up of flower. [MB & AK]; **e)** *Melicope denhamii* leaves and flowers. [WL]; **f)** *Phaleria nisidai* fruits and leaves, with inset showing flower. [AK & CT]; **g)** *Phyllanthus palauensis* with inset showing close-up of flowers. [SP]

f)

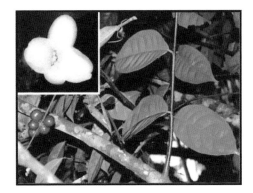

g)

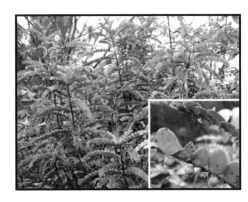

Local and Scientific names:
techellelachull*, *kukiut (Palauan); laurel dodder (English) - *Cassytha filiformis* L. (Lauraceae)

kobesos (Palauan) - *Dianella carolinensis* Laut. (Hemerocallidaceae)

iaml (Palauan); rice paddy herb (English) - *Limnophila chinensis* (Osb.) Merr. subsp. *aromatica* (Lam.) Yamazaki (Scrophulariaceae)

matakui (Palauan) - *Melastoma malabathricum* L. var. *mariannum* (Naudin) Fosb. & Sach. (Melastomataceae)

kertub (Palauan) - *Melicope denhamii* (Seem.) T.G. Hartley (Rutaceae)

ongael*, *delalakar (Palauan); mother of medicine (English) - *Phaleria nisidai* Kaneh. (Thymelaeaceae)

dudures*, *ukellelachedib (Palauan) - *Phyllanthus palauensis* Hosok. (Phyllanthaceae)

Descriptions
Cassytha filiformis L.: Herbaceous parasitic vine. In Palau it is found growing in savanna grassland and freshwater swamp forest (Hillmann Kitalong, DeMeo & Holm 2008). Tepals are white and the immature fruit is green, becoming yellow and at length white (Smith 1981).

Dianella carolinensis Laut.: A coarse herb, 1 m tall, with a subterranean rhizome, the leaves linear, crowded on stem base (Smith 1979). Flowers with racemiform branches, petals are bluish-gray and anthers are yellow. The fruit is a purple berry.

Limnophila chinensis (Osb.) Merr. subsp. *aromatica* (Lam.) Yamazaki: Herb, 5-50cm tall. Leaves opposite or in whorls of 3 or 4, sessile, ovate-lanceolate, 0.5-5.3 × 0.2-1.5 cm. Flowers solitary, purple-red or blue corolla, 1-1.5 cm. Capsule compressed, broadly ellipsoid, 5 mm (Wu & Raven 1994).

Melastoma malabathricum L. var. *mariannum* (Naudin) Fosb. & Sach.: Shrub or small tree to 2 m. Leaf blades entire, glossy green superior and pale green inferior side, 3-7 nerved, with conspicuous cross-veins. Solitary flowers, petals 4-5 white, pink to red carpels and stamens (Smith 1985). Red fruits.

Melicope denhamii (Seem.) T.G. Hartley: Understory tree up to 14 m tall, 33 cm dbh Stipules absent; leaves opposite, tri-foliolate compound, leaflets penni-veined, glabrous to hairy. Flowers 4 mm diameter, greenish white, placed in panicles. Fruits 5 mm diameter, greenish, dehiscent capsules [T. Flynn 6410].

Phaleria nisidai Kaneh.: A ca. 15 m tall tree with opposite leaves, 15-20 cm long, 7-8 cm wide; the corolla tube is white, 15 mm long

(Kanehira 1933). The drupe is red at maturity. It is native to Palau (Hillmann Kitalong, DeMeo & Holm 2008).

Phyllanthus palauensis Hosok.: Shrub to 1 m tall. Brown bracts; flowers and young fruits green. It is found growing in the savanna grassland (Hillmann Kitalong, DeMeo & Holm 2008).

Ranges

Cassytha filiformis L.: Cosmopolitan in tropical areas, occurring abundantly in most Pacific archipelagos (Smith 1981). It is native to Palau (Hillmann Kitalong, DeMeo & Holm 2008).

Dianella carolinensis Laut.: Species in this genus are found in tropical Asia to Australia, New Zealand, and the Pacific Islands (Smith 1979). This is the only species found in Palau, native, and found growing in the savanna grasslands (Hillmann Kitalong, DeMeo & Holm 2008).

Limnophila chinensis (Osb.) Merr. subsp. *aromatica* (Lam.) Yamazaki: The genus is paleotropical (Smith 1991). This species is native to Palau and found growing on marshes and areas of freshwater grasses, sedges, reeds, and other herbaceous plants (Hillmann Kitalong, DeMeo & Holm 2008).

Melastoma malabathricum L. var. *mariannum* (Naudin) Fosb. & Sach.: Southeastern Asia and the Seychelles through Malaysia into Australia and Polynesia (Smith 1985). Native to Palau and found growing on marshes that are areas of freshwater grasses, edges, reeds, and other herbaceous plants (Hillmann Kitalong, DeMeo & Holm 2008).

Melicope denhamii (Seem.) T.G. Hartley: Indonesia and the Philippines to New Guinea and the Western Pacific. Native to Palau and found growing in volcanic lowland forests (Hillmann Kitalong, DeMeo & Holm 2008).

Phaleria nisidai Kaneh.: Southeastern Asia and Ceylon through Malaysia to Micronesia,

Australia, and eastward in the Pacific to Samoa and Tonga (Smith 1981). In Palau, it grows in volcanic lowland forest and in freshwater swamp forest (Hillmann Kitalong, DeMeo & Holm 2008).

Phyllanthus palauensis Hosok.: Endemic to Palau (Hillmann Kitalong, DeMeo & Holm 2008).

Traditional Uses

Medicine used for cuts and strengthening. Chewing about 7 of *Melastoma malabathricum* (*matakui*) leaves and putting in on a wound can be used to stop blood flow; bandage it until the end of the day and check up on wound or until blood stops flowing. Leaves are chewed until they give an acrid taste, and it is said that plants that have an acrid taste have a medicinal purpose. *Matakui* is used in combination with *kobesos* for a heart strengthening remedy; it is used in combination with other herbs as a medicinal drink such as *Phaleria nisidai* (*ongael*), *Limnophila aromatica* (*iaml*), *Dianella carolinensis* (*kobesos*), *Cassytha filiformis* (*techelelachull*), *Melicope denhamii* (*kertub*), *Phyllanthus palauensis* (*dudurs*), and others. The plants are placed in a pot and just covered with water. This is boiled until the plants float. There is no name for this heart strengthening remedy. It is also used in the Ibobang ceremonial treatment; the number of leaves used is increased with the number of participants [Dirraklang Merei Ngirametuker].

Pharmacological Properties

Cassytha filiformis L.: No pharmacological reports relevant to this use were identified.

Dianella carolinensis Laut.: Crude extracts from the roots of the related species, *Dianella callicarpa,* show mild antimicrobial and antiviral activities (Dias, Silva & Urban 2009). Ethanolic extracts of the roots of the related species, *D. revoluta,* showed weak activity against Gram-negative bacteria but no activity against Gram-positive bacteria (Palombo & Semple 2001).

Limnophila chinensis (Osb.) Merr. subsp. *aromatica* (Lam.) Yamazaki: No pharmacological reports relevant to this use were identified.

Melastoma malabathricum L. var. *mariannum* (Naudin) Fosb. & Sach.: *Melastoma malabathricum* contains anti-inflammatory compounds such as flavonoids, quercetin, and pentacyclic triterpenes (Mazura, Susanti & Rasadah 2007). Ethanolic extracts of the whole plant demonstrated antinociceptive effect in mice at a dose of 30-300 mg/kg with a ED_{50} of 78-160 mg/kg (Sulaiman *et al.*, 2004). Aqueous extracts of *M. malabathricum* showed significant anti-inflammatory and antinociceptive activity *in vivo* (Zakaria *et al.*, 2006). An aqueous extract of *M. malabathricum* leaves had analgesic and antiinflammatory effects after subcutaneous injection in mice (Zakaria *et al.*, 2006). Aqueous extracts of the leaves had antimicrobial activity against Gram-positive and Gram-negative bacterial strains (Thatoi *et al.*, 2008).

Melicope denhamii (Seem.) T.G. Hartley: Several isolated compounds from related species, *Melicope semecarpifolia* and *Melicope confusa*, exhibited anti-platelet aggregating activities *in vitro* (Chen, K.S. *et al.*, 2000; Chen, I.S. *et al.*, 2001; Chou *et al.*, 2005).

Phaleria nisidai Kaneh.: A crude ethanolic extract of *Phaleria nisidai* increased the phagocytic activity of isolated RAW 264.7 macrophages *in vitro* (Matsuda *et al.*, 2005b).

Phyllanthus palauensis Hosok.: No pharmacological reports relevant to this use were identified.

Toxicology

Cassytha filiformis L.: A toxicological assessment of an aqueous extract of the stems and leaves revealed that a daily oral dose of 250-1,000 mg/kg for 28 days decreased levels of alkaline phosphatase and increased levels of serum cholesterol in rats. A decrease in relative weights of the heart and lung was also observed. The oral LD_{50} was determined to be greater than 500 mg/kg (Babayi *et al.*, 2007).

Dianella carolinensis Laut.: A related species, *Dianella revoluta,* is suspected in livestock poisoning and physiological disturbances in man when ingested. Isolation of the toxic compounds dianellidin, dianellinone, and stypandrol from *D. revoluta* indicates that possible caution should be exercised when ingesting this plant (Colegate, Dorling & Huxtable 1987, 1986). Stypandrol, isolated from *D. revoluta*, has been reported to induce toxicosis in goats and sheep, with acute intoxication causing weakness and paralysis of the hind limbs and sometimes leading to death (Dias, Silva & Urban 2009).

Limnophila chinensis (Osb.) Merr. subsp. *aromatica* (Lam.) Yamazaki: No reports of toxicity were identified.

Melastoma malabathricum L. var. *mariannum* (Naudin) Fosb. & Sach.: Oral doses up to 2,000 mg/kg of a cold water extract of *Melastoma malabathricum* leaves showed no signs of toxicity in mice (Sunilson *et al.*, 2009).

Melicope denhamii (Seem.) T.G. Hartley: No reports of toxicity were identified.

Phaleria nisidai Kaneh.: No reports of toxicity were identified.

Phyllanthus palauensis Hosok.: Aqueous extracts of the related species, *Phyllanthus amarus,* in rats at 400 mg/kg was toxic to blood cells, promoted weight loss, and caused testicular degeneration (Adedapo *et al.*, 2005; Adedapo, Adegbayibi & Emikpe 2005). Mice given 100 mg/kg of whole plant alcohol extracts of *P. amarus* were unable to get pregnant, possibly due to hormonal interference (Rao & Alice 2001). Chronic oral administration of the aqueous extract of the leaves of *P. amarus* caused hematological and histopathological changes indicative of potential toxicity in rats (Adedapo, Adegbayibi & Emikpe 2005).

a)

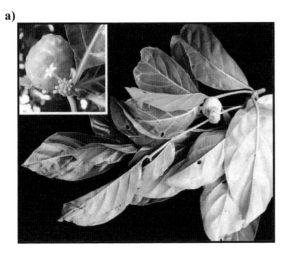

Figure 70. a) *Morinda citrifolia* leaves and fruit, with inset showing flower, flower buds, and fruit. [MB & AK]; **b)** *Opuntia cochenillifera.* [WL]

b)

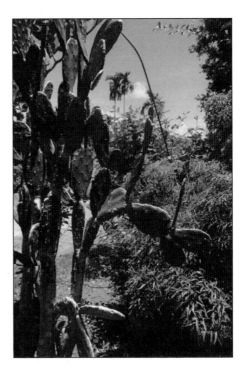

Local and Scientific names:
ngel (Palauan); noni (English) - *Morinda citrifolia* L. (Rubiaceae)
chesbocheb (Palauan); prickly pear (English) - *Opuntia cochenillifera* (L.) Mill. (Cactaceae)

Descriptions
Morinda citrifolia L.: A small tree 3 to 8 m in height, with a dbh of 10-30 cm and hairless, 4-angled stems. The simple, opposite, elliptic leaves are up to 45 cm long and 25 cm wide. The margins are entire, the surfaces are glossy, hairless and pliable, the stout petiole is up to 2 cm long. The flowers are borne in 75 to 90 flowered, oval to globe-like heads on a stalk about 3 cm long, with the calyx having a truncate rim with no lobes. The white corolla has 5 lobes that are slightly curled backward. The flower stalk is 1-3 cm long. The yellowish-white, fleshy, soft and odiferous, irregular heads are about 5 cm long and 3-4 cm wide. The fruits have a wart-

like appearance (Hillmann Kitalong, DeMeo & Holm 2008).

Opuntia cochenillifera (L.) Mill.: Plant 2.5 m tall, irregularly branching, pads green, slightly glaucous. Perianth tubular, pale red filaments to deep pinkish red, stigma yellowish green, exserted; fruits abortive [D.H. Lorence 5237, 5144].

Ranges
Morinda citrifolia L.: Indigenous to Indo-Malaysia, *Morinda citrifolia* ranges throughout the Pacific to Hawaiian Islands and other tropical regions around the world. In coastal forests, it is established as an understory plant often found near creeks, alongside the edge of mangrove swamps, and can be found growing up to 137 m above sea level (Smith 1988). In Palau, it is found along the volcanic forest edge and savanna (Hillmann Kitalong, DeMeo & Holm 2008).

Opuntia cochenillifera (L.) Mill.: Origin may be in Mexico. It was introduced to Palau and it is found growing in urban areas that typically have cultivated landscape and ornamental plants (Hillmann Kitalong, DeMeo & Holm 2008).

Traditional Uses
Medicine used for cuts and wounds. Scrape and apply on wound and place *Morinda citrifolia* (*ngel*) leaf on the fire to make it sturdy and cover the wound [Dr. Patrick Tellei]. Leaves and stems are mashed together and put on a deep cut to stop severe bleeding [Tadashi Belchal, Risao Bausouch, Scott Yano, Henry Yuri].

Pharmacological Properties
Morinda citrifolia L.: The fruit extract has potent antibacterial properties (Zaidan *et al.,* 2005). The ethanolic extract of the leaf of *Morinda citrifolia* improved wound healing parameters in rats following oral administration (Nayak *et al.*, 2009). The fruit extract of related species, *M. pubescens* Sm., accelerated wound healing in rats (Mathivanan *et al.,* 2006).

Opuntia cochenillifera (L.) Mill.: Hydroalcoholic and ethyl acetate extracts from the stem of the related species, *Opuntia humifusa*, exerted potent anti-inflammatory activities on macrophages *in vitro* (Cho *et al.*, 2006).

Toxicology
Morinda citrifolia L.: No toxicological reports relevant to the topical use of this plant have been identified.

Opuntia cochenillifera (L.) Mill.: No reports of toxicity were identified.

CHAPTER SEVEN: STRESS

Stress is a term that describes mechanical, physical, mental, and emotional strain. Sources of stress affect us on a daily basis and can be quite varied, ranging from external environmental factors, to increased demands on physical exertion or psychological/emotional/physical trauma. The catalyzing event unleashing a stress response can be perceived or real and is known as the "fight or flight" response. Exposure to stress over a prolonged period of time, usually months or years of daily stress or a sudden, startling or dramatic and disturbing event that creates an unforgettable lasting and stressful recurrent memory, can manifest into serious health conditions.

Acute and Chronic Disorders of Stress

Stress disorders can be acute or chronic. An acute stress disorder is defined as having occurred within four weeks of a traumatic or terrifying event and lasts only two to four weeks. Acute stress disorders can be experienced as a sense of numbness or distance from one's surroundings, a feeling that things are unreal or difficulty in remembering the traumatic/stressful event. In addition, there is a sense of heightened awareness.

In the short term stress can be useful, with the increase in awareness acting as an evolutionary response to help the person mobilize in a time of perceived danger. When we are faced with challenges or dangerous situations that require the body to respond quickly, the stress response immediately results in the body diverting precious resources to the vital organs, such as the heart and brain.

Stress lasting more than a month can lead to physiological changes that suppress the immune system, increase blood pressure, exacerbate pre-existing conditions such as diabetes and heart disease, and can disrupt effective digestion. Every day challenges from illness, surgery, work, depression, or other chronic disease can create a stress response as well (Thomas 1981). Physical symptoms can manifest as a result of both acute and chronic stress: sadness, anxiety and nervousness, lethargy and fatigue, chronic headaches, indigestion, irritability or excessive anger, and a general sense of ill-being.

Stress-induced conditions can also lead to substance abuse, suicidal feelings, or behavior and physical abuse. From the late 1970s until 2000 the suicide rate in the Federated States of Micronesia (FSM), Palau, and the Marshall Islands has hovered between twenty-five and thirty per 100,000, giving the area one of the highest rates in the world (Department of Public Health and Social Security).

Prevention of Stress

It is difficult to prevent stressful situations from occurring, but how an individual manages the stress, in general, is within her/his control. Leading an active, healthy lifestyle can improve the ability to handle stressful situations. Most stress experts suggest that stress can be alleviated by getting adequate amounts of sleep, eating wholesome nutritious foods, exercising, and remaining connected to family and loved ones for social and emotional support.

Treatment of Stress

Recovery from stress may require removing oneself from the situation, event, or trauma. In cases where stress has become chronic or debilitating, psychological support in the form of counseling can be extremely beneficial. In discussing or evaluating the situation, insight into potential solutions becomes possible. Certain harmful situations that create feelings of extreme anxiety may require more treatment and potentially medication. People who are having suicidal thoughts, difficulty concentrating or who are experiencing difficulty making decisions because they are overwhelmed with anxiety or depression should seek help from qualified healthcare professionals. Counseling or talking about stressful situations can serve as both prevention and treatment. There are also a variety of effective medications to help treat these ailments, but these must be prescribed by a licensed physician.

Taking plant remedies to reduce chronic stress may also alleviate harmful physical reactions from stress. Adaptogens are a class of medicine (often of a natural origin) with immunomodulatory properties. Panossian *et al*. (1999) define these remedies as:

• Non-specific in that the adaptogen increases resistance to a very broad spectrum of harmful factors ("stressors") of different physical, chemical and biological natures;
• An adaptogen is to have a normalizing effect, that is, it counteracts or prevents disturbances brought about by stressors;
• An adaptogen must be innocuous to have a broad range of therapeutical effects without causing any disturbance (other than very marginally) to the normal functioning of the organism.

Chapter Seven discusses seven different plant remedies used therapeutically to reduce stress and improve overall feelings of wellbeing.

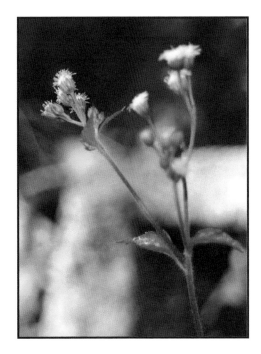

Figure 71. *Ageratum conyzoides* flowers. [RL]

Local names: *ngmak* (Palauan); goatweed, whiteweed (English)
Scientific name: *Ageratum conyzoides* L.
Family: Asteraceae (Daisy Family)

Description
Coarse herb 0.2-1 m high; opposite and simple leaves commonly subacute or obtuse to round at base; the corolla lobes and styles are white to pale lavender. Flowering heads usually 5-8 mm in diameter with 60-75 flowers. Flowering and fruiting seen throughout the year (Smith 1991).

Range
Mexico and the West Indies to South America, now often cultivated and established as an adventive in most warm countries. It was probably an early European introduction into the Pacific Islands as an ornamental (Smith 1991). Introduced to Palau and found growing in savanna grasslands and in urban areas that typically have cultivated landscape and ornamental

plants (Hillmann Kitalong, DeMeo & Holm 2008).

Traditional Uses
Stimulant and tonic. Used in an unspecified way (Del Rosario & Esguerra 2003).

Pharmacological Properties
Oral administration of an ethanolic leaf extract of *Ageratum conyzoides* for 90 days reduced subchronic and chronic inflammation in rats (Moura *et al.*, 2005). A single oral dose of an *A. conyzoides* ethanolic extract reduced gastric lesions in ibuprofen-, cold stress- and alcohol-induced ulcer models in rats (Shirwaikar *et al.*, 2003). A methanolic extract of this plant improved wound healing parameters in a rat model (Oladejo *et al.*, 2003).

Toxicology
No hepatotoxicity was observed with oral doses up to 500 mg/kg/day for 90 days in rats (Moura *et al.*, 2005).

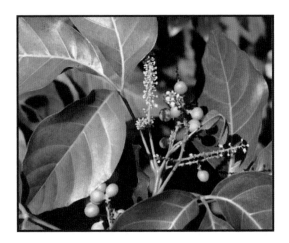

Figure 72. *Allophylus timoriensis* leaves, flowers, and fruits. [CT]

Local name: *chebeludes* (Palauan)
Scientific name: *Allophylus timoriensis* (DC.) Blume
Family: Sapindaceae (Soapberry Family)

Description
Small, sprawling tree 5 m tall with a narrow trunk. The leaves are three parted; the flowers are small and white with red fruits (Smith 1985).

Range
Allophylus timoriensis is widespread throughout the Pacific Islands, from Timor, Malaysia to Tonga and New Guinea. It is found growing mostly at sea level in dense forests, limestone forests, and in thickets (Smith 1985).

Traditional Uses
Energizer. Boil leaves as a decoction and drink (Hillmann Kitalong, DeMeo & Holm 2008).

Pharmacological Properties
The dichloromethane and ethyl acetate extracts of *Allophylus timoriensis* showed potent cytotoxicity against human colon and breast cancer cell lines (Bradacs, Maes & Heilmann 2010). The alcohol extract of the leaf of a related species, *A. serratus* Kurz., had an ulcer protective effect due to its anti-secretory and cytoprotective mechanisms (Dharmani *et al.,* 2005). A single oral dose of the crude methanolic extract of this same related species reduced gastric lesions in cold stress-, aspirin-, and ligation-induced models of stress ulcer (Dharmani *et al.,* 2005).

Toxicology
No reports of toxicity were identified.

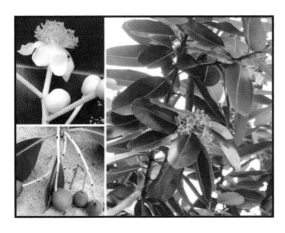

Figure 73. *Calophyllum inophyllum* branches, flowers, and fruits. [AK & CK]

Local names: *btaches* (Palauan); galip nut, beach mahogany (English)
Scientific name: *Calophyllum inophyllum* L.
Family: Clusiaceae (Clusia Family)

Description
Large and spreading tree 6-25 m high, with white latex and a massive trunk to 1.5 m in diameter. The fragrant flowers have white perianth segments and yellow anthers; the fruit is green to yellow, eventually becoming purplish or blackish (Smith 1981).

Range
Eastern Africa and India throughout Malaysia and eastward into the Tuamotus; it was presumably an aboriginal introduction into Hawaii (Smith 1981). It is native to Palau and found growing in volcanic lowland forests, savanna grasslands, and limestone forests, atolls and strand vegetation along the coasts (Hillmann Kitalong, DeMeo & Holm 2008).

Traditional Uses
Strengthening potion. Oil is extracted from nut and is used as strengthening potion.

Pharmacological Properties
A coumarin isolated from *Calophyllum inophyllum* exhibits anti-inflammatory properties (Bhalla *et al.*, 1980). A coumarin isolated from the aerial parts of *C. inophyllum* showed inhibition of TPA-induced tumor promotion in a two-stage skin tumor carcinogenesis model in mice over a study period of 20 weeks (Itoigawa *et al.*, 2001). Three xanthones isolated from the roots of *C. inophyllum* were strong inhibitors of platelet activating factor-induced hypertension in mice (Oku *et al.*, 2005). An oral dose of a methanolic stem bark extract protected mice from thermally-induced pain in the hot plate test (Mishra *et al.*, 2010). A methanol extract of the stem bark of *C. inophyllum* inhibited Gram-positive and Gram-negative bacteria *in vitro* (Mishra *et al.*, 2010). Calanolide-A, a major constituent of *C. inophyllum* was found to be a specific HIV-1 reverse transcriptase inhibitor, active aginst AZT- and pyridinone-resistant strains of the virus, *in vitro* (Kashman *et al.*, 1992). A hexane extract of *C. inophyllum* seeds was found to be active against the HIV-1 IIIB viral strain in C1866 cells (Spino, Dodier & Sotheeswaran 1998).

Toxicology
Oil extracted from the seed of *Calophyllum inophyllum* has been reported to cause contact dermatitis (Le Coz 2004). Rats fed *C. inophyllum* seed oil (5% of diet) for 8 weeks showed signs of liver, kidney and heart damage and demonstrated evidence of atherosclerosis (Ajayi *et al.*, 2008). After an oral dose of a stem bark methanolic extract at 2,000 mg/kg no acute toxicity was observed in mice (Mishra *et al.*, 2010). There are cases of contact dermatitis from the seed oil (Le Coz 2004). Anticoagulant properties of coumarins isolated from this plant may interfere with the intrinsic wound-healing

capacity of blood or potentiate the effect of anticoagulant and blood-thinning medications (Arora, Mathur & Seth 1962).

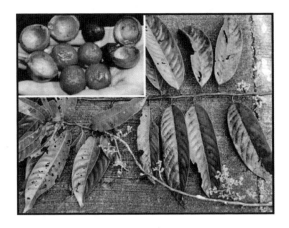

Figure 74. *Horsfieldia irya* leaves and flowers with inset showing fruits. [MB & AK]

Local name: *chemeklachel* (Palauan)
Scientific name: *Horsfieldia irya* (Gaertn.) Warb.
Family: Myristicaceae (Nutmeg Family)

Description

A large size tree growing up to 25 m in height, dbh of 1-1.4 m. The simple, alternate, oblong leaves are 20-30 cm long and 4-7 cm wide. The yellow flowers are unisexual, with male flowers borne in a hairy panicle 4-18 cm long and female flowers in clusters 2-3 cm long. The yellow, globe-like fruits are about 3.4 cm long × 3.2 cm wide with round seeds about 2.1 cm × 2.4 cm. (Hillmann Kitalong, DeMeo & Holm 2008).

Range

Horsfieldia irya is found in the swamp forests of Babeldaob and is distributed in Ceylon, Malaysia and the Solomon Islands (Hillmann Kitalong, DeMeo & Holm 2008).

Traditional Uses

Stimulant. Use leaves (Hillmann Kitalong, DeMeo & Holm 2008).

Medicine used to revive after fainting. Leaves are crushed and scent is used to revive someone who has fainted (Hillmann Kitalong, DeMeo & Holm 2008).

Pharmacological Properties

No relevant pharmacological reports were identified.

Toxicology

No reports of toxicity were identified.

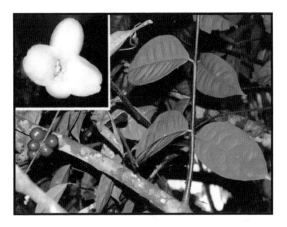

Figure 75. *Phaleria nisidai* fruits and leaves, with inset showing flower. [AK & CT]

Local names: *ongael*, *delalakar* (Palauan); mother of medicine (English)
Scientific name: *Phaleria nisidai* Kaneh.
Family: Thymelaeaceae (Mezereum Family)

Description

A ca. 15 m tall tree with opposite leaves, 15-20 cm long, 7-8 cm wide; the corolla tube is white, 15 mm long (Kanehira 1933). The drupe is red at maturity. It is native to Palau (Hillmann Kitalong, DeMeo & Holm 2008).

Range

Southeastern Asia and Ceylon through Malaysia to Micronesia, Australia, and eastward in the Pacific to Samoa and Tonga (Smith 1981). In Palau, it grows in volcanic lowland forest and in freshwater swamp forest (Hillmann Kitalong, DeMeo & Holm 2008).

Traditional Uses

Medicine for headaches, menstruation, and overall strengthening. Take 7 leaves, boil in 4 cups of water, and drink [Hiromi Nabeyama, Martha Nabeyama].

Energizing tonic. Boil 5-7 leaves in one gallon of water for 3 min and let cool. Drink throughout the day. Make new concoction everyday [Eriko Singeo, Dirraklang Merei Ngirametuker].

Pharmacological Properties

A crude ethanolic extract of *Phaleria nisidai* leaves inhibited a tumor-induced reduction of immunostimulatory cytokines and decreased tumor size in carcinoma-bearing mice (Matsuda *et al.*, 2005a). A crude ethanolic extract of *P. nisidai* increased the phagocytic activity of isolated RAW 264.7 macrophages *in vitro* (Matsuda *et al.*, 2005b). Oral administration of a crude ethanol extract of *P. nisidai* leaves decreased blood glucose levels and inhibited body weight gain in an obese-type non-insulin dependent diabetic mouse model. The crude ethanol extract, as well as mangiferin, isolated from this extract, inhibited rise of blood glucose levels in sucrose-loaded healthy mice and inhibited α-glucosidase (Matsuda *et al.*, 2004). A crude ethanolic extract of *P. nisidai* and mangiferin isolated from this extract increased immunostimulatory cytokines in an immunocompromised diabetic mouse model (Tokunaga *et al.*, 2006).

Toxicology

No reports of toxicity were identified.

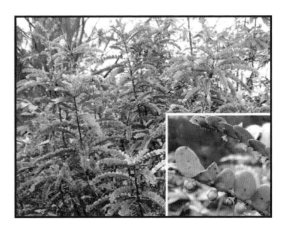

Figure 76. *Phyllanthus palauensis* with inset showing close-up of flowers. [SP]

Local names: *dudurs*, *ukellelachedib* (Palauan)
Scientific name: *Phyllanthus palauensis* Hosok.
Family: Phyllanthaceae (Phyllanthus Family)

Description

Shrub to 1 m tall. Brown bracts; flowers and young fruits green. It is found growing in the savanna grassland (Hillmann Kitalong, DeMeo & Holm 2008).

Range

It is endemic to Palau (Hillmann Kitalong, DeMeo & Holm 2008).

Traditional Uses

Medicine to flush out poison, drugs, etc. Boil plant and drink 3-5 days, 3 times daily [Clarence Kitalong].

Pharmacological Properties

Aqueous extracts of various species of *Phyllanthus* show hepatoprotective effects in rats. *Phyllanthus palauensis* was not tested, but the two most active species were *P. acidus* and *P. urinaria* (Lee *et al.*, 2006). An ethanol extract of *P. amarus* was shown to be hepatoprotective in mice and nephroprotective in rats (Naaz, Javed & Abdin 2007). An aqueous extract of *P. emblica* inhibited tumor promotion in a mouse skin carcinogenensis model and induced apoptosis and reduced tumor invasiveness *in vitro* (Ngamkitidechakul *et al.*, 2010). Oral administration of an aqueous extract of *P. fraternus* protected rats from bromobenzene-induced hepatic injury (Gopi & Setty 2010). An aqueous extract of *P. niruri* enhanced the maturation and antigen presentation of bone marrow-derived dendritic cells (Nworu *et al.*, 2010). Various extracts of the related plants, *P. polyphyllus*, *P. urinaria*, and *P. amarus*, showed anti-inflammatory effects on isolated gastric and hepatic cells, as well as, systemically through a PAF receptor-mediated mechanism (Rao, Fang & Tzeng 2006; Lai *et al.*, 2008; Kiemer *et al.*, 2003; Fang, Rao & Tzeng 2008; Lin *et al.*, 2008; Kassuya *et al.*, 2006). A butanol extract of the leaves of another related plant, *P. acidus*, decreased blood pressure in rats due to stimulation of nitric oxide release from the vascular endothelium (Leeya *et al.*, 2010).

Toxicology
Aqueous extracts of the related species, *Phyllanthus amarus,* in rats at 400 mg/kg was toxic to blood cells, promoted weight loss, and caused testicular degeneration (Adedapo *et al.*, 2005; Adedapo, Adegbayibi & Emikpe 2005). Mice given 100 mg/kg of whole plant alcohol extracts of *P. amarus* were unable to get pregnant, possibly due to hormonal interference (Rao & Alice 2001). Chronic oral administration of the aqueous extract of the leaves of *P. amarus* caused hematological and histopathological changes indicative of

potential toxicity in rats (Adedapo, Adegbayibi & Emikpe 2005).

COMBINATION THERAPY

a)
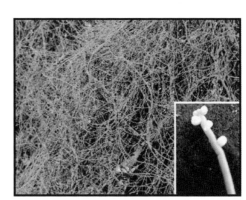

b)
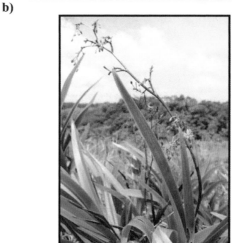

c)
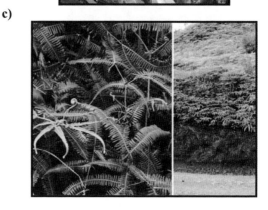

Figure 77. a) *Cassytha filiformis* with inset showing flowers. [MB]; **b)** *Dianella carolinensis*. [CT]; **c)** *Dicranopteris linearis* var. *ferruginea*. [MB];

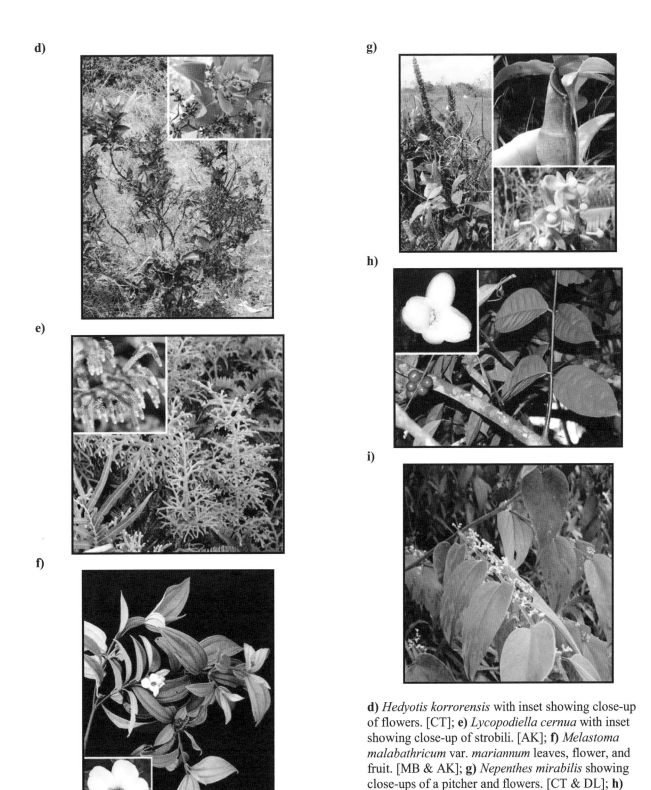

d) *Hedyotis korrorensis* with inset showing close-up of flowers. [CT]; **e)** *Lycopodiella cernua* with inset showing close-up of strobili. [AK]; **f)** *Melastoma malabathricum* var. *mariannum* leaves, flower, and fruit. [MB & AK]; **g)** *Nepenthes mirabilis* showing close-ups of a pitcher and flowers. [CT & DL]; **h)** *Phaleria nisidai* fruits and leaves, with inset showing flower. [AK & CT]; **i)** *Trema* sp. leaves and flowers. [AK]

Local and Scientific names:

techellachull (Palauan); laurel dodder (English) - *Cassytha filiformis* L. (Lauraceae)

kobesos (Palauan) - *Dianella carolinensis* Laut. (Xanthorrhoeaceae)

itouch (Palauan); Old World forked fern (English) - *Dicranopteris linearis* (Burm. f.) Und. var. *ferruginea* (Blume) Rac. (Gleicheniaceae)

chemudelach (Palauan) - *Hedyotis korrorensis* (Val.) Hosok. (Rubiaceae)

olcheiulabeab (Palauan); staghorn clubmoss (English) - *Lycopodiella cernua* (L.) Pic. Serm (Lycopodiaceae)

matakui (Palauan) - *Melastoma malabathricum* L. var. *mariannum* (Naudin) Fosb. & Sach. (Melastomataceae)

meliik (Palauan); common swamp pitcher-plant (English) - *Nepenthes mirabilis* (Lour.) Druce (Nepenthaceae)

ongael, delalakar (Palauan); mother of medicine (English) - *Phaleria nisidai* Kaneh. (Thymelaeaceae)

cheludechoel (Palauan); trema (English) - *Trema* sp. (Cannabaceae)

Descriptions

Cassytha filiformis L.: Herbaceous parasitic vine. In Palau it is found growing in savanna grassland and freshwater swamp forest (Hillmann Kitalong, DeMeo & Holm 2008). Tepals are white and the immature fruit is green, becoming yellow and at length white (Smith 1981).

Dianella carolinensis Laut.: A coarse herb, 1 m tall, with a subterranean rhizome, the leaves linear, crowded on stem base (Smith 1979). Flowers with racemiform branches, petals are bluish-gray and anthers are yellow. The fruit is a purple berry.

Dicranopteris linearis (Burm. f.) Und. var. *ferruginea* (Blume) Rac.: Terrestrial fern with scrambling, dichotomizing fronds reaching 1-2 m high and 2-2.5 m long,

forming dense tangles; pinnae dark medium green above; rachis yellow, below glaucous blue-green; sporangia golden yellow [T. Flynn 6252, 7031; D.H. Lorence 7764].

Hedyotis korrorensis (Val.) Hosok.: Shrub 1.5 m tall; large purple stipules; leaf margins sinuate, leaves discolorous, stems and petioles yellowish green; hypanthium purplish black, corolla lavender color [D.H. Lorence 8207; C. Trauernicht 332].

Lycopodiella cernua (L.) Pic. Serm: Herb up to 1 m tall, spreading by horizontal stolons; stems erect; strobili pendant; branchlets are green to yellow-green, covered with whorls of tiny leaves. The leaves are shiny, narrowly triangular and curved toward the stem tip [D.H. Lorence 9388].

Melastoma malabathricum L. var. *mariannum* (Naudin) Fosb. & Sach.: Shrub or small tree to 2 m. Leaf blades entire, glossy green superior and pale green inferior side, 3-7 nerved, with conspicuous cross-veins. Solitary flowers, petals 4-5 white, pink to red carpels and stamens (Smith 1985). Red fruits.

Nepenthes mirabilis (Lour.) Druce: Herbs erect or climbing, 0.5-2 m tall. Basal leaves about 10 cm, margin usually denticulate. Pitcher narrowly ovoid to subcylindric, variable in size, 2-7 cm, pubescent with simple and stellate hairs. Leaf blade dotted purple-red on both surfaces, oblong to lanceolate, 10-25 cm. Raceme 20-50 cm, tepals 4, red to purplish red, elliptic or oblong. Capsule brown, 1.5-3 cm; valves 4, lanceolate (Wu & Raven 1994).

Phaleria nisidai Kaneh.: See earlier in this chapter.

Trema sp.: Species in this genus are usually monoecious trees or shrubs; stipules free, extrapetiolar; leaf blades triplinerved at base, serrate, subglabrous to variously pilose; inflorescence axillary, paniculate, racemose, or thyrsoid, multi-flowered; male flowers globular, 4- or 5-lobed; female flowers ovoid. The fruit a drupe (Smith 1981).

Ranges

Cassytha filiformis L.: Cosmopolitan in tropical areas, occurring abundantly in most Pacific archipelagos (Smith 1981). Native to Palau (Hillmann Kitalong, DeMeo & Holm 2008).

Dianella carolinensis Laut.: Species in this genus are found in tropical Asia to Australia, New Zealand, and the Pacific Islands (Smith 1979). There is only one species found in Palau, which is native and found growing in the savanna grasslands (Hillmann Kitalong, DeMeo & Holm 2008).

Dicranopteris linearis (Burm. f.) Und. var. *ferruginea* (Blume) Rac.: This species has a pantropical distribution. It is native to Palau and found growing in the savanna grasslands (Hillmann Kitalong, DeMeo & Holm 2008).

Hedyotis korrorensis (Val.) Hosok.: Endemic to Palau, found growing in savanna grasslands (Hillmann Kitalong, DeMeo & Holm 2008).

Lycopodiella cernua (L.) Pic. Serm: Distributed across tropical and subtropical regions of the world (Schelpe 1970). It is native to Palau and it grows in savanna grasslands (Hillmann Kitalong, DeMeo & Holm 2008).

Melastoma malabathricum L. var. *mariannum* (Naudin) Fosb. & Sach.: Southeastern Asia and the Seychelles through Malaysia into Australia and Polynesia (Smith 1985). Native to Palau and found growing on marshes that are areas of freshwater grasses, sedges, reeds, and other herbaceous plants (Hillmann Kitalong, DeMeo & Holm 2008).

Nepenthes mirabilis (Lour.) Druce: Distributed across southern China, southeast Asia, northern Australia, and Western Pacific islands (Wu & Raven 1994). It is native to Palau and it is found growing in savanna grasslands, volcanic lowland forests, and in limestone forests, atolls, and strand vegetation along the coasts (Hillmann Kitalong, DeMeo & Holm 2008).

Phaleria nisidai Kaneh.: See earlier in this chapter.

Trema sp.: This genus is distributed throughout the tropics, extending into warm temperate areas northward and southward, with 10-15 species (Smith 1981). The species of this genus are native to Palau and are found growing in volcanic lowland forests, and in limestone forests, atolls, and strand vegetation along the coasts (Hillmann Kitalong, DeMeo & Holm 2008).

Traditional Uses

Medicine used to cleanse and rid body of unhealthy things. A remedy consumed once a day in a 12 fl oz bottle includes the following herbs: *Dianella carolinensis* (*kobesos*), *Phaleria nisidai* (*ongael*), *Melastoma malabathricum* L. var. *mariannum* (*matakui*), *Nepenthes mirabilis* (*meliik*), leaves of *Lycopodiella cernua* (*olcheiulabeab*), *Dicranopteris linearis* (Burm. f.) Und. var. *ferruginea* (Blume) Rac. (*itouch*), *Cassytha filiformis* (*techelelachull, kukiut*), *Trema* sp. (*chelodechoel*) and *Hedyotis korrorensis* (Val.) Hosok. (*chemudelach*), boiled in water [Dirraklang Merei Ngirametuker].

Pharmacological Properties

Cassytha filiformis L.: A 50% ethanolic extract of *Cassytha filiformis* showed selective cytotoxicity against malignant human hepatoma cell lines (Prayong, Barusrux & Weerapreeyakul 2008) and alkaloids isolated from this plant showed activity against HeLa, Mel-5 and HL-60 cancer cell lines (Stévigny *et al.*, 2002). Compounds isolated from this plant showed inhibition of platelet aggregation induced by arachidonic acid, collagen, ADP and platelet-activating factor (Chang *et al.*, 1998).

Dianella carolinensis Laut.: Crude extracts from the roots of the related species, *Dianella callicarpa,* show mild antimicrobial and antiviral activities (Dias, Silva & Urban 2009). Ethanolic extracts of the roots of the related species, *D. revoluta,* showed weak activity against Gram-negative bacteria but no activity against Gram-positive bacteria (Palombo & Semple 2001). Chrysophanic acid from the related species, *D. longifolia,* inhibits the replication of the poliovirus *in vitro* (Semple *et al.*, 2001; Semple *et al.*, 1998).

Dicranopteris linearis (Burm. f.) Und. var. *ferruginea* (Blume) Rac.: Leaf extracts of *Dicranopteris linearis* (Burm.) Underwood var. *linearis* showed antibacterial activity (Lai, Lim & Tan 2009). Aqueous leaf extracts of *D. linearis* showed significant antinociceptive, anti-inflammatory and antipyretic activity in mice with subcutaneous injected doses (Zakaria *et al.*, 2008). Ethanol extracts of leaves show slight antifungal activity (Davvamani *et al.*, 2005).

Hedyotis korrorensis (Val.) Hosok.: Oral administration of the methanolic extract of the related species, *Hedyotis puberula*, protected rats against indomethacin-, ethanol- and pyloric ligation-induced gastric ulcers (Joseph, Sowndhararajan & Manian 2010a) and had anti-inflammatory and analgesic effects in mice (Joseph, Sowndhararajan & Manian 2010b). The methanolic extract of the related species, *H. corymbosa*, protected rats against paracetamol-induced liver damage (Sadasivan *et al.*, 2006). An ethanolic extract of the related species, *H. diffusa*, induced apoptosis in a human colon cancer cell line via a mitochondria-dependent pathway (Lin *et al.*, 2010).

Lycopodiella cernua (L.) Pic. Serm: The methanolic extract of the whole plant of *Lycopodiella cernua* showed minimal antibacterial and antifungal activity (Wiart *et al.*, 2004). Two compounds present in an ethanolic extract of *L. cernua* leaves inhibited growth of *Candida albicans* (Zhang *et al.*, 2002).

Melastoma malabathricum L. var. *mariannum* (Naudin) Fosb. & Sach.: *Melastoma malabathricum* contains anti-inflammatory compounds such as flavonoids, quercetin, and pentacyclic triterpenes (Mazura, Susanti & Rasadah 2007). Interaperitoneal doses of ethanolic extracts of the whole plant demonstrated analgesic effects in mice, which may be due to an opioid-dependent pathway (Sulaiman *et al.*, 2004). Aqueous extracts of *M. malabathricum* showed significant anti-inflammatory, antinociceptive, and antipyretic effects (Zakaria *et al.*, 2006). Aqueous extracts of the leaves had antimicrobial activity against Gram-positive and Gram-negative bacterial strains (Thatoi *et al.*, 2008) and a methanolic extract had antiviral activity against HSV-1 and poliovirus (Lohezic-Le Devehat *et al.*, 2002). A cold water extract of *M. malabathricum* leaves reduced fecal output in a castor oil-induced model of diarrhea and reduced magnesium sulfate-induced intestinal fluid secretion in mice (Sunilson *et al.*, 2009). Pretreatment with a *M. malabathricum* aqueous extract reduced ethanol-induced gastric lesions and reduced gastric mucosal damage, edema and leukocyte infiltration in mice (Hussain *et al.*, 2008). An aqueous extract of *M. malabathricum* leaves had analgesic, antiinflammatory and antipyretic effects after subcutaneous injection in mice (Zakaria *et al.*, 2006). Flavonoids isolated from *M. malabathricum* inhibited proliferation of breast cancer cells *in vitro* (Susanti *et al.*, 2007).

Nepenthes mirabilis (Lour.) Druce: No pharmacological reports relevant to treatment or management of stress were identified.

Phaleria nisidai Kaneh.: A crude ethanolic extract of *Phaleria nisidai* inhibited a tumor-induced reduction of immunostimulatory cytokines and decreased tumor size in carcinoma-bearing mice (Matsuda *et al.*, 2005a). A crude ethanolic extract of *P. nisidai* increased the phagocytic activity of isolated RAW 264.7 macrophages *in vitro* (Matsuda *et al.*, 2005b). A crude ethanolic extract of *P. nisidai* and mangiferin isolated from this extract increased immunostimulatory cytokine levels in an immunocompromised diabetic mouse model (Tokunaga *et al.*, 2006).

Trema sp.: No relevant pharmacological studies were identified.

Toxicology

Cassytha filiformis L.: A toxicological assessment of an aqueous extract of the stems and leaves revealed that a daily oral dose of 250-1,000 mg/kg for 28 days decreased levels of alkaline phosphatase and increased levels of serum cholesterol in rats. A decrease in relative weights of the heart and lung was also observed. The oral LD_{50} was determined to be greater than 500 mg/kg (Babayi *et al.*, 2007).

Dianella carolinensis Laut.: A related species, *Dianella revoluta* is suspected in livestock poisoning and physiological disturbances in man when ingested. Isolation of the toxic compounds dianellidin, dianellinone, and stypandrol from *D. revoluta* indicates that possible caution should be exercised when ingesting this plant (Colegate, Dorling & Huxtable 1987, 1986). Stypandrol, isolated from *D. revoluta*, has been reported to induce toxicosis in goats and sheep, with acute intoxication causing weakness and paralysis of the hind limbs and sometimes leading to death (Dias, Silva & Urban 2009).

Dicranopteris linearis (Burm. f.) Und. var. *ferruginea* (Blume) Rac.: Some people may be allergic to *Dicranopteris linearis* spores (Chew *et al.*, 2000).

Hedyotis korrorensis (Val.) Hosok.: No reports of toxicity have been identified.

Lycopodiella cernua (L.) Pic. Serm: No reports of toxicity have been identified.

Melastoma malabathricum L. var. *mariannum* (Naudin) Fosb. & Sach.: Oral doses up to 2,000 mg/kg of a cold water extract of *Melastoma malabathricum* leaves showed no signs of toxicity in mice (Sunilson *et al.*, 2009).

Nepenthes mirabilis (Lour.) Druce: No reports of toxicity were identified.

Phaleria nisidai Kaneh.: No reports of toxicity were identified.

Trema sp.: No reports of toxicity were identified.

CHAPTER EIGHT: PAIN

Pain is a sensation that everyone experiences at some point in their lives. Some estimates on chronic pain number the suffering at rates higher than heart disease, diabetes and cancer combined (Tsang *et al.*, 2008). The sensation of pain can range from mild and occasional to severe and constant (Thomas 1981).

General Pain

Pain is a sensation that is triggered in the nervous system. It affects nearly every part of the body, including skin, joints, bones, and muscles. Acute pain is a normal sensation that alerts you to a possible injury and that you need to take care of yourself. Chronic pain, however, is different in that the pain signals are repeatedly fired in the nervous system for weeks, months, and even years. Chronic pain can persist well after the body has healed and can lead to chronically tense muscles, decreased mobility, depression, anger, fear, and/or loss of energy.

Back and Joint Pain

Back pain is defined as any pain in the back. The sensation of pain can vary, but is generally characterized by a dull or throbbing ache and most commonly occur in the muscle attachments of the lumbar, lumbosacral, or sacroiliac regions of the lower back (Thomas 1981). **Patients with low back pain require immediate evaluation by a medical doctor if their symptoms include any of the following:**

- History of cancer
- Unexplained weight loss >10 kg within 6 months
- Age over 50 years or under 17 years old
- Failure to improve with therapy

- Pain persisting for more than 4 to 6 weeks
- Night pain or pain at rest
- Persistent fever (temperature over 100.4° F)
- History of IV drug abuse
- Recent bacterial infection
- Immunocompromised states
- Saddle anesthesia
- Anal sphincter tone decreased or fecal incontinence
- Bilateral lower extremity weakness or numbness
- Progressive neurologic deficit
- Kidney/renal problems

Due to their locations, joints tend to be susceptible to injury, stress, and inflammation. Although joints are affected by general wear and tear, serious injuries such as contusions, sprains, dislocations, wounds, and diseases, such as rheumatoid arthritis, rheumatoid fever, gout, and osteoarthritis can occur (Thomas 1981). **Any patient presenting rapid onset monoarticular joint inflammation (joint pain, swelling, warmth, erythema, and significantly decreased joint range of motion) should be evaluated immediately by a medical doctor**.

Headaches

Headaches can be either acute or chronic, with pain sensations varying from tight pressure, or dull achiness, to pounding, sharp or unbearable pain. Headaches can be located in the temporal, frontal, or occipital lobes of the head or may be more diffuse and generalized. Headaches may result from a variety of diseases, problems relating to sinuses, ears, eyes, teeth, and throat, as well as trauma or injury to the head and neck. **Acute, intense (described as worst ever of** one's life) headaches can be the herald of a severe, potentially fatal problem with the blood vessels in the brain and requires immediate emergency medical care (Thomas 1981).

Earaches and Toothaches

Earaches are a common condition in most children and are usually due to viral or bacterial infections. Ear infections in adults are far less common. Most often, pain in the adult ear is due to referred pain from another location such as the temporamandibular joint (TMJ), teeth, or throat. Children and adults may also get "swimmer's ear," an outer ear canal infection. Both outer and inner infections can be very painful and should be examined by a physician. Signs of an ear infection in children include fever, irritability, increased crying, fussiness, and ear pain. If you suspect an infection, seek professional medical attention.

Toothaches are characterized by pain in the tooth or gums usually resulting from inflammation or infection. Tooth decay is a common cause of toothaches. Dental work such as extractions, root canals, etc., can also cause pain. Pain can also be derived from injury to the TMJ or ear pain (Thomas 1981). Tooth decay can be prevented by practicing proper dental hygiene, brushing and flossing daily and getting annual cleanings.

Chapter Eight introduces 15 traditional plant remedies used in the treatment for general pain including back pain, joint pain, earaches, headaches, and miscellaneous inflammation based on the combined interviews with healers where no specific condition was determined.

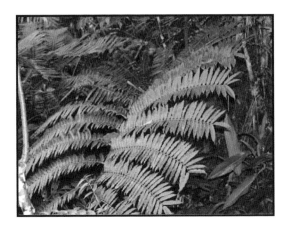

Figure 78. *Angiopteris evecta.* [AK]

Local names: *dermarm* (Palauan); Oriental vessel fern, mule's foot fern (English)
Scientific name: *Angiopteris evecta* (G. Forst.) G.F. Hoffm.
Family: Marattiaceae (Giant Fern Family)

Description
Terrestrial fern with massive rhizome convex, conical, 50 cm diameter; stipes 1 m or more, 5-7 cm diameter, smooth or with brown scurf ramentum along lower portion, rachis up to 2 m with about 20 pinnae, alternate, about 70 cm long × 30 cm wide, with 60-80 pinnules, dark green above, paler beneath with brown sporangia [D.H. Lorence 9018; K.R. Wood 10476].

Range
Distributed from Madagascar through tropical Asia to northeastern Australia and the Western Pacific [K.R. Wood 10476]. Native to Palau; it grows in volcanic lowland forests (Hillmann Kitalong, DeMeo & Holm 2008).

Traditional Uses
Medicine used to cure headaches. Leaves are tied around the head (DeFilipps, Maina & Pray 1988).

113

Pharmacological Properties
No pharmacological reports relevant to this use were identified.

Toxicology
No reports of toxicity were identified.

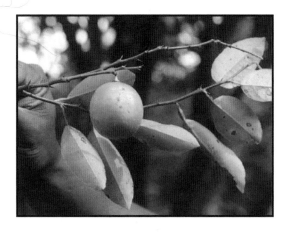

Figure 79. *Citrus aurantiifolia* leaves and fruit. [WL]

Local names: *malchianged* (Palauan); bitter orange (English)
Scientific name: *Citrus aurantiifolia* (Christm.) Swingle
Family: Rutaceae (Citrus Family)

Description
A tree, 4-8 m tall, usually with many short spines; petioles narrowly winged, leaf blades ovate-elliptic, 4-12 × 2-7 cm. Flowers are small, 2-2.5 cm in diameter, have pale pink to white petals, and the fruits are ovoid, 3-6 cm in diameter and greenish yellow when ripe, with thin, adherent peel and greenish, very acid fruit (Smith 1985).

Range
Probably indigenous to Malaysia, and has spread throughout the tropics and subtropics (Smith 1985).

Traditional Uses
Medicine used for headaches. Component of an unspecified preparation [Tadashi Belchal].

Pharmacological Properties
A pill containing a combination of *Citrus sinsensis* peel and *Phellodendron amurense* bark significantly reduced joint pain and increased joint movement in overweight and normal patients suffering from osteoarthritis (Oben *et al.*, 2009). Flavonoids from *C. sinensis* peel improved inflammation and joint mobility in a Freud's complete adjuvant-induced arthritis model in mice due to suppression of inflammatory mediators (Chen, Yin & Zheng 2010). Oral doses of a methanolic extract of *C. sinensis* peel had analgesic, antipyretic and wound healing properties in mice (Anbu *et al.*, 2008).

Toxicology
A daily oral dose of a cold water extract of *Citrus sinensis* peel for 10 days produced hepatotoxicity in mice (Parmar & Kar 2008). Acute toxicity was observed with high one-time oral doses of a methanolic extract of *C. sinensis* peel (Anbu *et al.*, 2008). Ingestion of 2.5 L/day of *C. sinensis* juice for 3 weeks led to hyperkalemia and associated paralysis of the limbs in a 51-year-old man (Javed *et al.*, 2007). Other species in the *Citrus* genus have been shown to interfere with the metabolism of drugs by cytochrome P450 3A4 (CYP3A4). CYP3A4 is an enzyme involved in the intestinal absorption and metabolism of many drugs in use today. Chemicals that inhibit CYP3A4 can increase the bioavailability of the drug *in vivo*. Flavonoids found in grapefruit (*C. paradisi*), pomelo (*C. maxima*), and bitter orange (*C. aurantiifolia*) have all been shown to inhibit CYP3A4 (Adepoju & Adeyemi 2010; Egashira *et al.*,

2004; Grenier *et al.*, 2006; Hanley *et al.*, 2011; Xu, Go & Lim 2003).

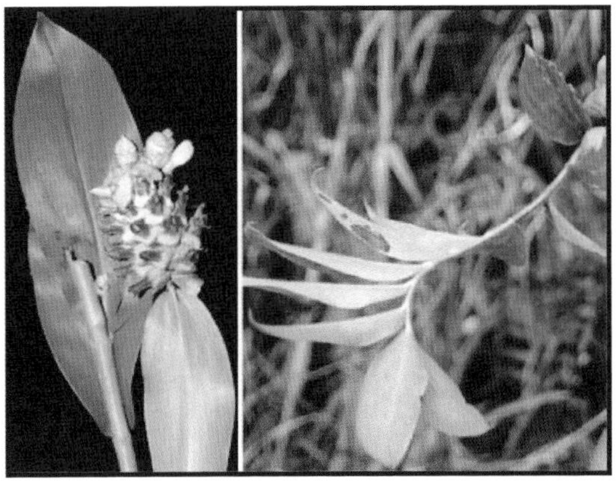

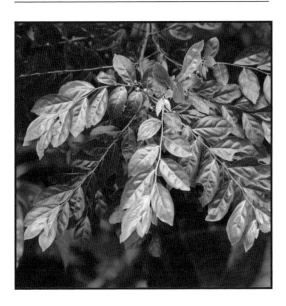

Figure 80. *Cheilocostus speciosus* leaves and flowers. [MB & KS]

Local names: *isebab* (Palauan); Malay ginger, spiral flag (English)
Scientific name: *Cheilocostus speciosus* (J. Koenig) C. Specht
Family: Costaceae (Costus Family)

Description
Coarse herb 1-4 m high. Its ovoid inflorescence is 5-10 cm long, with bracts green to red or red-purple; the outer perianth segments are purplish, the inner ones white; the labellum is white with a yellow center and 5 cm long or more; the filament is white; and the fruit is bright red (Smith 1979).

Range
Indo-Malaysia from the Himalayas to New Guinea, but widely cultivated and sometimes naturalized elsewhere (Smith 1979). Introduced to Palau, now naturalized; found growing in the volcanic lowland forests (Hillmann Kitalong, DeMeo & Holm 2008).

Traditional Uses
Medicine used for sore legs. Cut a small piece of leaf and stem and put it in the sun so it becomes wilted. Then pound and mix with coconut oil and apply to bruise. Alternatively, you can take the leaf and stem and boil in water until the water is nearly gone and wash the sore leg or bruise with it [Elin Rebluud].

Pharmacological Properties
No pharmacological reports relevant to this use were identified.

Toxicology
No reports of toxicity were identified.

Figure 81. *Glochidion ramiflorum* leaves and fruits. [MB]

Local names: *ngolm* (Palauan)
Scientific name: *Glochidion ramiflorum* J.R. Forst. & G. Forst.
Family: Phyllanthaceae (Phyllanthus Family)

Description
A small tree about 10 m in height, dbh 6-32 cm. The simple, alternate, elliptic to spear-

115

shaped leaves are 3-18 cm long, often unequally sided. The long-stalked yellow female flower is 4 mm wide and grows singly at the base of the male raceme. The male flowers grow on the axis of a long simple flower cluster up to 15 cm long. The green, flattened capsule is 5-15 mm in diameter, with unequal lobes, and grows on a stalk about 1 cm long. Fruits look like miniature pumpkins (Hillmann Kitalong, DeMeo & Holm 2008).

Range
Glochidion ramiflorum (*ngolm*) is found in both limestone and volcanic primary and secondary forests of Palau. *Ngolm* is native in Palau and is distributed throughout Micronesia and Polynesia (Hillmann Kitalong, DeMeo & Holm 2008).

Traditional Uses
Medicine used for toothaches. Pulp from young unopened leaves placed on painful tooth.

Pharmacological Properties
No pharmacological reports relevant to this use were identified.

Toxicology
No reports of toxicity were identified.

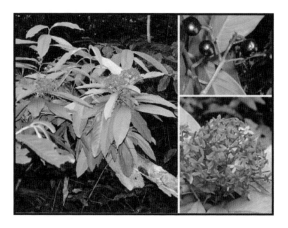

Figure 82. *Ixora casei* with close-ups of fruits and flowers. [DL]

Local names: *kerdeu* (Palauan); ixora, spear palm (English)
Scientific name: *Ixora casei* Hance
Family: Rubiaceae (Coffee Family)

Description
A large shrub 6 m in height, with 1-5 stems 4-8 cm in diameter. The branches are dark brown and smooth. The simple, opposite, oblong to lance-shaped leaves are 21-30 cm long and 6-12 cm wide. The flowers are in rounded clusters 12-18 cm across at the end of the stem. The red corolla is 4-lobed, with lance-shaped lobes about 1 cm long and a slender tube 2.4-3.5 cm long. The dark red, fleshy and smooth berries are 6-9 mm in diameter (Hillmann Kitalong, DeMeo & Holm 2008).

Range
Ixora casei (*kerdeu*) is an understory shrub that grows in limestone and volcanic forests. It is also distributed in Kosrae, Yap, Pohnpei, and Chuuk. It was introduced to Australia, the Marianas Islands and the Marshall Islands as an ornamental shrub (Hillmann Kitalong, DeMeo & Holm 2008).

Traditional Uses
Medicine used for healing internal injuries after a fall. A flower bud is mixed with other unspecified plants and ingested [Johnson Emesiochel].

Pharmacological Properties
The aqueous leaf extract of the related species, *Ixora coccinea* L., has demonstrated fast-onset analgesic properties with a long duration in male rats in tail flick-, hot plate- and formalin-nocicieption assays (Ratnasooriya *et al.*, 2005).

Toxicology
No reports of toxicity were identified.

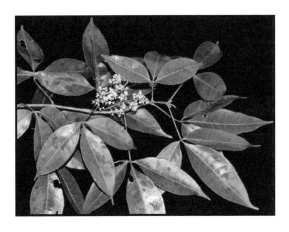

Figure 83. *Melicope denhamii* leaves and flowers. [WL]

Local name: *kertub* (Palauan)
Scientific name: *Melicope denhamii* (Seem.) T. G. Hartley
Family: Rutaceae (Citrus Family)

Description
Understory tree up to 14 m tall, 33 cm dbh. Leaves opposite, trifoliolate compound, leaflets penni-veined, glabrous to hairy. Flowers 4 mm diameter, greenish-white, placed in panicles. Fruits 5 mm diameter, greenish, dehiscent capsules [T. Flynn 6410].

Range
Indonesia and the Philippines to New Guinea and the Western Pacific. Native to Palau and found growing in volcanic lowland forests (Hillmann Kitalong, DeMeo & Holm 2008).

Traditional Uses
Medicine used to prevent major bodyaches and other pain. Boil 8 leaves and drink unspecified amount [Gloria Emesiochel, Bedebii Chiokai].

Pharmacological Properties
Oral administration of an ethanolic extract of the related species, *Melicope ptelefolia*, demonstrated significant dose-dependent analgesic effects in mice and rats in a formalin-induced paw licking test and acetic acid-induced writhing test, respectively (Sulaiman *et al.*, 2010).

Toxicology
No reports of toxicity have been identified. Single oral doses of up to 5 g/kg of the related species, *Melicope ptelefolia*, did not cause any signs of toxicity in both rats and mice (Sulaiman *et al.*, 2010).

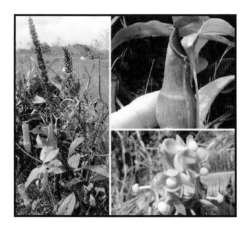

Figure 84. *Nepenthes mirabilis* showing close-ups of a pitcher and flowers. [CT & DL]

Local names: *meliik* (Palauan); common swamp pitcher-plant (English)
Scientific name: *Nepenthes mirabilis* (Lour.) Druce
Family: Nepenthaceae (Pitcher-Plant Family)

Description
Herbs erect or climbing, 0.5-2 m tall. Basal leaves about 10 cm, margin usually denticulate. Pitcher narrowly ovoid to subcylindric, variable in size, 2-7 cm, pubescent with simple and stellate hairs. Leaf blade dotted purple-red on both surfaces, oblong to lanceolate, 10-25 cm. Raceme 20-50 cm, tepals 4, red to purplish-red, elliptic or oblong. Capsule brown, 1.5-3 cm; valves 4, lanceolate (Wu & Raven 1994).

Range
Distributed across southern China, Southeast Asia, Northern Australia, and Western Pacific Islands (Wu & Raven 1994). Native to Palau and found growing in savanna grasslands, volcanic lowland forests, and in limestone forests, atolls, and strand vegetation along the coasts (Hillmann Kitalong, DeMeo & Holm 2008).

Traditional Uses
Medicine used for toothaches. Collect the apex of the plant where the young leaves are forming. Grind this part and hold onto the toothache whenever it hurts. Or, alternatively, you can chew this with your teeth and then put in the area where it is painful. Said to have a spicy taste [Clarence Kitalong].

Pharmacological Properties
No pharmacological reports relevant to the treatment of pain were identified.

Toxicology
No reports of toxicity were identified.

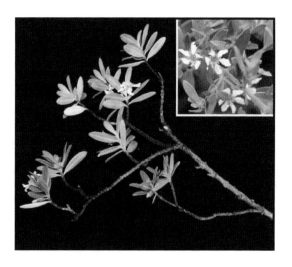

Figure 85. *Pemphis acidula* with inset showing close-up of flowers. [AP & AK]

Local name: *ngis* (Palauan)
Scientific name: *Pemphis acidula* J. R. Forst.
Family: Lythraceae (Loosestrife Family)

Description
A small tree 4 m or more in height with smooth, white bark. The simple, opposite, narrow, oval to inversely egg-shaped leaves are 2-2.5 cm long and 4-10 mm wide. The

white flowers are 1-1.5 cm in diameter. The egg-shaped, reddish-brown capsule is 6-7 mm long, with a cap that splits off releasing the numerous seeds (Hillmann Kitalong, DeMeo & Holm 2008).

Range
Often found along coastal strand vegetation. It is also on coralline substrate and sometimes at the mangrove interface exposed to tidal influence. *Ngis* is distributed from East Africa to the Pacific and is native to the Caroline and Mariana Islands (Hillmann Kitalong, DeMeo & Holm 2008).

Traditional Uses
Medicine used for toothaches. Place mashed leaves on affected tooth [Hillmann Kitalong, DeMeo & Holm 2008].

Pharmacological Properties
No pharmacological reports relevant to the treatment of pain were identified.

Toxicology
Based on reports of potential abortifacient activity, pregnant women may want to avoid using *Pemphis acidula* (Bourdy *et al.*, 1996).

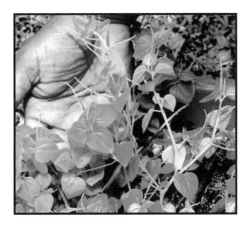

Figure 86. *Peperomia pellucida*. [MB]

Local name: *rtertiil* (Palauan)
Scientific name: *Peperomia pellucida* (L.) Kunth
Family: Piperaceae (Pepper Family)

Description
A terrestrial or occasionally epiphytic herb usually 20-45 cm high. Occurring at elevations of sea level to about 400 m as a weed along roadsides, in plantations, on damp ground in shady places near houses, and occasionally along forest trails. Flowering and fruiting throughout the year (Smith 1981).

Range
Tropical America, but now widely dispersed as a weed throughout tropical areas (Smith 1981). It was introduced to Palau (Hillmann Kitalong, DeMeo & Holm 2008).

Traditional Uses
Medicine used for healing arthritis & gout. Boil 1 handful of the whole plant, without roots, with 1 gal of water for 15-25 min. Drink 8 oz in the morning and evening every day [Ingas Spesungel].

Pharmacological Properties
The methanol extract of the aerial parts of *Peperomia pellucida* showed analgesic activity in mice when given orally (Aziba *et al.*, 2001). An aqueous extract of the aerial parts of *P. pellucida* exhibited antiinflammatory and analgesic activity in rats and mice, respectively, after oral administration (de Fatima Arrigoni-Blank *et al.*, 2004).

Toxicology
The LD_{50} was determined to be 5 g/kg orally, indicating low toxicity (de Fatima Arrigoni-Blank *et al.*, 2004).

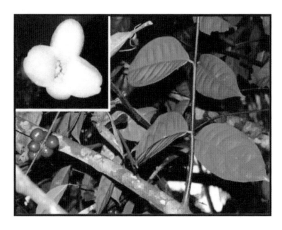

Figure 87. *Phaleria nisidai* fruits and leaves, with inset showing flower. [AK & CT]

Local names: *ongael*, *delalakar* (Palauan); mother of medicine (English)
Scientific name: *Phaleria nisidai* Kaneh.
Family: Thymelaeaceae (Mezereum Family)

Description
A ca. 15 m tall tree with opposite leaves, 15-20 cm long, 7-8 cm wide; the corolla tube is white, 15 mm long (Kanehira 1933). The drupe is red at maturity. It is native to Palau (Hillmann Kitalong, DeMeo & Holm 2008).

Range
Southeastern Asia and Ceylon through Malaysia to Micronesia, Australia, and eastward in the Pacific to Samoa and Tonga (Smith 1981). In Palau, it grows in volcanic lowland forest and in freshwater swamp forest (Hillmann Kitalong, DeMeo & Holm 2008).

Traditional Uses
Medicine used for headaches, menstruation, and body aches. Boil 7 leaves in 4 cups of water, and drink [Hiromi Nabeyama, Martha Nabeyama].

Pharmacological Properties
No pharmacological reports relevant to this use were identified.

Toxicology
No reports of toxicity were identified.

COMBINATION THERAPIES

a)

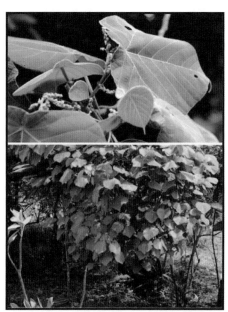

b)

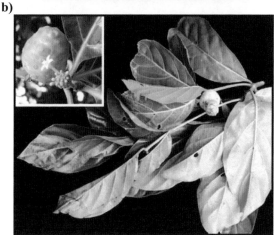

c)

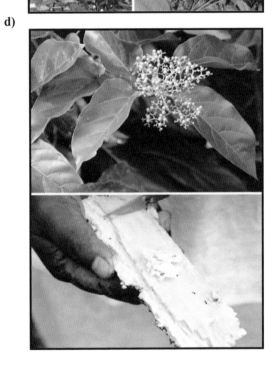

d)

Figure 88. a) *Macaranga carolinensis* leaves and flowers (above); view of tree (below). [AK]; **b)** *Morinda citrifolia* leaves and fruit, with inset showing flower, flower buds, and fruit. [MB & AK]; **c)** *Pangium edule* branch showing leaves and fruits (left); fallen fruit and leaves (right). [AK & MB]; **d)** *Premna serratifolia* leaves, flowers, and inner bark. [MB]

Local and Scientific names:

bedel (Palauan) - *Macaranga carolinensis* Volk. (Euphorbiaceae)

ngel (Palauan); noni (English) - *Morinda citrifolia* L. (Rubiaceae)

riamel (Palauan); false durian (English) - *Pangium edule* Reinw. ex Blume (Achariaceae)

chosm (Palauan) - *Premna serratifolia* L. (Lamiaceae)

Descriptions

Macaranga carolinensis Volk.: A small tree 3-10 m in height with a dbh of 3-40 cm. The simple, alternate leaves are 20-41 cm long, with hairy surfaces. Male and female flowers both lack corollas and are found on separate plants (dioecious). The convex or flat-topped female cluster is enclosed by a serrated triangular modified leaf and is borne on a stalk about 15 cm long. The male flowers are borne in a slender axillary compound cluster with the youngest flowers at the tip. The solitary, globe-like, fuzzy capsules are about 5 mm across (Hillmann Kitalong, DeMeo & Holm 2008).

Morinda citrifolia L.: A small tree 3 to 8 m in height, with a dbh of 10-30 cm and hairless, 4-angled stems. The simple, opposite, elliptic leaves are up to 45 cm long and 25 cm wide. The margins are entire, the surfaces are glossy, hairless and pliable, the stout petiole is up to 2 cm long. The flowers are borne in 75 to 90 flowered, oval to globe-like heads on a stalk about 3 cm long, with the calyx having a truncate rim with no lobes. The white corolla has 5 lobes that are slightly curled backward. The flower stalk is 1 to 3 cm long. The yellowish-white, fleshy, soft and odiferous, irregular heads are about 5 cm long and 3 to 4 cm wide. The fruits have a wart-like appearance (Hillmann Kitalong, DeMeo & Holm 2008).

Pangium edule Reinw. ex Blume: Tree 12-20 m tall; dbh 30 cm; leaves with blades shiny dark green above, paler beneath. Flowers with yellow stamens, anthers orange, perianth green; flowers with strong, sweet odor. The fruit is 15 cm long, ovoid shape with brown, warty skin [D.H. Lorence 9646; M.J. Balick 3805].

Premna serratifolia L.: *Premna serratifolia* is a low shrub or small tree, growing to 10 m in height, with compressed branchlets. The leaves are opposite, round to oval in shape, and 0.5-8 cm in length. The inflorescences are up to 2 cm in length, with small white cup-shaped calyces. The fruits are round, 2-4 mm in diameter, green ripening to black (Smith 1991).

Ranges

Macaranga carolinensis Volk.: *Macaranga carolinensis* (*bedel*) is a fast-growing species common along forest edges, disturbed forests and secondary forests. It ranges from Indo-Malaya to Kosrae (Hillmann Kitalong, DeMeo & Holm 2008).

Morinda citrifolia L.: Indigenous to Indo-Malaysia, *Morinda citrifolia* ranges throughout the Pacific to the Hawaiian Islands and other tropical regions around the world. In coastal forests, it is established as an understory plant often found near creeks, alongside the edge of mangrove swamps, and can be found growing up to 137 m above sea level (Smith 1988). In Palau, it is found along the volcanic forest edge and savanna (Hillmann Kitalong, DeMeo & Holm 2008).

Pangium edule Reinw. ex Blume: Native to Southeast Asia. It was introduced and now naturalized in Palau and found growing on volcanic lowland forests (Hillmann Kitalong, DeMeo & Holm 2008).

Premna serratifolia L.: Lowland species ranging from eastern Africa to Sri Lanka, southeastern Asia, the Ryuku Islands, Taiwan, Malaysia, and tropical Australia to the southern Pacific Islands. Found growing in beach thickets, dry lowland forest, along rocky shores, on the edges of mangrove swamps, and in agroforest areas (Balick 2009; Smith 1991). Native to Palau (Hillmann Kitalong, DeMeo & Holm 2008).

Traditional Uses

Medicine used for muscle pain. Get four large, mature, undamaged leaves of *Premna serratifolia* (*chosm*), leaves of *Macaranga carolinensis* var. *carolinensis* (*bedel*), *Pangium edule* (*riamel*), and *Morinda citrifolia* var. *citrifolia* (*ngel*). Boil together with 4 gal water for 25-40 min and pour into basin and mix with cool water, warm enough but not burning to the skin, and use for bath to relieve muscle pain [Siabal L. Kitalong].

Pharmacological Properties

Macaranga carolinensis Volk.: No pharmacological reports relevant to this use were identified.

Morinda citrifolia L.: No pharmacological reports relevant to this use were identified.

Pangium edule Reinw. ex Blume: No pharmacological reports relevant to this use were identified.

Premna serratifolia L.: An alcoholic leaf extract of the related species, *Premna tomentosa*, demonstrated analgesic properties in rats (Devi *et al.*, 2003).

Toxicology

Macaranga carolinensis Volk.: No toxicological reports were identified.

Morinda citrifolia L.: No toxicological reports relevant to the topical use of *Morinda citrifolia* were identified.

Pangium edule Reinw. ex Blume: A toxic cyanogenic glycoside, gynocardine, occurs in the leaves, bark, roots, and kernels. In addition, the seed, fruit, leaves, and bark possess narcotic properties if orally ingested at excessive doses; sleepiness, headaches, intoxication and delirium may occur (Henty 1980).

Premna serratifolia L.: Isolated compounds from the chloroform extract of the leaves of the related species, *Premna tomentosa*, demonstrated potential carcinogenic effects in a healthy human cell line (Chin *et al.*, 2006).

a)

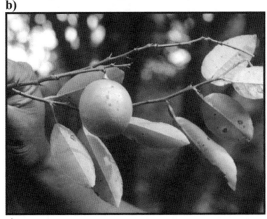

b)

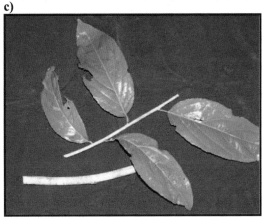

c)

Figure 89. a) *Allophylus timoriensis* leaves, flowers, and fruits. [MB]; **b)** *Citrus aurantiifolia* leaves and fruit. [WL]; **c)** *Lophopyxis maingayi.* [MB]

Local and Scientific names:
chebeludes (Palauan) - *Allophylus timoriensis* (DC.) Blume (Sapindaceae)
malchianged (Palauan); bitter orange (English) - *Citrus aurantiifolia* (Christm.) Swingle (Burm. ex Rumph.) Merr. (Rutaceae)
iutekill (Palauan) - *Lophopyxis maingayi* Hook. f. (Lophophyxidaceae)

Descriptions
Allophylus timoriensis (DC.) Blume: Small, sprawling tree 5 m tall with a narrow trunk. The leaves are three parted; the flowers are small and white with red fruits (Smith 1985).
Citrus aurantiifolia (Christm.) Swingle: See earlier in this chapter.
Lophopyxis maingayi Hook. f.: A climbing liana up to 30 m long; the stem is up to 7 cm in diameter; it has tendrils that can be strong and woody; leaves are spirally arranged, simple, ovate to oblong; inflorescences are axillary or terminal spike-like, pendant raceme; bracts at base transform into tendrils; petals of flowers are white, male flowers with free stamens, female flowers with a superior ovary; the fruit is an obovoid or ellipsoid 5-winged samara (Lemmens & Bunyapraphatsara 2003).

Ranges
Allophylus timoriensis (DC.) Blume: Widespread throughout the Pacific Islands, from Timor, Malaysia to Tonga and New Guinea. It is found growing mostly at sea level in dense forests, limestone forests, and in thickets (Smith 1985).
Citrus aurantiifolia (Christm.) Swingle: See earlier in this chapter.

Lophopyxis maingayi Hook. f.: Found from Malaysia and Indonesia to the Solomon and Caroline Islands (Lemmens & Bunyapraphatsara 2003). It is native to Palau and grows in volcanic lowland forests, and urban areas that typically have cultivated landscape and ornamental plants (Hillmann Kitalong, DeMeo & Holm 2008).

Traditional Uses
Medicine for headaches. The leaves of *Allophyllus timoriensis* (*chebeludes*), *Lophopyxis maingayi* (*iutekill*), and *Citrus aurantiifolia* (*malchianged*) are crushed and sniffed [Gloria Emesiochel, Tadashi Belchal].

Pharmacological Properties
Allophyllus timoriensis (DC.) Blume: No pharmacological reports relevant to the treatment of pain were identified.
Citrus aurantiifolia (Christm.) Swingle: The dried methanolic extract of the related species, *Citrus sinensis*, demonstrated significant analgesic activity when administered orally to mice in the writhing reflux assay (Anbu *et al.*, 2008).
Lophopyxis maingayi Hook. f.: No pharmacological reports relevant to this use were identified.

Toxicology
Allophyllus timoriensis (DC.) Blume: No reports of toxicity were identified.
Citrus aurantiifolia (Christm.) Swingle: Flavonoids found in *Citrus aurantiifolia* and other *Citrus* species have been shown to inhibit CYP3A4 (Adepoju & Adeyemi 2010; Egashira *et al.*, 2004; Grenier *et al.*, 2006; Hanley *et al.*, 2011; Xu, Go & Lim 2003). Compounds that inhibit this enzyme can increase the bioavailability of drugs metabolized by this enzyme *in vivo*, such as warfarin and many other pharmaceuticals (Adepoju & Adeyemi 2010).
Lophopyxis maingayi Hook. f.: No reports of toxicity were identified.

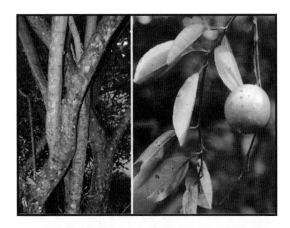

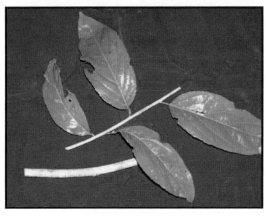

Figure 90. *Citrus aurantiifolia* branches, leaves, and fruit. [WL] (top); *Lophopyxis maingayi*. [MB] (bottom).

Local names and scientific names:
malchianged (Palauan); bitter orange (English) - *Citrus aurantiifolia* (Christm.) Swingle (Rutaceae)
iutekill (Palauan) - *Lophopyxis maingayi* Hook. f. (Lophophyxidaceae)

Descriptions
Citrus aurantiifolia (Christm.) Swingle: See earlier in this chapter.

Lophopyxis maingayi Hook. f.: See earlier in this chapter.

Ranges
Citrus aurantiifolia (Christm.) Swingle: See earlier in this chapter.
Lophophyxis maingayi Hook. f.: See earlier in this chapter.

Traditional Uses
Medicine used for sinus headaches and migraines. Young leaves of *iutekill* (*Lophopyxis maingayi*) and *malchianged* (*Citrus aurantiifolia*) are pounded together. This mixture is chewed and swallowed as you immerse your face in the river, blowing air out of your nose. Alternatively, one can chew and swallow leaves while drinking plenty of water [Tadashi Belchal, Risao Bausoch, Scott Yano].

Pharmacological Properties
Citrus aurantiifolia (Christm.) Swingle: The dried methanolic extract of the related species, *Citrus sinensis*, demonstrated significant analgesic activity when administered orally to mice in the writhing reflux assay (Anbu *et al.*, 2008).
Lophophyxis maingayi Hook. f.: No pharmacological reports relevant to this use were identified.

Toxicology
Citrus aurantiifolia (Christm.) Swingle: Flavonoids found in *Citrus aurantiifolia* and other *Citrus* species have been shown to inhibit CYP3A4 (Adepoju & Adeyemi 2010; Egashira *et al.*, 2004; Grenier *et al.*, 2006; Hanley *et al.*, 2011; Xu, Go & Lim 2003). Compounds that inhibit this enzyme can increase the bioavailability of drugs metabolized by this enzyme *in vivo*, such as warfarin and many other pharmaceuticals (Adepoju & Adeyemi 2010).

Lophophyxis maingayi Hook. f.: There are no known studies examining the toxicity of *Lophopyxis maingayi*.

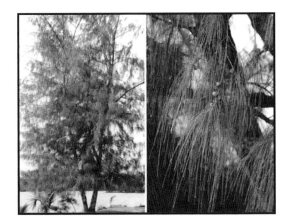

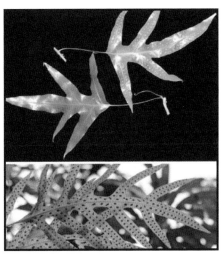

Figure 91. *Casuarina equisetifolia* showing close-up of leaves and female cones. [MB] (top); *Microsorum scolopendria* fronds and rhizomes, and close-up of sori. [MB & AK] (bottom).

Local and Scientific names:
ngas (Palauan); ironwood (English) - *Casuarina equisetifolia* L. (Casuarinaceae)
chebechab (Palauan) - *Microsorum scolopendria* (Burm. f.) Copel. Synonym: *Phymatosorus scolopendria* (Burm. f.) Pic. Serm. (Polypodiaceae)

Descriptions

Casuarina equisetifolia L.: A large tree 20 to 30 m in height. This tree has a symmetrical conical crown with erect branches and weeping needle-like branchlets. The true leaves are minute scales just visible on the green branchlets that are in whorls of 6-8. The rounded female cones are 1 to 2 cm in diameter. The male spikes have numerous flowers and are borne on branches on which the female cones are borne. (Hillmann Kitalong, DeMeo & Holm 2008).

Microsorum scolopendria (Burm. f.) Copel.: Fern, epiphytic or terrestrial; creeping rhizome up to 10 mm in diameter. The deeply pinnatifid, leathery fronds, up to 0.9 m long, are widely spaced along the rhizome. The stipe (leaf stalk) is up to 4 cm long. The leaf blade is divided into narrowly oblong lobes. The somewhat sunken sori are round to oval, 2-3 mm in diameter and occur in 1 or 2 rows on either side of the costa (Roux 2005).

Ranges

Casuarina equisetifolia L.: A coastal tree common in sand and coral rubble near the highwater mark and in coastal strand vegetation. In Palau, it is commonly found on the limestone islands, atoll islands, and along the coastal areas of the volcanic island of Babeldaob. The genus is distributed from Southeast Asia throughout the Pacific (Hillmann Kitalong, DeMeo & Holm 2008).

Microsorum scolopendria (Burm. f.) Copel.: Widespread in the Old World, occurring from Australia, throughout Polynesia and Asia and extending to Madagascar and Africa (Roux 2005). Native to Palau and found growing on volcanic lowland forests, as well as in cultivated landscapes as ornamental plants (Hillmann Kitalong, DeMeo & Holm 2008). It can grow beside saltwater beaches and shady moist forest (Roux 2005).

Traditional Uses

Medicine used for toothaches. Take a teaspoon of bark from the young part of the *Casuarina* branch and pound with the tip of *chebechab* (*Microsorum scolopendria*). Tie mixture in cloth and apply to tooth [Flora Wasisang]. Tip of root is used to treat toothaches [Tadashi Belchal, Risao Bausoch, Scott Yano].

Pharmacological Properties

Casuarina equisetifolia L.: No pharmacological reports relevant to this use were identified.

Microsorum scolopendria (Burm. f.) Copel.: No pharmacological reports relevant to this use were identified.

Toxicology

Casuarina equisetifolia L.: No reports of toxicity were identified.

Microsorum scolopendria (Burm. f.) Copel.: No reports of toxicity were identified.

---

a)

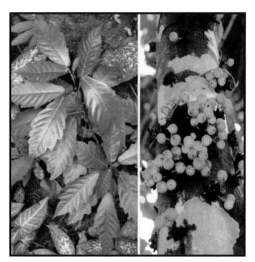

b)

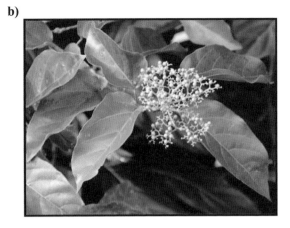

c)

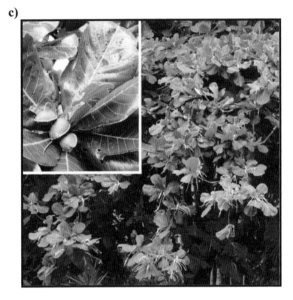

Figure 92. a) *Ficus copiosa* leaves and fruits [AK];
b) *Premna serratifolia* leaves and flower buds. [MB];
c) *Terminalia catappa* with inset showing fruits. [AK & MB]

Local and Scientific names:

uosech (Palauan) - *Ficus copiosa* Steud. (Moraceae)

chosm (Palauan) - *Premna serratifolia* L. (Lamiaceae)

miich (Palauan); Indian almond (English) - *Terminalia catappa* L. (Combretaceae)

Descriptions

Ficus copiosa Steud.: Tree with trunk 20 cm dbh, bark exudate clear but usually turning brownish or pinkish brown on exposure. Leaf blades large, 10-25 × 5-12 cm, petioles with a sandpaper feel. Tepals long and narrow, pink when fresh, apices with bristle-like hairs. Male flowers produced around the ostiole. Stigma pink when fresh and receptive. Figs pedunculate, depressed globular, about 30-40 × 40-50 mm (Hyland, Whiffin & Zich 2010).

Premna serratifolia L.: *Premna serratifolia* is a low shrub or small tree, growing to 10 m in height, with compressed branchlets. The leaves are opposite, round to oval in shape, and 0.5-8 cm in length. The inflorescences are up to 2 cm in length, with small white cup-shaped calyces. The fruits are round, 2-4 mm in diameter, green ripening to black (Smith 1991).

Terminalia catappa L.: A large tree, normally up to 30 m tall. Leaves in whorls at ends of branches, broad and inversely oval, generally dark green and glossy. Older leaves turn brilliant shades of red and orange before dropping. Flowers small in whitish-yellow clusters with racemes (or spikes) 5-15 cm long. Fruits are flattened and egg-shaped, green when young but turn reddish yellow when ripe. Edible cylindrical seeds are encased in a tough fibrous husk with a fleshy outer layer (Hillmann Kitalong, DeMeo & Holm 2008).

Ranges

Ficus copiosa Steud.: It occurs in Malaysia, Australia, and many Pacific islands (Hyland, Whiffin & Zich 2010). Native to Palau, growing in volcanic lowland forests (Hillmann Kitalong, DeMeo & Holm 2008).

Premna serratifolia L.: Lowland species ranging from eastern Africa to Sri Lanka, southeastern Asia, the Ryuku Islands, Taiwan, Malaysia, and tropical Australia to the southern Pacific Islands. Found growing in beach thickets, dry lowland forest, along rocky shores, on the edges of mangrove swamps, and in agroforest areas (Balick 2009; Smith 1991). Native to Palau (Hillmann Kitalong, DeMeo & Holm 2008).

Terminalia catappa L.: Usually found in atoll forests, inland from ocean beaches near river mouths and around coastal areas in general. Native to coastal areas of Eastern India, Indochina, Malaysia, Indonesia, Northern Australia, Oceania, the Philippines and Taiwan. Widely planted and naturalized in the lowland tropical regions of the rest of the world (Hillmann Kitalong, DeMeo & Holm 2008).

Traditional Uses

Medicine used for toothaches. 2 or 4 leaves and fruit of *Ficus copiosa* (*uosech*) are mixed with young leaves of *Terminalia catappa* (*miich*), pounded together and held on toothache. Let the juice drip onto the painful area. Two young leaves, or 4 mature leaves of *chosm* (*Premna serratifolia*) can be added to recipe as well [Henry Yuri].

Pharmacological Properties

Ficus copiosa Steud.: The alcohol extract of the stem bark of the related species, *Ficus religiosa* L., has potent anti-inflammatory activity (Vinutha *et al.*, 2007). Analgesic activity is displayed by the alcohol extracts of the leaves and bark of another related species, *F. glomerata* Roxb. (Malairajan *et al.*, 2006). The alcohol extract of the stem bark of *F. religiosa* L. has potent anti-inflammatory activity (Vinutha *et al.*, 2007). Analgesic activity is displayed by the alcohol extracts of the leaves and bark of another related species, *F. glomerata* Roxb. (Malairajan *et al.*, 2006).

Premna serratifolia L.: Oral administration of a methanolic leaf extract of the related species, *Premna tomentosa,* demonstrated analgesic properties in rats (Devi *et al.*, 2003).

Terminalia catappa L.: No pharmacological reports relevant to the treatment of pain were identified.

Toxicology

Ficus copiosa Steud.: Direct contact with the latex of related species, *Ficus benjamina* L., causes rhinitis and asthma in some people (Delbourg *et al.*, 1995). Delbourg *et al.* (1995) suggests that there is an increased risk of sensitization and allergy to the widely used latex devices and the extensive exposure to *Ficus* species in households and offices. Latex-allergic patients are at higher risk of becoming sensitized to *Ficus* species (Chen, Z. *et al.*, 2000).

Premna serratifolia L.: Isolated compounds from the chloroform extract of the leaves of the related species, *Premna tomentosa,* demonstrated potential carcinogenic effects in a healthy human cell line (Chin *et al.*, 2006).

Terminalia catappa L.: No reports of toxicity were identified.

CHAPTER NINE: WOMEN'S HEALTH

> Women's health refers to a state of "complete mental, physical, spiritual and social well-being" for all female infants, girls and women regardless of age, socioeconomic class, race, ethnicity and geographic location (WHO).

Palauan women have a life expectancy rate of 77 years (WHO 2011). The total fertility rate (women age 15-49 years) is 1.70 and the adolescent pregnancy/birth rate is 27.00 per 1,000. The contraceptive prevalence rate (using modern methods) is 22.26%. About 29% of all women aged 15-44 used any method of birth control in 1993. An estimated 974 persons used family planning services (from 2005 or earlier) (Office of Women's Health: http://www.womenshealth.gov/about-us/who-we-are/regional-offices/9/#palau).

Women play a key role in overall health because they make up the majority of health care workers and consumers and also serve as the "health guardians" of their families.

Palauan women are at significantly higher risk of developing cervical cancer than women in the United States. Nevertheless, there has been reluctance to undertake cancer screening which, up to the mid-1990's, only succeeded in screening less than 15% of the target population. There has also been an upsurge of breast cancer in Palauan women, and as a response, a community women's group called "Ekei" has been actively and effectively involved in promoting participation in cervical and breast cancer screening. The hospital outreach program provides breast and cervical cancer screenings at the dispensaries for patients with limited or no access to the hospital.

Urinary Tract Infection

Many women suffer from urinary infections. Sometimes the only symptoms are painful urination and the need to urinate often. Other common signs are blood in the urine and pain in the lower belly. Pain in the mid or lower back, often spreading around the sides below the ribs, with fever, indicates a more serious problem. Many minor urinary infections can be cured by simply drinking a lot of water, without the need for medicine. If a patient does not continually improve by drinking lots of water, a doctor should be consulted for treatment with an antibiotic. **Painful urination during pregnancy could indicate a urinary tract infection (UTI) and should be treated immediately by a physician**.

Vaginal Discharge

All women normally have a small amount of vaginal discharge, which is clear, milky, or slightly yellow. If there is no itching or bad smell, there is probably no problem. But many women, especially during pregnancy, suffer from a discharge often with itching in the vagina. This discharge may be caused by various infections. Most of them are bothersome, but not dangerous. However, an infection caused by gonorrhea or chlamydia can harm a baby at birth and can cause infertility in women if left untreated. Other infections can also cause changes in vaginal discharge. These changes should be evaluated by a medical doctor for proper treatment.

Menstrual Problems

Most girls have their first 'period' or monthly bleeding between the ages of 11 and

16. This means that they are now old enough to become pregnant. The normal period comes once every 28 days or so, and lasts three to six days. However, this can vary amongst different women. Irregular or painful periods are common in adolescent (teenage) girls. This does not usually mean there is anything wrong.

Irregularity in the length of time between periods is normal for certain women, but for others it may be a sign of chronic illness, anemia, malnutrition, tuberculosis, worsening HIV infection, or possibly an infection or tumor in the womb. If a period does not come when it should, this may be a sign of pregnancy. For many girls who have recently begun to menstruate, and for women over 40, it is often normal to miss or have irregular periods. Worry or emotional upset (stress or long-term strenuous exercise) may also cause a woman to miss her period. If the bleeding comes later than expected, is more severe, and lasts longer, it may be a miscarriage. If the menstrual period lasts more than 6 days, results in unusually heavy bleeding, or comes more than approximately once a month, the woman should be seen by a medical doctor. Abnormal vaginal bleeding and or persistent pain may indicate a more serious illness such as hemorrhage, and/or uterine, cervical, or ovarian cancers and requires immediate medical attention.

For painful periods, it may help to take aspirin or ibuprofen and use warm compresses on the belly. During menstruation, a woman should take care to keep clean, get enough sleep, and eat a well balanced diet. She can eat everything she normally eats and can continue to do her usual work. It is not harmful to have sex during the menstrual period.

Chapter Nine discusses 18 botanical treatments for women's health in Palau.

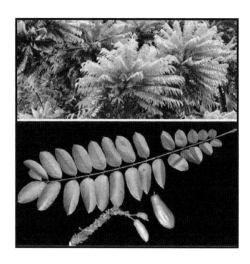

Figure 93. *Averrhoa bilimbi* showing close-up of leaves and fruits. [AK & MB]

Local names: *imekurs* (Palauan); bilimbi (English)
Scientific name: *Averrhoa bilimbi* L.
Family: Oxalidaceae (Wood Sorrel Family)

Description
Shrub or small tree 4-15 m high, with yellowish red to purple sepals and red petals. It is usually cauliflorous and ramiflorous, the leaves having 15-41 leaflets with predominant oblong blades usually 3-7 × 1.5-2.5 cm, acute at apex, a few proximal ones smaller than the distal ones. Fruits are green, terete to obtusely angled, ellipsoid to obovoid, up to 10 × 5 cm, with seeds 6-8 × 4-6 mm and lacking arils (Smith 1985).

Range
Exact origin unknown, but often seen as a relict of former cultivation in eastern Melanesia (Smith 1985). Introduced to Palau, it is found growing in agricultural and agroforest areas, as well as in urban areas that typically have cultivated landscape and ornamental plants (Hillmann Kitalong, DeMeo & Holm 2008).

Traditional Uses
Medicine used for menstrual cramps. Take a handful of leaves and twist them. Swallow with water [Eriko Singeo].

Pharmacological Properties
An ethanolic extract of *Averrhoa bilimbi* showed antimicrobial activity with a MIC range of 100-800 µg/ml (Mackeen *et al.*, 1997).

Toxicology
Feeding of the fruit at daily oral doses of 250-1,000 mg/kg for fourteen days did not result in any obvious toxicity in rats (Ambili, Subramoniam & Nagarajan 2009).

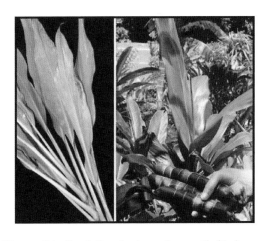

Figure 94. *Cordyline fruticosa* leaves (left); leaves used to wrap food (right). [MB & WL]

Local names: *ditmechei, siselianged* (Palauan); ti plant, good luck plant (English)
Scientific name: *Cordyline fruticosa* L. Chev.
Family: Laxmanniaceae (Laxmannia Family)

Description
Cordyline fruticosa (*ditmechei* local variety) is a shrub growing 2-4 m in height. The leaves are oppositely arranged and spear- shaped. They range from 30-50 cm in length and red or green in color with purplish margins and underside with purplish midvein and lateral veins. The flower is a raceme of small purple or red flowers. The fruits are red, fleshy berries (Burkill 1935; Lee Ling 1998).

Range
Cordyline fruticosa is indigenous to the Himalayas, Southeast Asia, Malaysia and northern Australia and has become naturalized in the Pacific Islands (Smith 1991). Throughout its range, *C. fruticosa* has been widely cultivated as an ornamental for its colorful leaves (Burkill 1935).

Traditional Uses
Medicine used for menstrual cramps and to help with menstrual flow. Only the specific local variety of *Cordyline fruticosa* called "*ditmechei*" will work for this remedy. The variety can be distinguished by having pink venation and midvein on the underside of the leaf. Leaf has pink margins and is not as wide as *sis*. Two young leaf tips are rubbed together with 8 oz of water until the juice comes out and then drink [Ingas Spesungel].

Pharmacological Properties
No relevant reports of pharmacological properties were identified.

Toxicology
No reports of toxicity were identified.

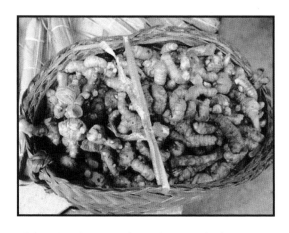

Figure 95. *Curcuma longa* harvested tubers. [AK]

Local name: *kesol, reng, telab* (Palauan); turmeric (English)
Scientific name: *Curcuma longa* L.
Family: Zingiberaceae (Ginger Family)

Description
An herb 1 m high with a spike of pale yellow flowers surrounded by white bracts. The tuber is orange brown on the outside and bright yellow orange on the inside (Smith 1979).

Range
Cultivated throughout the tropical regions of China, India, and Indo-Malaysia. The origin is thought to be South Asia; the species is so widely naturalized throughout the Pacific Islands that it appears indigenous (Smith 1979). Introduced to Palau, it is found growing in agricultural and agroforest areas (Hillmann Kitalong, DeMeo & Holm 2008).

Traditional Uses
Medicine used to protect and heal skin during hotbath. To prepare this medicine, grind the roots of the *telab*, (*Curcuma longa*) enough for ½ gal and combine with ½ gal of *lius* (*Cocos nucifera*) oil (*cheluch er Belau*) and boil at low heat for about 45 min or until it turns yellow, constantly stirring the mixture. This mixture is then applied to the whole body of a woman who is going through her first hot/steam bath. This ointment is used to reduce the appearance of stretch marks and darkened skin areas. Also used regularly as a skin oil [Ingas Spesungel, Flora Wasisang, Bedebii Chiokai].

Pharmacological Properties
No pharmacological effects relevant to women's health have been identified.

Toxicology
No reports of toxicity for *Curcuma longa* were identified. One study reported no effects of turmeric oil intake on weight and blood pressure of healthy volunteers (between 20 and 33 years of age) for up to 12 weeks; there was no clinical, hematological, renal, or hepatotoxicity at months 1 and 3 (Joshi *et al.*, 2003).

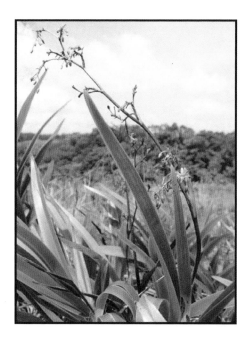

Figure 96. *Dianella carolinensis* leaves and flowers. [CT]

Local name: *kobesos* (Palauan)
Scientific name: *Dianella carolinensis* Laut.
Family: Xanthorrhoeaceae (Hemerocallis Family)

Description
A coarse herb, 1 m tall, with a subterranean rhizome, the leaves linear, crowded on stem base. Flowers with racemiform branches, petals are bluish-gray and anthers are yellow. The fruit is a purple berry (Smith 1979).

Range
Species in this genus are found in tropical Asia to Australia, New Zealand, and the Pacific Islands (Smith 1979). There is only one species found in Palau, which is native and found growing in the savanna grasslands (Hillmann Kitalong, DeMeo & Holm 2008).

Traditional Uses
Medicine used to strengthen body during hotbath. On last day of the steam bath, boil whole plant without roots with unspecified other herbs. This is consumed to strengthen the body. The plants are boiled together until the liquid is light yellow-green. The resulting decoction is bitter. It can be taken hot or cold, but tastes less bitter if taken warm. It can be kept at room temperature or cold. The treatment is usually taken in the morning, after food. The remaining liquid can be reheated without adding new leaves, with the addition of more water, until the liquid turns green again. The decoction is thrown away when the bitter flavor becomes weak [Dirraklang Merei Ngirametuker].

Pharmacological Properties
Crude extracts from the roots of the related species, *Dianella callicarpa,* show mild antimicrobial and antiviral activities (Dias, Silva & Urban 2009). Ethanolic extracts of the roots of the related species, *D. revoluta,* showed weak activity against Gram-negative bacteria but no activity against Gram-positive bacteria (Palombo & Semple 2001).

Toxicology
A related species, *Dianella revoluta,* is suspected in livestock poisoning and physiological disturbances in humans when ingested. Isolation of the toxic compounds dianellidin, dianellinone, and stypandrol from *D. revoluta* indicates that possible caution should be exercised when ingesting this plant. It is unclear how these chemicals react, and what quantities would produce a toxic reaction (Colegate, Dorling & Huxtable 1987, 1986). Stypandrol, isolated from *D. revoluta*, has been reported to induce toxicosis in goats and sheep, with acute intoxication causing weakness and paralysis of the hind limbs and sometimes leading to death (Dias, Silva & Urban 2009).

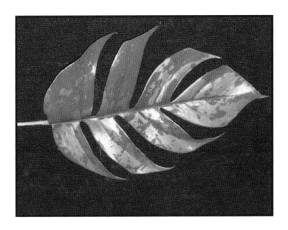

Figure 97. *Epipremnum pinnatum* leaf. [MB]

Local names: *toilalech* (Palauan); pothos, taro vine, devil's ivy (English)
Scientific name: *Epipremnum pinnatum* (L.) Engl.
Family: Araceae (Arum Family)

Description

High-climbing liana; sheath soon withering but leaving a mat of intertwined venation; blade pinnatisect (adult) to entire (juvenile), to 1 × 0.5 m, often with tiny perforations along midrib; spathe cream; spadix sessile, to 17 × 3 cm (Smith 1979).

Range

Southeastern Asia through Malaysia and into Oceania, occasionally cultivated and naturalizing (Smith 1979). It was introduced to Palau and is found growing in areas that typically have cultivated landscape and ornamental plants (Hillmann Kitalong, DeMeo & Holm 2008).

Traditional Uses

Medicine used to cleanse the system during menstruation, especially when periods are abnormal. Five leaves are collected and submerged in cold water until the juices seep out and the water turns a greenish color. Then it is consumed [Tadashi Belchal, Risao Baosauch].

Pharmacological Properties

One study screening several plants found that the leaves and stems of *Epipremnum pinnatum* extracted in ethanol, water, or boiled in water showed no antimicrobial activity (Chan *et al.*, 2008).

Toxicology

A related species, *Epipremnum aureum* has been shown to be a contact irritant (Paulsen, Skov & Andersen 1998). There were 725 cases reported to the American Association of Poison Control Center in 2004 from *E. aureum* exposure. The cases do not indicate the severity of reactions nor do they assume that this plant is an ingestible poison (Watson *et al.*, 2005).

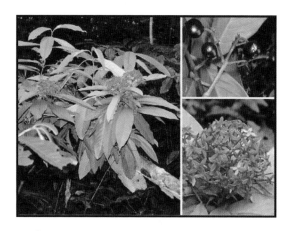

Figure 98. *Ixora casei* with close-ups of fruits and flowers. [DL]

Local names: *kerdeu* (Palauan); ixora (English)
Scientific name: *Ixora casei* Hance
Family: Rubiaceae (Coffee Family)

Description

A large shrub 6 m in height, with 1-5 stems 4-8 cm in diameter. The branches are dark brown and smooth. The simple, opposite, oblong to lance-shaped leaves are 21-30 cm long and 6-12 cm wide. The flowers are in rounded clusters 12-18 cm across at the end of the stem. The red corolla is 4-lobed, with lance-shaped lobes about 1 cm long and a slender tube 2.4-3.5 cm long. The dark red, fleshy and smooth berries are 6-9 mm in diameter (Hillmann Kitalong, DeMeo & Holm 2008).

Range

Ixora casei is an understory shrub which grows in limestone and volcanic forests. It is also distributed in Kosrae, Yap, Pohnpei and Chuuk. It was introduced to Australia, the Mariana Islands and the Marshall Islands as an ornamental shrub (Hillmann Kitalong, DeMeo & Holm 2008).

Traditional Uses

Medicine used for a mother after birth of first child. Chew 4-5 flower buds and leaves, then drink with water for stomach and headaches [Johnson Emesiochel].

Medicine for menstrual cramps. One bunch of unopened flower buds are chewed and washed down with water. They taste bitter and must be chewed quickly before drinking water. This will help with the menstrual cramps (Ingas Spesungel).

Pharmacological Properties

No pharmacological reports relevant to this use were identified.

Toxicology

No reports of toxicity were identified.

Description

Herb up to 1 m tall, spreading by horizontal stolons; stems erect; strobili pendant; branchlets are green to yellow-green, covered with whorls of tiny leaves. The leaves are shiny, narrowly triangular and curved toward the stem tip [D.H. Lorence 9388].

Range

Distributed across tropical and subtropical regions of the world (Schelpe 1970). It is native to Palau and it grows in savanna grasslands (Hillmann Kitalong, DeMeo & Holm 2008).

Traditional Uses

Medicine used in hotbath for healing body. One of the components of hotbath mixture for first birth ceremony [Clarence Kitalong, Kiblas Soaladaob].

Pharmacological Properties

Two compounds isolated from the ethanolic extract of *Lycopodiella cernua* leaves showed inhibition of *Candida albicans* (Zhang *et al.*, 2002). Screening of 50 plants showed the methanolic extract of the whole plant of *L. cernua* to have only minimal and insignificant antibacterial and antifungal activity (Wiart *et al.*, 2004).

Toxicology

No reports of toxicity were identified.

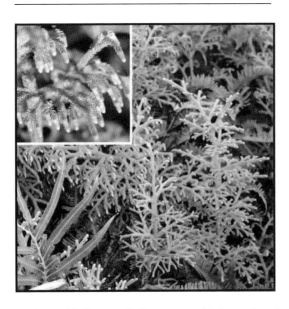

Figure 99. *Lycopodiella cernua* with inset showing close-up of strobili. [AK]

Local names: *olcheiulabeab* (Palauan); staghorn clubmoss (English)
Scientific name: *Lycopodiella cernua* (L.) Pic. Serm
Family: Lycopodiaceae (Clubmoss Family)

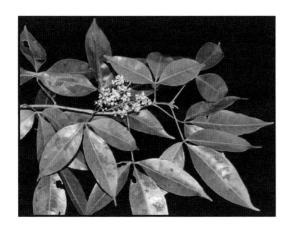

Figure 100. *Melicope denhamii* leaves and flowers. [WL]

Local name: *kertub* (Palauan)
Scientific name: *Melicope denhamii* (Seem.) T. G. Hartley
Family: Rutaceae (Citrus Family)

Description
Understory tree up to 14 m tall, 33 cm dbh. Leaves opposite, tri-foliolate compound, leaflets penni-veined, glabrous to hairy. Flowers 4 mm diameter, greenish-white, placed in panicles. Fruits 5 mm diameter, greenish, dehiscent capsules [T. Flynn 6410].

Range
Indonesia and the Philippines to New Guinea and the Western Pacific. Native to Palau and found growing in volcanic lowland forests (Hillmann Kitalong, DeMeo & Holm 2008).

Traditional Uses
Hotbath. One of the components of the final steam bath mixture for first birth ceremony [Elin Rebluud, David Ngirakesau, Dirraklang Merei Ngirametuker].
Medicine used for prevention of major bodyaches and other pain. Take 8 leaves, boil, and drink unspecified amount [Gloria Emesiochel, Bedebii Chiokai].

Medicine used for a mother after birth of first child. Boil 8 leaves in water and drink three times daily [Flora Wasisang].

Pharmacological Properties
No pharmacological reports relevant to this use were identified.

Toxicology
No reports of toxicity have been identified.

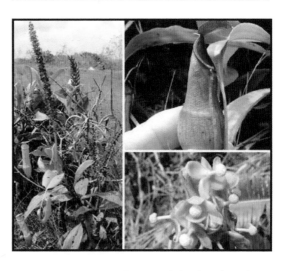

Figure 101. *Nepenthes mirabilis* showing close-ups of a pitcher and flowers. [CT & DL]

Local names: *meliik* (Palauan); pitcher-plant (English)
Scientific names: *Nepenthes mirabilis* (Lour.) Druce
Family: Nepenthaceae (Pitcher-Plant Family)

Descriptions
Herbs erect or climbing, 0.5-2 m tall. Basal leaves about 10 cm, margin usually denticulate. Pitcher narrowly ovoid to subcylindric, variable in size, 2-7 cm, pubescent with simple and stellate hairs. Leaf blade dotted purple-red on both surfaces, oblong to lanceolate, 10-25 cm. Raceme 20-50 cm, tepals 4, red to purplish-red, elliptic or

oblong. Capsule brown, 1.5-3 cm; valves 4, lanceolate (Wu & Raven 1994).

Ranges
Distributed across southern China, southeast Asia, northern Australia, and Western Pacific islands (Wu & Raven 1994). It is native to Palau and it is found growing in savanna grasslands, volcanic lowland forests, and in limestone forests, atolls, and strand vegetation along the coasts (Hillmann Kitalong, DeMeo & Holm 2008).

Traditional Uses
Medicine used in hotbath to heal body after first birth. After the birth of a woman's first child, a 3-10 day long (varies according to clan) hotbath treatment is given. *Nepenthes mirabilis* (*meliik*) is used on the last day of this treatment. Some use the flowers; some use the whole plant, combining them with unspecified other herbs. *Meliik* has a fragrance which also contributes to its use in the steam bath [Yvonne Singeo, Sariang Timulech, Demei Otobed, Dirraklang Merei Ngirametuker].

Pharmacological Properties
No pharmacological effects relevant to this use were identified.

Toxicology
No reports of toxicity were identified.

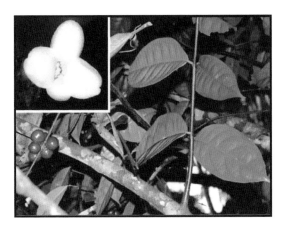

Figure 102. *Phaleria nisidai* fruits and leaves, with inset showing flower. [AK & CT]

Local names: *ongael*, *delalakar* (Palauan); mother of medicine (English)
Scientific name: *Phaleria nisidai* Kaneh.
Family: Thymelaeaceae (Mezereum Family)

Description
A ca. 15 m tall tree with opposite leaves, 15-20 cm long, 7-8 cm wide; the corolla tube is white, 15 mm long (Kanehira 1933). The drupe is red at maturity. It is native to Palau (Hillmann Kitalong, DeMeo & Holm 2008).

Range
Southeastern Asia and Ceylon through Malaysia to Micronesia, Australia, and eastward in the Pacific to Samoa and Tonga (Smith 1981). In Palau, it grows in volcanic lowland forest and in freshwater swamp forest (Hillmann Kitalong, DeMeo & Holm 2008).

Traditional Uses
Medicine used for headaches, menstruation, and overall strengthening from bodyache. Take 7 leaves, boil in 4 cups of water, and drink [Hiromi Nabeyama, Martha Nabeyama].

Pharmacological Properties
No pharmacological reports relevant to this use were identified.

Toxicology
No reports of toxicity were identified.

COMBINATION THERAPIES

a)

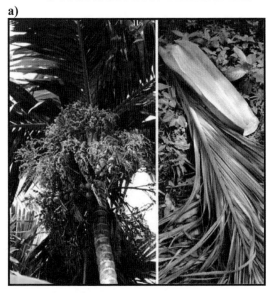

b)

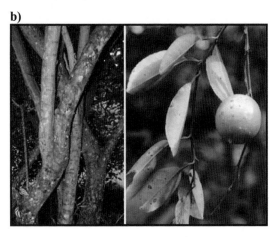

c)

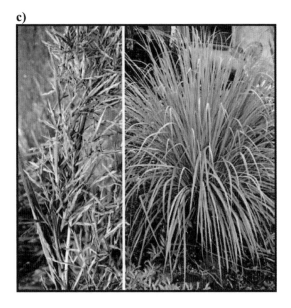

d)

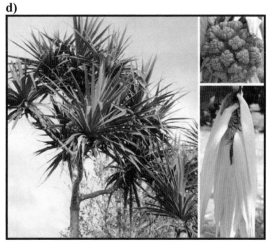

Figure 103. a) *Areca catechu* flowers, fruits, and a dried, fallen leaf. [AK]; **b)** *Citrus aurantiifolia* branches, leaves, and fruit. [WL]; **c)** *Cymbopogon citratus* showing close-up of panicle, and leaf blades. [AK]; **d)** *Pandanus tectorius* tree, showing aggregate fruit and male flower. [MB & AK]

Local and Scientific names:
buuch (Palauan); betel nut (English) - *Areca catechu* L. (Arecaceae)
malchianged (Palauan) - *Citrus aurantiifolia* (Christm.) Swingle (Rutaceae)
keskus (Palauan); lemon grass (English) - *Cymbopogon citratus* (DC. ex Nées) Stapf (Poaceae)
ongor (Palauan); pandanus, screwpine (English) - *Pandanus tectorius* Parkinson ex Du Roi (Pandanaceae)

Descriptions

Areca catechu L.: Small palm tree with solitary, green, and prominently ringed stem, about 10-30 m high, dbh 15-20 cm. Leaves about 2 m long with 12 pinnae on each side, and usually 2-3 ribbed. Inflorescence with staminate and pistillate flowers with small sepals. The fruit is oblong to ovoid in shape 4-5 cm long, dull orange to red (Smith 1979).

Citrus aurantiifolia (Christm.) Swingle: A tree, 4-8 m tall, usually with many short spines; petioles narrowly winged, leaf blades ovate-elliptic, 4-12 × 2-7 cm. Flowers are small, 2-2.5 cm in diameter, have pale pink to white petals, and the fruits are ovoid, 3-6 cm in diameter and greenish yellow when ripe, with thin, adherent peel and greenish, very acid fruit (Smith 1985).

Cymbopogon citratus (DC. ex Nees) Stapf: Perennial, shortly rhizomatous. Culms tufted, robust, up to 2 m tall, about 4 mm in diameter. Leaf sheaths glabrous, greenish inside; leaf blades glaucous, 30-90 × 0.5-2 cm, both surfaces scabrid, base gradually narrowed, apex long acuminate; ligule about 1 mm. Spathate compound panicle large, lax, up to 50 cm, drooping, branches slender; spatheoles reddish or yellowish-brown, 1.5-2 cm; racemes 1.5-2 cm; rachis internodes and pedicels 2.5-4 mm, loosely villous on margins. Sessile spikelet linear-lanceolate, 5-6 × 0.7 mm; lower glume flat or slightly concave toward base, sharply 2-keeled, keels wingless (Wu & Raven 1994).

Pandanus tectorius Parkinson ex Du Roi: Small tree to about 10 m in height, dbh 18-23 cm, with forked branches and aerial prop roots. The spirally arranged leaves are clustered at the branch tips and are approximately 2 m long × 8 cm wide. They have a stiff glossy surface and short, curved thorns along the margin and midrib. The male and female flowers grow on separate plants. The female flower forms a head with several modified leaves at the base. The fragrant male flowers form spikes of many stamens with cream colored modified leaves. The woody, bright orange, nearly spherical aggregate fruit consists of about 50 fruitlets (Hillmann Kitalong, DeMeo & Holm 2008).

Ranges

Areca catechu L.: The origin of *Areca catechu* is uncertain. It is distributed across India and Sri Lanka to southeastern Asia, Indonesia, and the Philippines. It is widely cultivated in the Asiatic tropics, including Pohnpei Island (Smith 1979).

Citrus aurantiifolia (Christm.) Swingle: Probably indigenous to Malaysia, and has spread throughout the tropics and subtropics (Smith 1985).

Cymbopogon citratus (DC. ex Nees) Stapf: The origin is Southeast Asia. This species has been widely cultivated in tropical Asia and South America (Smith 1979). Introduced and cultivated in Palau (Hillmann Kitalong, DeMeo & Holm 2008).

Pandanus tectorius Parkinson ex Du Roi: *Pandanus tectorius* grows mainly on marshy ground and along sea coasts, from Africa and the islands of the eastern Indian Ocean to the Pacific Islands. It is widely cultivated for its edible fruits, fragrant flowers and useful leaves (Burkill 1935; Ghazanfar 1994; Lemmens & Bunyapraphatsara 2003). It is a common component of savanna grassland vegetation in Palau (Hillmann Kitalong, DeMeo & Holm 2008).

Traditional Uses

Medicine used for first menstruation. Use 5 segments from female fruit and a light-yellow flower with bract from the male *Pandanus tectorius* (*ongor*) tree, 1 tip of newly emerged leaf of *Areca catechu* (*buuch*), about 1 ft of the roots of *Citrus aurantiifolia* (*malchianged*) and 1 handful of

Cymbopogon citratus (*keskus*) and drink once after first menstruation. For one year you must avoid eating *Carica papaya* (*bobai*), *Psidium guajava* (*kuabang*) and *Pangium edule* (*riamel*), stingray (*ruul*), shark (*edeng*), sea urchin (*ualsch*), or fish paste [Flora Wasisang].

Pharmacological Properties

Areca catechu L.: No pharmacological effects relative to this use were identified.

Citrus aurantiifolia (Christm.) Swingle: Essential oil and extracts of the related species, *Citrus maxima* demonstrated anti-fungal activity against *Aspergillus flavus* and *Saccharomyce cerevisiae* (Singh, F. *et al.*, 2010; Tao *et al.*, 2010).

Cymbopogon citratus (DC. ex Nees) Stapf: No pharmacological reports relevant to this use were identified.

Pandanus tectorius Parkinson ex Du Roi: No pharmacological reports relevant to this use were identified.

Toxicology

Areca catechu L.: A study undertaken with mice where arecoline from *Areca catechu* seed (170 mg/ml) was administered in the drinking water (each mouse consumed 1 mg of arecoline per day) for 15 days, showed greater frequencies of cancers in oral tissues and organs such as the kidneys and the liver (Chatterjee & Deb 1999), though it is not clear that arecoline is present in the fronds of this plant.

Citrus aurantiifolia (Christm.) Swingle: Flavonoids found in *Citrus aurantiifolia* and other *Citrus* species have been shown to inhibit CYP3A4 (Adepoju & Adeyemi 2010; Egashira *et al.*, 2004; Grenier *et al.*, 2006; Hanley *et al.*, 2011; Xu, Go & Lim 2003). Compounds that inhibit this enzyme can increase the bioavailability of drugs metabolized by this enzyme *in vivo*, such as warfarin and many other pharmaceuticals (Adepoju & Adeyemi 2010).

Cymbopogon citratus (DC. ex Nees) Stapf: The essential oil of the leaves has the following main components: citral A (32%), citral B (34%), myrcene (20%), and terpinen-4-ol (3%). A complete dose-dependent toxicology profile of this oil was examined *in vivo* and in postmortem histological analyses in rats; results showed that consumption of the oil was safe at doses lower than 1,500 mg/kg body weight, though significant functional damages to stomach and liver occurred at higher doses. It was concluded that the oil is safe for humans at low concentrations (Fandohan *et al.*, 2008). The no observed adverse effect level for rat embryo-fetotoxicity is 0.5 g myrcene/kg body weight (Delgado *et al.*, 1993).

Pandanus tectorius Parkinson ex Du Roi: Doses of 2 g of guaiacol, found in *Pandanus tectorius*, are hazardous when applied to skin and ingestion of 5 ml was fatal in 9 year old girl (Clayton & Clayton 1981-1982). Guaiacol may interact with the absorption and metabolism of ibuprofen (Catanese, Interdonato & Barillari 1979). The LD_{50} for guaiacol in rats is 50 mg/kg (Council 1977).

a)

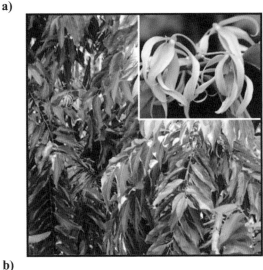

b)

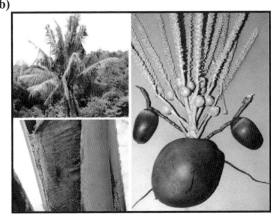

c)

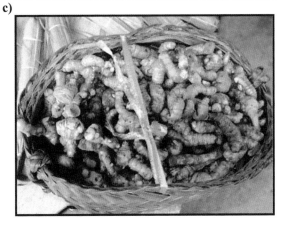

d)

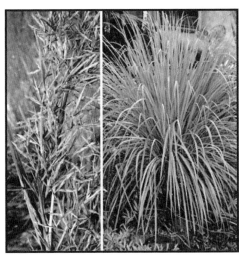

e)

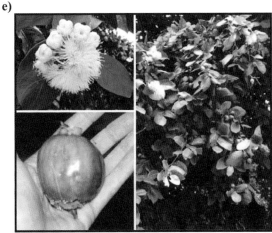

Figure 104. a) *Cananga odorata* with inset showing close-up of flowers. [AK]; **b)** *Cocos nucifera* leaves, husk, and fruits. [DL & WL]; **c)** *Curcuma longa* showing harvested tubers [AK]; **d)** *Cymbopogon citratus* showing close-up of panicle, and leaf blades. [AK]; **e)** *Syzygium samarangense* flowers, matured fruit, and branches. [CT & AK]

Local and Scientific names:
irang irang (Palauan); ylang-ylang (English) - *Cananga odorata* (Lam.) Hook. f. & Thomson (Annonaceae)

lius (Palauan); coconut (English) - *Cocos nucifera* L. (Arecaceae)

kesol (Palauan); turmeric (English) - *Curcuma longa* L. Zingiberaceae (Ginger Family)

keskus (Palauan); lemon grass (English) - *Cymbopogon citratus* (DC. ex Nees) Stapf (Poaceae)

rebotel (Palauan) - *Syzygium samarangense* (Blume) Merr. & Perry (Myrtaceae)

141

Descriptions
Cananga odorata (Lam.) Hook. f. & Thomson: A tree 6-20 m high; the fragrant flowers with conspicuous petals, pale green to yellowish-green or pale yellow, the maturing carpels, at first green, eventually become black, with pale brown seeds embedded in yellowish, oily pulp (Smith 1981).

Cocos nucifera L.: *Cocos nucifera* is a tall palm, reaching heights of 20-30 m. It bears a terminal crown of leaves. The trunk is grayish-brown in color and is 20-40 cm in diameter. The fruits are green, yellow or red depending on the variety. This species may live up to 80-100 years (Purseglove 1988; Smith 1979).

Cucurma longa L.: See earlier in this chapter.

Cymbopogon citratus (DC. ex Nees) Stapf: See earlier in this chapter.

Syzygium samarangense (Blume) Merr. & Perry: Shrub or tree 1-15 m high. Leaves are often subsessile, the petioles 1-7 mm long, the blades 10-25 × 5-12 cm, cordate to rounded at base; inflorescences terminal, axillary, or in axils of fallen leaves; flowers 3-5 cm across expanded stamens, petals and filaments are white; the fruits are borne on branches and when mature are red and as large as 15 × 8 cm (Smith 1985).

Ranges
Cananga odorata (Lam.) Hook. f. & Thomson: Presumably indigenous to southeastern Asia, northern Australia, and perhaps even as far east as the Solomon and Caroline Islands. Elsewhere in the Pacific, it is cultivated and abundantly naturalized eastward to the Societies and the Marquesas (Smith 1981). It is an introduction to Palau and grows in urban areas that typically have cultivated landscape and ornamental plants (Hillmann Kitalong, DeMeo & Holm 2008).

Cocos nucifera L.: A pantropical species, *Cocos nucifera* is native to the Old World tropics, most likely the Pacific Islands (*Cocos nucifera*, TRAMIL 2008). It has been cultivated extensively throughout the tropics as an important economic crop. Due to its wide distribution, commonness, and unwieldy size, few voucher collections are made of this species (Smith 1979).

Curcuma longa L.: See earlier in this chapter.

Cymbopogon citratus (DC. ex Nees) Stapf: See earlier in this chapter.

Syzygium samarangense (Blume) Merr. & Perry: Indigenous to the Indo-Malaysia region, but has long been cultivated and naturalized so its precise origin is unknown (Smith 1985). Similarly, it is introduced to Palau and found growing on agricultural and agroforest areas, as well as urban areas that typically have cultivated landscape and ornamental plants (Hillmann Kitalong, DeMeo & Holm 2008).

Traditional Uses
Medicine used in last steam bath to heal a first time mother. *Cananga odorata* (*irang irang*), *Cymbopogon citratus* (*keskus*), *Curcuma longa* (*kesol*), *Cocos nucifera* (*lius*) oil, and *Syzygium samarangense* (*rebotel*) are combined and boiled to create a fragrant steam for the final steam bath of the first birth ceremony [Kerengel Tesei].

Pharmacological Properties
Cananga odorata (Lam.) Hook. f. & Thomson: No pharmacological reports relevant to this use were identified.

Cocos nucifera L.: The oil from the nut is valued as an emollient (Aburjai & Natcheh 2003; Mendonça-Filho *et al.*, 2004).

Curcuma longa L.: No pharmacological reports relevant to this use were identified.

Cymbopogon citratus (DC. ex Nees) Stapf: No pharmacological reports relevant to this use were identified.

Syzygium samarangense (Blume) Merr. & Perry: No pharmacological reports relevant to this use were identified.

Toxicology

Cananga odorata (Lam.) Hook. f. & Thomson: Available reports indicate that the oil possesses a low order of acute oral and dermal contact reactions in animals and humans, but it is unclear what chemical constituents within the oil may cause these allergic reactions (Burdock & Carabin 2008). A 50% ethanolic extract of the root bark was orally administered to male albino rats at 1g/kg body weight/day for a period of 60 days. The results suggest that this plant species may possess spermatotoxic effects (Anitha & Indira 2006). Similar results were shown in another study by Pankajakshy and Madambath (2009).

Cocos nucifera L.: No reports of toxicity were identified.

Curcuma longa L.: No reports of toxicity were identified.

Cymbopogon citratus (DC. ex Nees) Stapf: No toxicological reports relevant to this use were identified.

Syzygium samarangense (Blume) Merr. & Perry: No reports of toxicity were identified.

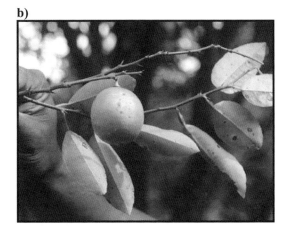

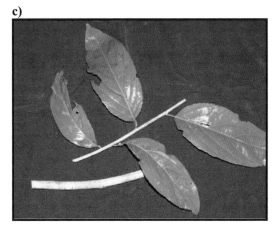

Figure 105. a) *Carica papaya* leaves, flowers, and fruits. [AK]; **b)** *Citrus aurantiifolia* leaves and fruit. [AK]; **c)** *Lophopyxis maingayi*. [MB]

Local and Scientific names:

bobai (Palauan); papaya (English) - *Carica papaya* L. (Caricaceae)

malchianged (Palauan); bitter orange (English) - *Citrus aurantiifolia* (Christm.) Swingle (Rutaceae)

iuetekill (Palauan) - *Lophopyxis maingayi* Hook. f.: (Lophopyxidaceae)

Descriptions

Carica papaya L.: *Carica papaya* is a fast growing tree, reaching 2-10 m in height. The trunk is soft and fibrous with large leaf scars. The fruit is a fleshy berry, weighing up to 9 kg. The skin may be yellow or green when ripe and the flesh is orange. The seeds are numerous, black and wrinkled (Smith 1981).

Citrus aurantiifolia (Christm.) Swingle: See earlier in this chapter.

Lophopyxis maingayi Hook. f.: A climbing liana up to 30 m long; the stem is up to 7 cm in diameter; it has tendrils that can be strong and woody; leaves are spirally arranged, simple, ovate to oblong; inflorescences are axillary or terminal spike-like, pendant raceme; bracts at base transform into tendrils; petals of flowers are white, male flowers with free stamens, female flowers with a superior ovary; the fruit is an obovoid or ellipsoid 5-winged samara (Lemmens & Bunyapraphatsara 2003).

Ranges

Carica papaya L.: *Carica papaya* probably originated from Central America and spread to other tropical regions during the European colonial period. Currently, it is cultivated extensively throughout the tropical regions for its edible fruit (Smith 1981).

Citrus aurantiifolia (Christm.) Swingle: See earlier in this chapter.

Lophopyxis maingayi Hook. f.: Found from Malaysia and Indonesia to the Solomon and Caroline Islands (Lemmens & Bunyapraphatsara 2003). It is native to Palau and grows in volcanic lowland forests, and areas that typically have cultivated landscape and ornamental plants (Hillmann Kitalong, DeMeo & Holm 2008).

Traditional Uses

Medicine used to heal a new mother. *Iuetekill* (*Lophopyxis maingayi*) leaves are picked and combined with young leaves of *malchianged* (*Citrus aurantiifolia*). They are pounded together and placed in the mouth. While the leaves are chewed, the new mother dives into a stream or river. This will relieve headaches, and/or sinus discomfort. If there is no river nearby, leaves can be chewed while drinking water. Some people combine *iuetekill* leaves with *bobai* (*Carica papaya*) leaves for the same purpose [Ngiraklang Merei Ngirametuker].

Pharmacological Properties

Carica papaya L.: No pharmacological reports relevant to this use were identified.

Citrus aurantiifolia (Christm.) Swingle: The dried methanolic extract of the related species, *Citrus sinensis*, demonstrated significant analgesic activity when administered orally to mice in the writhing reflux assay (Anbu *et al.*, 2008).

Lophopyxis maingayi Hook. f.: No pharmacological reports relevant to this use were identified.

Toxicology

Carica papaya L.: Due to the powerful effects of some of the compounds in *Carica papaya*, oral use should be avoided by young children and pregnant women. Use of *C. papaya* should also be limited to no more than 7 consecutive days (Germosen-Robineau 1998). *Carica papaya* may possess abortifacient activity (Anuar *et al.*, 2008). Allergic reactions to *C. papaya* are common, with anaphylaxis occuring in 1% of the patients studied (Iwu 1993). People allergic to latex may have an allergic reaction to papain, an enzyme that degrades polypeptides (Quarre *et al.*, 1995). Change in the structure or function of the esophagus in humans may occur with an oral dose of 71 mg/kg (Davis, Thomas & Guice 1987).

Citrus aurantiifolia (Christm.) Swingle: Flavonoids found in *Citrus aurantiifolia* and other *Citrus* species have been shown to inhibit CYP3A4 (Adepoju & Adeyemi 2010; Egashira *et al.*, 2004; Grenier *et al.*, 2006; Hanley *et al.*, 2011; Xu, Go & Lim 2003). Compounds that inhibit this enzyme can increase the bioavailability of drugs metabolized by this enzyme *in vivo*, such as warfarin and many other pharmaceuticals (Adepoju & Adeyemi 2010).

Lophophyxis maingayi Hook. F.: No reports of toxicity were identified.

c)

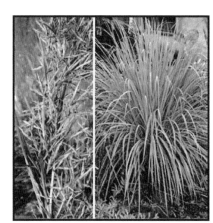

d)

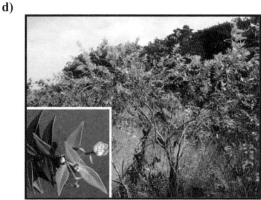

e)

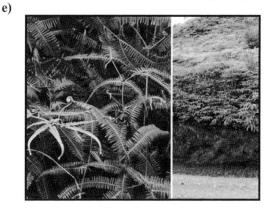

a)

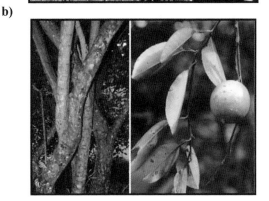

b)

Figure 106. a) *Cassytha filiformis* with inset showing flowers. [MB]; **b)** *Citrus aurantiifolia* branches, leaves, and fruit. [WL]; **c)** *Cymbopogon citratus* showing close-up of panicle, and leaf blades. [AK]; **d)** *Decaspermum parviflorum* with inset showing close-up of flowers. [CT]; **e)** *Dicranopteris linearis* var. *ferruginea* growing on the roadside. [MB];

f)

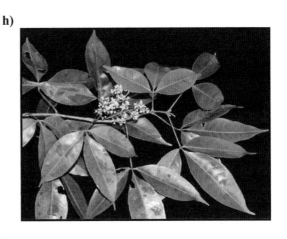

h)

g)

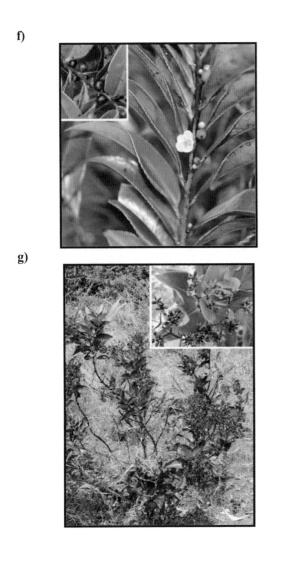

i)

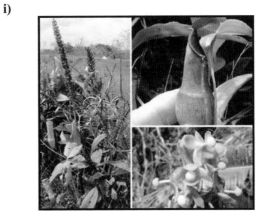

j)

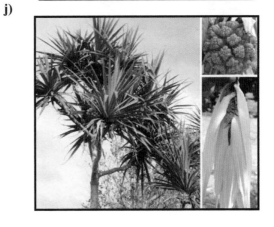

Figure 106. f) *Eurya japonica* var. *nitida* leaves and flowers, with inset showing close-up of fruits. [AK]; **g)** *Hedyotis korrorensis* with inset showing close-up of flowers. [CT]; **h)** *Melicope denhamii* leaves and flowers. [WL]; **i)** *Nepenthes mirabilis* showing close-ups of a pitcher and flowers. [CT & DL]; **j)** *Pandanus tectorius* tree, showing aggregate fruit and male flower. [MB & AK]

Local and Scientific names:
techellelachull (Palauan); laurel dodder (English) - *Cassytha filiformis* L. (Lauraceae)
malchianged (Palauan); bitter orange (English) - *Citrus aurantiifolia* (Christm.) Swingle (Rutaceae)

146

keskus (Palauan); lemon grass (English) - *Cymbopogon citratus* (DC. ex Nees) Stapf (Poaceae)

kertaku (Palauan) - *Decaspermum parviflorum* (Lam.) A. J. Scott (Myrtaceae)

itouch (Palauan); Old World forked fern (English) - *Dicranopteris linearis* (Burm. f.) Und. var. *ferruginea* (Blume) Rac. (Gleicheniaceae)

cheskiik (Palauan) - *Eurya japonica* Thunb. var. *nitida* (Korth.) This.-Dyer (Theaceae)

chemudelach (Palauan) - *Hedyotis korrorensis* (Val.) Hosok. (Rubiaceae)

kertub (Palauan) - *Melicope denhamii* (Seem.) T.G. Hartley (Rutaceae)

meliik (Palauan); common swamp pitcher-plant (English) - *Nepenthes mirabilis* (Lour.) Druce (Nepenthaceae)

ongor (Palauan); pandanus, screwpine (English) - *Pandanus tectorius* Parkinson ex Du Roi (Pandanaceae)

Descriptions

Cassytha filiformis L.: Herbaceous parasitic vine. In Palau it is found growing in savanna grassland and freshwater swamp forest (Hillmann Kitalong, Demeo & Holm 2008). Tepals are white and the immature fruit is green, becoming yellow and at length white (Smith 1981).

Citrus aurantiifolia (Christm.) Swingle: See earlier in this chapter.

Cymbopogon citratus (DC. ex Nees) Stapf: See earlier in this chapter.

Decaspermum parviflorum (Lam.) A. J. Scott: Shrubs or trees, to 20 m tall. Branchlets terete, grayish tomentose or sericeous. Petiole 3-7 mm, pubescent or glabrous; leaf blade elliptic, ovate, oblong, or lanceolate, 4-13 × 1.2-6 cm, glabrous or sparsely pubescent. Inflorescences axillary or terminal, when axillary then thyrses or rarely some flowers in racemes in more basal axils, when terminal then paniculately arranged and

to 9 cm; flowers bisexual or staminate, (4- or) 5-merous; bracteoles lanceolate, 1-1.5 mm, caducous. Hypanthium sericeous, 1-1.5 mm. Petals white or pink, orbicular, 3-4 mm, margin ciliate. Stamens 3-4 mm; filaments pink or white. Fruit 3-5 mm in diameter, sparsely pubescent (Wu & Raven 1994).

Dicranopteris linearis (Burm. f.) Und. var. *ferruginea* (Blume) Rac.: Terrestrial fern with scrambling, dichotomizing fronds reaching 1-2 m high and 2-2.5 m long, forming dense tangles; pinnae dark medium green above; rachis yellow, below glaucous blue-green; sporangia golden yellow [T. Flynn 6252, 7031; D.H. Lorence 7764].

Eurya japonica Thunb. var. *nitida* (Korth.) This.-Dyer: Shrub 5 m tall. Branches striate, glabrous. Petiole 4 mm, leaf blade narrow elliptic or oblanceolate, serrate, above acute or shortly accuminatate, 3-6 × 1-2.5 cm. Flowers small, dioecious, sessile or shortly pedicelled in axillary fascicles. Sepals 5, glabrous. Petals 5, united at base (Hooker 1875).

Hedyotis korrorensis (Val.) Hosok.: Shrub 1.5 m tall; large purple stipules; leaf margins sinuate, leaves discolorous, stems and petioles yellowish green; hypanthium purplish black, corolla lavender color [D.H. Lorence 8207; C. Trauernicht 332].

Melicope denhamii (Seem.) T. G. Hartley: See earlier in this chapter.

Nepenthes mirabilis (Lour.) Druce: See earlier in this chapter.

Pandanus tectorius Parkinson ex Du Roi: See earlier in this chapter.

Ranges

Cassytha filiformis L.: Cosmopolitan in tropical areas, occurring abundantly in most Pacific archipelagos (Smith 1981). It is native to Palau (Hillmann Kitalong, Demeo & Holm 2008).

Citrus aurantiifolia (Christm.) Swingle: See earlier in this chapter.

Cymbopogon citratus (DC. ex Nees) Stapf: See earlier in this chapter.

Decaspermum parviflorum (Lam.) A. J. Scott: Distributed across southern China, northeastern India, Southeast Asia, and the Pacific Islands (Wu & Raven 1994). Native to Palau and found growing in volcanic lowland forests (Hillmann Kitalong, DeMeo & Holm 2008).

Dicranopteris linearis (Burm. f.) Und. var. *ferruginea* (Blume) Rac.: This species has a pantropical distribution. It is native to Palau and found growing in the savanna grasslands (Hillmann Kitalong, DeMeo & Holm 2008).

Eurya japonica Thunb. var. *nitida* (Korth.) This.-Dyer: Borneo, Sumatra, Java (Hooker 1875). Native to Palau and found growing in savanna grasslands (Hillmann Kitalong, Demeo & Holm 2008).

Hedyotis korrorensis (Val.) Hosok.: It is endemic to Palau and it is found growing in savanna grasslands (Hillmann Kitalong, DeMeo & Holm 2008).

Melicope denhamii (Seem.) T. G. Hartley: See earlier in this chapter.

Nepenthes mirabilis (Lour.) Druce: See earlier in this chapter.

Pandanus tectorius Parkinson ex Du Roi: See earlier in this chapter.

Traditional Uses
Medicine to heal the body. For use during steambath on last day of first birth ceremony or for bath during girl's first menstrual period. Combine grass blades of *keskus* (*Cymbopogon citratus*) with the fleshy stems of *kukiut* (*Cassytha filiformis*), the flowers of *meliik* (*Nepenthes mirabilis*), ripe fruit and light yellow flowers and bracts (*redechel a ongor ma bachiei*) of *Pandanus tectorius* (*ongorraked*), leaves of *Decaspermum parviflorum* (*kertaku*), fronds of

Dicranopteris linearis var. *linearis* (*itouch*), leaves of *Citrus aurantiifolia* (*malchianged*), leaves and flowers of *Hedyotis korrorensis* var. *korrorensis* (*chemudelach*), leaves of *kertub* (*Melicope denhamii*) and leaves of *cheskiik* (*Eurya japonica* var. *nitida*). Boil the plants in 30 gal of water for 2 hours. After boiling, put 2-4 gal of water and herbs from the pot into a basin to be used for the steambath in the hut (*bliukell*) [Sariang Timulech].

Pharmacological Properties
Cassytha filiformis L.: No pharmacological reports relevant to this use were identified.

Citrus aurantiifolia (Christm.) Swingle: See earlier in this chapter.

Cymbopogon citratus (DC. ex Nees) Stapf: No pharmacological reports relevant to this use were identified.

Decaspermum parviflorum (Lam.) A.J. Scott: No pharmacological reports relevant to this use were identified.

Dicranopteris linearis (Burm. f.) Und. var. *ferruginea* (Blume) Rac.: Ethanol extracts of leaves show slight antifungal activity at as low as 100 µl/ml (Davvamani *et al.*, 2005).

Eurya japonica Thunb. var. *nitida* (Korth.) This.-Dyer: No pharmacological reports relevant to this use were identified.

Hedyotis korrorensis (Val.) Hosok.: No pharmacological reports relevant to this use were identified.

Melicope denhamii (Seem.) T. G. Hartley: No pharmacological effects relevant to this use were identified.

Nepenthes mirabilis (Lour.) Druce: No pharmacological effects relevant to this use were identified.

Pandanus tectorius Parkinson ex Du Roi: No pharmacological effects relevant to this use were identified.

Toxicology

Cassytha filiformis L.: No toxicological reports relevant to this use were identified.

Citrus aurantiifolia (Christm.) Swingle: There are many case reports of photosensitization known to occur with topical exposure to compounds present in the leaves and fruits of *Citrus aurantiifolia* in combination with sunlight. Symptoms are similar to severe sunburn (Goskowicz, Friedlander & Lawrence 1994; Pomeranz & Karen 2007; Thomson *et al.*, 2007). Lemon juice, (unspecified related species, *Citrus* sp.) has been shown to be toxic to a vaginal cell line and inhibited the growth of healthful *Lactobacillus* spp. bacteria *in vitro* (Anukam & Reid 2009). Lime juice (unspecified related species, *Citrus* sp.) demonstrated time- and dose-dependent toxicity toward human cervicovaginal tissue explants (Fletcher *et al.*, 2008). Epidemiological studies have shown a correlation between douching with lime juice and cervical dysplasia (Sagay *et al.*, 2009).

Cymbopogon citratus (DC. ex Nees) Stapf: No toxicological reports relevant to this use have been identified.

Decaspermum parviflorum (Lam.) A. J. Scott: No reports of toxicity have been identified.

Dicranopteris linearis (Burm. f.) Und. var. *ferruginea* (Blume) Rac.: Some patients may be allergic to spores of *Dicranopteris linearis* (Chew *et al.*, 2000).

Eurya japonica Thunb. var. *nitida* (Korth.) This.-Dyer: No reports of toxicity were identified.

Hedyotis korrorensis (Val.) Hosok.: No reports of toxicity have been identified.

Melicope denhamii (Seem.) T. G. Hartley: No reports of toxicity have been identified.

Nepenthes mirabilis (Lour.) Druce: No reports of toxicity have been identified.

Pandanus tectorius Parkinson ex Du Roi: Doses of 2 g of guaiacol, found in *Pandanus tectorius*, are hazardous when applied to skin and ingestion of 5 ml was fatal in a 9-year-old girl (Clayton & Clayton 1981-1982). Guaiacol may interact with the absorption and metabolism of ibuprofen (Catanese, Interdonato & Barillari 1979). The LD_{50} for guaiacol in rats is 50 mg/kg (Council 1977).

a)

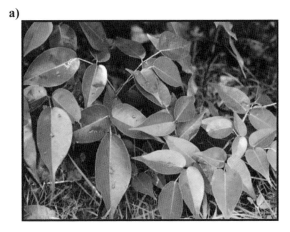

b)

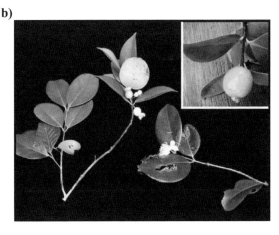

Figure 107. a) Leaves of *Derris trifoliata*. [MB]; **b)** *Eugenia reinwardtiana* leaves and flowers, with inset showing fruit. [MB];

c)

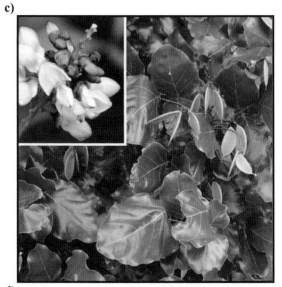

d)

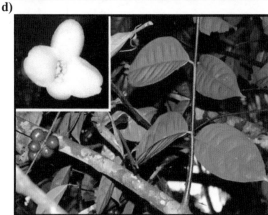

e)

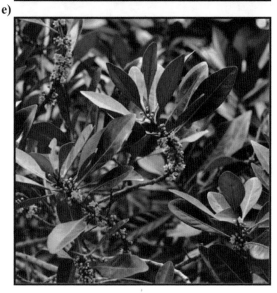

Figure 107. c) *Millettia pinnata* leaves and immature fruits, with inset showing close-up of flowers. [AK]; **d)** *Phaleria nisidai* fruits and leaves, with inset showing flower. [AK & CT]; **e)** *Pouteria obovata* leaves and flowers. [AK]

Local and Scientific names:

kemokem (Palauan); common derris (English) - *Derris trifoliata* Lour. (Fabaceae)
kesiil (Palauan); cedar bay cherry, mountain stopper (English) - *Eugenia reinwardtiana* (Blume) DC. (Myrtaceae)
kisaks (Palauan); Indian beech, pongame oiltree (English) - *Millettia pinnata* (L.) Panigraphi (Fabaceae)
ongael, ***delalakar*** (Palauan) - *Phaleria nisidai* Kaneh. (Thymelaeceae)
chelangel (Palauan); northern yellow boxwood (English) - *Pouteria obovata* (R. Br.) Baehni (Sapotaceae)

Descriptions

Derris trifoliata Lour.: Woody vine or liana, frequent near sea level, sometimes on limestone cliffs and on the edges of mangrove swamps. The calyx is pale green; the petals are pale pink or greenish white. The fruits are subreniform to oblong, usually 3-4.5 × 2-3.5 cm, with a wing 1-2 mm broad along the upper suture, and the 1 or 2 seeds are 1.5-2.5 cm long (Smith 1985).
Eugenia reinwardtiana (Blume) DC.: Tree or shrub 1-5 m high, often spreading or slender, never far inland. Young branchlets, foliage, and inflorescences are short-pale-sericeous. Leaves are broadly ovate to elliptic or obovate blades 4-8 × 2-6.5 cm, rounded to acute at base, obtuse to rounded at apex. Flowers have white petals; fruits are subglobose, 12-20 mm in diameter, yellow to bright orange to brownish, with persistent sepals (Smith 1985).
Millettia pinnata (L.) Panigraphi: Spreading tree 4-25 m high, with a trunk to 1 m in diameter. The leaves, 13-30 cm long, have 3,

5, or 7 leaflets, these with ovate to oblong, acuminate blades 6-25 × 2.5-15 cm. The petals are white to pinkish without and rich pink or purple within; fruits turn from greenish to dull brown and are ellipsoid, beaked, 3-8.5 × 1.5-3 cm, thick at maturity (Smith 1985).

Phaleria nisidai Kaneh.: See earlier in this chapter.

Pouteria obovata (R. Br.) Baehni: A shrubby to tall tree about 18 m in height, with a dbh of 30-60 cm. The simple, alternate elliptic-oblong leaves are 8-12 cm long and 3.5-5 cm wide, with a distinct coppery underside. Greenish- white flowers grow in axilliary clusters of 1-5. The young fruits are green for over a month and turn black as they ripen. The black, flattened, kidney-shaped, fleshy fruits are 3-5 cm long, and contain one large seed (Hillmann Kitalong, DeMeo & Holm 2008).

Ranges

Derris trifoliata Lour.: Eastern Africa to tropical Asia, eastward through Malaysia to Australia and into the Pacific as far as Tonga and Samoa, sometimes cultivated and naturalized elsewhere (Smith 1985). Native to Palau (Hillmann Kitalong, DeMeo & Holm 2008).

Eugenia reinwardtiana (Blume) DC.: It is distributed across Borneo and the Kangean Islands eastward through Malaysia to Micronesia, the Tuamotus, and Hawaii (Smith 1985). Native to Palau and grows in volcanic lowland forests, as well as in limestone forests, atolls, and strand vegetation along the coasts (Hillmann Kitalong, DeMeo & Holm 2008).

Millettia pinnata (L.) Panigraphi: Tropical Asia, throughout Malaysia to Australia and eastward to Samoa (Smith 1985). Native to Palau; it is found growing in volcanic lowland forests, as well as in limestone forests, atolls, and strand vegetation along the coasts (Hillmann Kitalong, DeMeo & Holm 2008).

Phaleria nisidai Kaneh.: See earlier in this chapter.

Pouteria obovata (R. Br.) Baehni: Commonly found in both volcanic and limestone forests of Palau. It is broadly distributed in the tropics from India and Malaysia to Australia and the Pacific Islands (Hillmann Kitalong, DeMeo & Holm 2008).

Traditional Uses

Hotbath to heal the body after the first birth. Two leaves from the middle of the branch (*chedesaoch*) of *Phaleria nisidai* (*ongael*) are placed on the bottom of a pot large enough to hold 30 gal of water. Then 20 leaves of *Pouteria obovata* (*chelangel*), 2 handfuls of *Derris trifoliata* (*kemokem*), and 10 leaves of *Eugenia reinwardtiana* (*kesiil*) are added in layers to the pot. Continue layering these three plants until all 240 leaves (12 layers) of *Pouteria obovata* are gone. Top off with two leaves of *Phaleria nisidai* (*ongael*). Then fill with water and boil for 4 hours. If the water becomes low, add more water, but do not let it overflow. After boiling, take 1 gal of water from the pot to be consumed by the woman having the hotbath for internal healing after labor and delivery. The rest of the 30 gal of water and leaves are for the hotbath for the woman [Sariang Timulchel].

Pharmacological Properties

Derris trifoliata Lour.: An ethanolic extract of the related species, *Derris brevipes,* demonstrated anti-implantation and reduced litter numbers in female rats, suggesting antifertility activity (Badami *et al.,* 2003). The powdered root of *D. brevipes,* also exhibited anti-implanatation and abortifacient activity when given to female rats orally during mating and through the first seven days of pregnancy (Badami *et al.*, 2003).

Eugenia reinwardtiana (Blume) DC.: No pharmacological reports relevant to women's health were identified.

Millettia pinnata (L.) Panigraphi: No pharmacological reports relevant to women's health were identified.

Phaleria nisidai Kaneh.: No pharmacological reports relevant to women's health were identified.

Pouteria obovata (R. Br.) Baehni: No pharmacological reports relevant to women's health were identified.

Toxicology

Derris trifoliata Lour.: There was a case report of contact dermatitis in a 27-year-old due to derris root (Dorne & Friedman 1940).

Eugenia reinwardtiana (Blume) DC.: No toxicological reports relevant to this use were identified.

Millettia pinnata (L.) Panigraphi: No toxicological reports relevant to this use were identified.

Phaleria nisidai Kaneh.: No reports of toxicity were identified.

Pouteria obovata (R. Br.) Baehni: No toxicological reports relevant to this use were identified.

a)

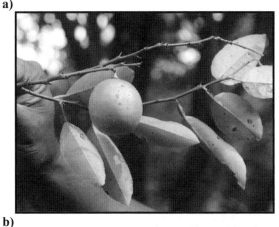

b)

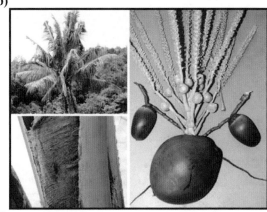

c)

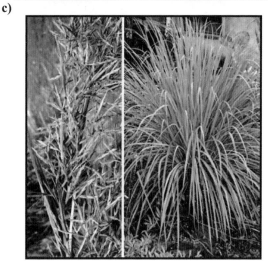

d)

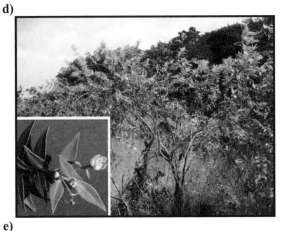

e)

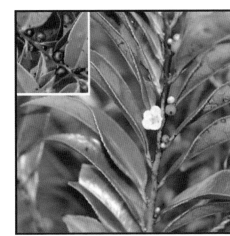

Figure 108. a) *Citrus aurantiifolia* leaves and fruit.
[WL]; **b)** *Cocos nucifera* leaves, husk, and fruits. [DL
& WL]; **c)** *Cymbopogon citratus* showing close-up of
panicle, and leaf blades. [AK]; **d)** *Decaspermum
parviflorum* with inset showing close-up of flowers.
[CT]; **e)** *Eurya japonica* var. *nitida* leaves and flowers,
with inset showing close-up of fruits. [AK]

Local and Scientific names:

malchianged (Palauan); bitter orange
(English) - *Citrus aurantiifolia* (Christm.)
Swingle (Rutaceae)
lius (Palauan); coconut (English) - *Cocos
nucifera* L. (Arecaceae)
keskus (Palauan); lemon grass (English) --
Cymbopogon citratus (DC. ex Nees) Stapf
(Poaceae)
kertaku (Palauan) - *Decaspermum
parviflorum* (Lam.) A. J. Scott (Myrtaceae)

cheskiik (Palauan) - *Eurya japonica* Thunb.
var. *nitida* (Korth.) This.-Dyer (Theaceae)

Descriptions
Citrus aurantiifolia (Christm.) Swingle: See
earlier in this chapter.
Cocos nucifera L.: See earlier in this chapter.
Cymbopogon citratus (DC. ex Nees) Stapf:
See earlier in this chapter.
Decaspermum parviflorum (Lam.) A. J.
Scott: See earlier in this chapter.
Eurya japonica Thunb. var. *nitida* (Korth.)
This.-Dyer: See earlier in this chapter.

Ranges
Citrus aurantiifolia (Christm.) Swingle: See
earlier in this chapter.
Cocos nucifera L.: See earlier in this chapter.
Cymbopogon citratus (DC. ex Nees) Stapf:
See earlier in this chapter.
Decaspermum parviflorum (Lam.) A. J.
Scott: See earlier in this chapter.
Eurya japonica Thunb. var. *nitida* (Korth.)
This.-Dyer: See earlier in this chapter.

Traditional Uses
Bath for first menstruation. The following
plants are used for the first menstruation
bath: leaves of *Cymbopogon citratus*, roots of
Citrus aurantiifolia, leaves of *Eurya japonica*
var. *nitida* and *Decaspermum parviflorum*,
and roasted *Cocos nucifera* meat
(endosperm) [Gloria Emesiochel].

Pharmacological Properties
Citrus aurantiifolia (Christm.) Swingle: No
pharmacological reports relevant to this use
were identified.
Cocos nucifera L.: The oil from the nut is
valued as an emollient (Aburjai & Natcheh
2003; Mendonça-Filho *et al.*, 2004).
Decaspermum parviflorum (Lam.) A. J.
Scott: No pharmacological reports relevant to
this use were identified.

Eurya japonica Thunb. var. *nitida* (Korth.) This.-Dyer: No relevant pharmacological reports were identified.

Toxicology

Citrus aurantiifolia (Christm.) Swingle.: There are many case reports of photosensitization known to occur with topical exposure to compounds present in the leaves and fruits of *Citrus aurantiifolia* in combination with sunlight. Symptoms are similar to severe sunburn (Goskowica, Friedlander & Lawrence 1994; Pomeranz & Karen 2007; Thomson *et al.*, 2007). Lemon juice, (unspecified related species, *Citrus* sp.) has been shown to be toxic to a vaginal cell line and inhibit the growth of healthful *Lactobacillus* spp. bacteria *in vitro* (Anukam & Reid 2009). Lime juice (unspecified related species, *Citrus* sp.) demonstrated time- and dose-dependent toxicity toward human cervicovaginal tissue explants (Fletcher *et al.*, 2008). Epidemiological studies have shown a correlation between douching with lime juice and cervical dysplasia (Sagay *et al.*, 2009).

Cocos nucifera L.: No reports of toxicity were identified.

Decaspermum parviflorum (Lam.) A. J. Scott: No reports of toxicity were identified.

Eurya japonica Thunb. var. *nitida* (Korth.) This.-Dyer: No reports of toxicity were identified.

a)

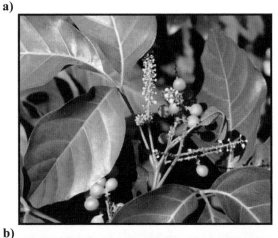

b)

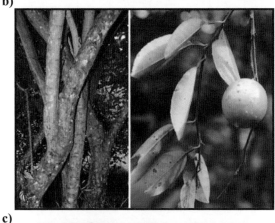

c)

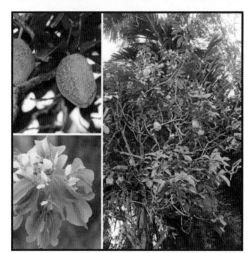

d)

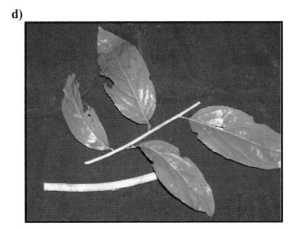

Figure 109. a) *Allophylus timoriensis* leaves, flowers, and fruits. [CT]; **b)** *Citrus aurantiifolia* branches, leaves, and fruit. [WL]; **c)** *Crateva religiosa* with close-ups of fruits and flowers. [AK]; **d)** *Lophopyxis maingayi*. [MB]

Local and Scientific names:
chebeludes (Palauan) - *Allophylus timoriensis* (DC.) Blume (Sapindaceae)
malchianged (Palauan); bitter orange (English) - *Citrus aurantiifolia* (Christm.) Swingle (Rutaceae)
chedebsungel (Palauan) - *Crateva religiosa* G. Forst. (Capparaceae)
iuetekill (Palauan) - *Lophopyxis maingayi* Hook. f. (Lophophyxidaceae)

Descriptions
Allophylus timoriensis (DC.) Blume: Small, sprawling tree 5 m tall with a narrow trunk. The leaves are three parted; the flowers are small and white with red fruits (Smith 1985).
Citrus aurantiifolia (Christm.) Swingle: See earlier in this chapter.
Crateva religiosa G. Forst.: Tree, usually 5-15 m high. Sepals are green, the petals white, becoming cream-colored or yellowish, the filaments distally pink or purple, and the fruit pale green, up to 20 × 9.5 cm but usually smaller, drying grayish (Smith 1981).
Lophopyxis maingayi Hook. f.: See earlier in this chapter.

Ranges
Allophylus timoriensis (DC.) Blume: *Allophylus timoriensis* is widespread throughout the Pacific Islands, from Timor, Malaysia to Tonga and New Guinea. It is found growing mostly at sea level in dense forests, limestone forests, and in thickets (Smith 1985).
Citrus aurantiifolia (Christm.) Swingle: See earlier in this chapter.
Crateva religiosa G. Forst.: Himalayan India and Burma eastward through Micronesia and Malaysia to the Gambier Islands in the Tuamotus (Smith 1981). Native to Palau and found growing in the savanna grassland (Hillmann Kitalong, DeMeo & Holm 2008).
Lophopyxis maingayi Hook. f.: See earlier in this chapter.

Traditional Uses
Medicine used to heal the body after the first birth. Get 4 tips with young leaves (*cheberdil*) and combine the same amount and stages of leaves from each plant, *Allophylus timorensis* (*chebeludes*), *Crateva religiosa* (*chedubsungel*), *Citrus aurantiifolia* (*malchianged*), and *Lophophyxis maingayi* (*iuetekill*), then chew and drink with about 4 oz water, while simultaneously diving in a river or while showering with cold water. Let the water splash on your head or keep your head underwater for at least 1 min while chewing and swallowing the remedy. This medicine is only for women who have just had their first born child. The new mother must do this once a week before sunrise until the first day of hotbath. This remedy is to help avoid the feeling of dizziness from heat of hot/steam bath and the heat of the sun [Ingas Spesungel].

Pharmacological Properties

Allophylus timoriensis (DC.) Blume: No pharmacological reports relevant to this use were identified.

Citrus aurantiifolia (Christm.) Swingle: The dried methanolic extract of the related species, *Citrus sinensis*, demonstrated significant analgesic activity when administered orally to mice in the writhing reflux assay (Anbu *et al.*, 2008).

Cymbopogon citratus (DC. ex Nees) Stapf: No pharmacological reports relevant to this use were identified.

Crateva religiosa G. Forst.: No pharmacological reports relevant to this use were identified.

Lophopyxis maingayi Hook. f.: No pharmacological reports relevant to this use were identified.

Toxicology

Allophylus timoriensis (DC.) Blume: No reports of toxicity were identified.

Citrus aurantiifolia (Christm.) Swingle: Flavonoids found in *Citrus aurantiifolia* and other *Citrus* species have been shown to inhibit CYP3A4 (Adepoju & Adeyemi 2010; Egashira *et al.*, 2004; Grenier *et al.*, 2006; Hanley *et al.*, 2011; Xu, Go & Lim 2003). Compounds that inhibit this enzyme can increase the bioavailability of drugs metabolized by this enzyme *in vivo*, such as warfarin and many other pharmaceuticals (Adepoju & Adeyemi 2010).

Cymbopogon citratus (DC. ex Nees) Stapf: No toxicological reports relevant to this use were identified.

Crateva religiosa G. Forst.: No toxicological reports relevant to this use were identified.

Lophopyxis maingayi Hook. f.: No reports of toxicity were identified.

a)

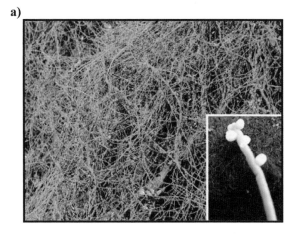

b)

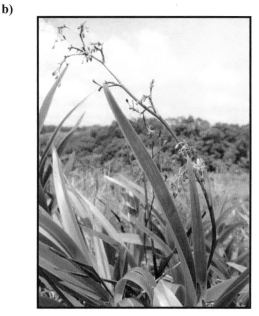

c)

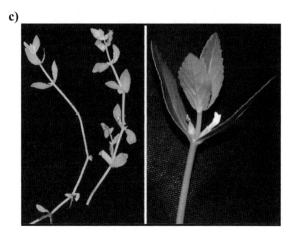

d)

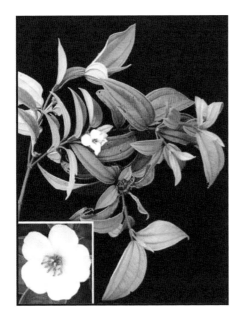

e)

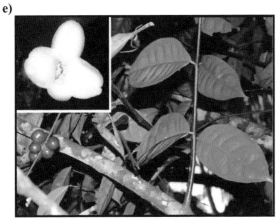

f)

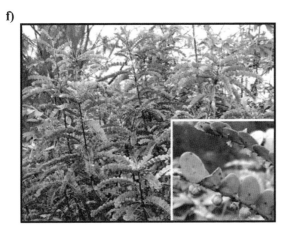

Figure 110. a) *Cassytha filiformis* with inset showing flowers. [MB]; **b)** *Dianella carolinensis* leaves and flowers. [CT]; **c)** *Limnophila chinensis* subsp. *aromatica* leaves and close-up of flowers. [MB & WL]; **d)** *Melastoma malabathricum* var. *mariannum* leaves, flower, and fruit, with inset showing close-up of flower. [MB & AK]; **e)** *Phaleria nisidai* fruits and leaves, with inset showing flower. [AK & CT]; **f)** *Phyllanthus palauensis* with inset showing flowers. [SP]

Local and Scientific names:

techellachull (Palauan); laurel dodder (English) - *Cassytha filiformis* L. (Lauraceae)

kobesos (Palauan) - *Dianella carolinensis* Laut. (Xanthorrhoeaceae)

iaml (Palauan); rice paddy herb (English) - *Limnophila chinensis* (Osb.) Merr. subsp. *aromatica* (Lam.) Yamazaki (Scrophulariaceae)

matakui (Palauan) - *Melastoma malabathricum* L. var. *mariannum* (Naudin) Fosb. & Sach. (Melastomataceae)

ongael, *delalakar* (Palauan); mother of medicine (English) - *Phaleria nisidai* Kaneh. (Thymelaeaecea)

dudurs, *ukellelachedib* (Palauan) - *Phyllanthus palauensis* Hosok. (Phyllanthaceae)

Descriptions

Cassytha filiformis L.: See earlier in this chapter.

Dianella carolinensis Laut.: See earlier in this chapter.

Limnophila chinensis (Osb.) Merr. subsp. *aromatica* (Lam.) Yamazaki: Herb, 5-50 cm tall. Leaves opposite or in whorls of 3 or 4, sessile, ovate-lanceolate, 0.5-5.3 × 0.2-1.5 cm. Flowers solitary, purple-red or blue corolla, 1-1.5 cm. Capsule compressed, broadly ellipsoid, 5 mm (Wu & Raven 1994).

Melastoma malabathricum L. var. *mariannum* (Naudin) Fosb. & Sach.: Shrub or small tree to 2 m. Leaf blades entire, glossy green superior and pale green inferior side, 3-7 nerved, with conspicuous cross-veins. Solitary flowers, petals 4-5 white, pink to red carpels and stamens (Smith 1985). Red fruits.

Phaleria nisidai Kaneh.: See earlier in this chapter.

Phyllanthus palauensis Hosok.: Shrub to 1 m tall. Brown bracts; flowers and young fruits green. It is found growing in the savanna grassland (Hillmann Kitalong, DeMeo & Holm 2008).

Ranges

Cassytha filiformis L.: See earlier in this chapter.

Dianella carolinensis Laut.: See earlier in this chapter.

Limnophila chinensis (Osb.) Merr. subsp. *aromatica* (Lam.) Yamazaki: The genus is paleotropical (Smith 1991). This species is native to Palau and found growing on marshes that are areas of freshwater grasses, sedges, reeds, and other herbaceous plants (Hillmann Kitalong, DeMeo & Holm 2008).

Melastoma malabathricum L. var. *mariannum* (Naudin) Fosb. & Sach.: Southeastern Asia and the Seychelles through Malaysia into Australia and Polynesia (Smith 1985). It is native to Palau and found growing on marshes that are areas of freshwater grasses, sedges, reeds, and other herbaceous plants (Hillmann Kitalong, DeMeo & Holm 2008).

Phaleria nisidai Kaneh.: See earlier in this chapter.

Phyllanthus palauensis Hosok.: It is endemic to Palau (Hillmann Kitalong, DeMeo & Holm 2008).

Traditional Uses
Medicine used to heal the body after the first birth. The following plants are commonly combined with other plants for the steam bath on the last day of the first birth ceremony: *Phaleria nisidai* (*ongael*), *Phyllanthus palauensis* (*dudurs*), *Dianella carolinensis* (*kebesos*), *Limnophila aromatica* (*iaml*), *Cassytha filiformis* (*techellachull*), and *Melastoma malabathricum* var. *mariannum* (*matakui*) [Dirraklang Merei Ngirametuker].

Pharmacological Properties
Cassytha filiformis L.: No pharmacological effects relevant to this use were identified.

Dianella carolinensis Laut.: Crude extracts from the roots of the related species, *Dianella callicarpa,* show mild antimicrobial and antiviral activities (Dias, Silva & Urban 2009). Ethanolic extracts of the roots of the related species, *Dianella revoluta,* showed weak activity against Gram-negative bacteria but no activity against Gram-positive bacteria (Palombo & Semple 2001).

Limnophila chinensis (Osb.) Merr. subsp. *aromatica* (Lam.) Yamazaki: No pharmacological reports relevant to this use were identified.

Melastoma malabathricum L. var. *mariannum* (Naudin) Fosb. & Sach.: Flavonoids isolated from *M. malabathricum* inhibited proliferation of breast cancer cells *in vitro* (Susanti *et al.*, 2007).

Phaleria nisidai Kaneh.: No pharmacological reports relevant to this use were identified.

Phyllanthus palauensis Hosok.: No pharmacological reports relevant to this use were identified.

Toxicology
Cassytha filiformis L.: No toxicological reports relevant to this use were identified.

Dianella carolinensis Laut.: *Dianella carolinensis* Laut.: A related species, *Dianella revoluta,* is suspected in livestock poisoning and physiological disturbances in man when ingested. Isolation of the toxic compounds dianellidin, dianellinone, and stypandrol from *D. revoluta* indicates that possible caution should be exercised when ingesting this plant (Colegate, Dorling & Huxtable 1987, 1986). Stypandrol, isolated from *D. revoluta*, has been reported to induce toxicosis in goats and sheep, with acute intoxication causing weakness and paralysis of the hind limbs and sometimes leading to death (Dias, Silva & Urban 2009).

Limnophila chinensis (Osb.) Merr. subsp. *aromatica* (Lam.) Yamazaki: No reports of toxicity were identified.

Melastoma malabathricum L. var. *mariannum* (Naudin) Fosb. & Sach.: Oral doses up to 2,000 mg/kg of a cold water extract of *Melastoma malabathricum* leaves showed no signs of toxicity in mice (Sunilson *et al.*, 2009).

Phaleria nisidai Kaneh.: No reports of toxicity were identified.

Phyllanthus palauensis Hosok.: No toxicological reports relevant to this use were identified.

NOTES

CHAPTER TEN: MEN'S HEALTH

For male babies in Palau, when his bellybutton falls, it is wrapped in coconut sheath (*techiir ra lius*) and placed between one of the frond bases. This is believed to make the boy grow up to be a man and a good provider [Rechelulk ra Kleuang Walter Ringang].

This symbol was created and approved by the 3rd Men's Health Conference Organizing Committee to serve as an image to represent men's 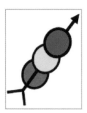 health in the Republic of Palau. The 3rd Men's Health conference was attended by 334 men representing various age groups, ethnicities and career/educational backgrounds and signifies the changing role of men in the healthcare arena. The three circles and their colors represent the different stages of life, while the arrow symbolizes the fish spear, which is a traditional Palauan symbol of manhood. The spear's tip and the third circle then combine to form the international symbol of males.

Men in Palau have a higher mortality rate in the top 15 leading causes of death in comparison to women and are more prone to suffer from injury, chronic diseases, and HIV than women. Men also exercise less, consume fewer dietary supplements such as vitamins, and have a lower life expectancy than women in Palau. Statistics on the cause of death in 2008 reveal 17 injury deaths (14 of them are male) with the leading causes being drowning and suicide. In 2010, the top 5 causes of male mortality (from most to least) were cardio/cerebrovascular disease, cancer, respiratory disease, injury, kidney disease. In 2007, the top 5 causes of male deaths were injury, heart disease, stroke, cancer, and chronic obstructive pulmonary disease (COPD). Of the diabetics on the island, 42% are male and of the hypertensives (high blood pressure), 37% are male. There is suspicion that the numbers are lower than the female rates because men traditionally avoid regular check ups. Females have higher rates at Outpatient Department, but males have higher rates at the Emergency Room (WHO 2011).

Urinary Tract Infection

Painful urination could indicate a urinary tract infection (UTI) or a sexually transmitted infection (STI) that requires medical treatment. If a man experiences painful urination or discharge from the penis, he should seek immediate medical attention.

Infertility

Male infertility can have many causes, but problems with the number or quality of sperm being made are the most common cause. Coping with male infertility can be very difficult: men can become stressed and frustrated. In nearly half of cases, doctors can find no reason why sperm are not being made normally. Certain causes, such as a varicocele, can be treated by a doctor.

Prostate Cancer

Prostate cancer is the most common type of cancer in Palau and often occurs with no symptoms. Men should speak with their doctor about risks and benefits of testing by rectal examination and Prostate Specific Antigen (PSA) test. Prostate cancer can be treated with surgery, radiation therapy, and in certain cases, 'watchful waiting'.

Testicular Cancer

Testicular cancer is the second most common cancer in men aged from 18 to 39. When found early, nearly all men (over 95%) are cured. A hard, painless lump in the testicle is the most common sign, but the testicle may also feel painful and tender. In a few men, constant backache, coughing or breathlessness, and swollen or tender breasts can mean the cancer has spread to other parts of the body. Removing the cancerous testicle by surgery is the first treatment for all testicular cancer and therefore all men with testicular lumps should be referred to their doctors. This surgery does not usually change sexual performance or the ability to get an erection.

Erectile Dysfunction

In some cases, erectile dysfunction is a sign of another serious disease such as diabetes or heart problems. There are many treatments for erectile dysfunction, including medications. A thorough examination by a medical doctor is the most important first step.

Prostate Enlargement

The most common prostate disease is a non-cancerous growth (enlargement) of the prostate called Benign Prostatic Hyperplasia (BPH). This condition is usually not life-threatening but can make urination difficult and can affect quality of life. In more severe cases, surgery and drugs can improve the symptoms of prostate disease. Not all urination problems are caused by the prostate, and patients with urinary difficulties should be seen by a medical doctor.

Chapter Ten discusses two botanical treatments for men's health in Palau.

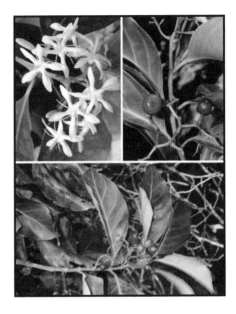

Figure 111. *Aidia racemosa* flowers, fruits, and leaves. [CT]

Local name: *kerumes* (Palauan); archer cherry (English)
Scientific name: *Aidia racemosa* (Cavanilles) Tirvengadum
Family: Rubiaceae (Coffee Family)

Description

A small tree 2-6 m in height with spreading branches. Simple, opposite leaves. Flowers are white, showy, fragrant, occurring on long pedicels in dense axillary cymes along the branches; corolla is 2-4 cm wide; petals oblong-obovate shaped, sometimes twisted or curved toward apex. Small rounded, red fruits, 1-2.5 cm in diameter (Hillmann Kitalong, DeMeo & Holm 2008).

Range

It is native to Palau, and found growing in the limestone forests of the Rock Islands and other limestone areas. It also occurs from tropical Asia eastward through the islands of the Western Pacific (Hillmann Kitalong, DeMeo & Holm 2008).

Traditional Uses
Medicine used for virility in older men.
Gather one handful of leaves, boil in a pot of water, about ½ gal for each handful of leaves, for 10 min, until the water turns light green-brown. Drink warm or cool when fatigued, to make a person stronger [Van-Ray Tadao 2010]. Also, when men go away to the Rock Islands for a couple of days, and drink *kerumes* tea the entire time, on their return home, women cannot resist them [Clarence Kitalong 2010].

Pharmacological Properties
No pharmacological reports relevant to men's health were identified.

Toxicology
No reports of toxicity were identified.

COMBINATION THERAPIES

a)

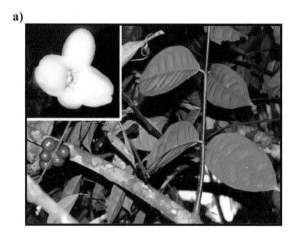

b)

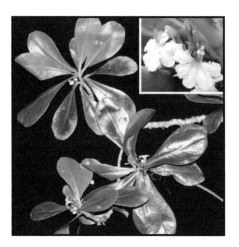

c)

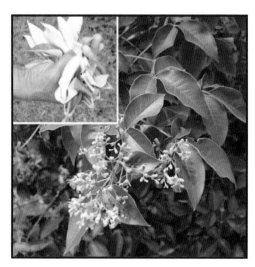

Figure 112. a) *Phaleria nisidai* fruits and leaves, with inset showing flower. [AK & CT]; **b)** *Scaevola taccada* leaves, with inset showing flowers. [MB & AK]; **c)** *Vitex trifolia* var. *trifolia* leaves and flowers, with inset showing four harvested branch tips. [CT & AK]

Local and scientific names:
ongael*, *delalakar (Palauan) - *Phaleria nisidai* Kaneh. (Thymelaeaceae)
kirrai*, *korrai (Palauan); beach naupaka (English) - *Scaevola taccada* (Gaertn.) Roxb. (Goodeniaceae)
kelsechedui (Palauan); simple-leaf chastetree, Arabian lilac (English) - *Vitex trifolia* L. var. *trifolia* (Lamiaceae)

Descriptions
Phaleria nisidai Kaneh.: A ca. 15 m tall tree with opposite leaves, 15-20 cm long, 7-8 cm wide; the corolla tube is white, 15 mm long (Kanehira 1933). The drupe is red at

maturity. It is native to Palau (Hillmann Kitalong, DeMeo & Holm 2008).

Scaevola taccada (Gaertn.) Roxb.: Freely branching, spreading shrub 0.5-5 m high. The vegetative parts and inflorescences soft-white-sericeous to glabrous (but with hair tufts in leaf axils); petioles winged to base; leaf blades obovate to spathulate, variable in size 8-26 cm long, 4-12 cm broad. Inflorescences axilary, few-flowered, 2-5 cm long, corolla 12-22 mm long, the tube white to greenish or purplish; fruit white, globose to ovoid, 10-18 mm in diameter when fresh (Smith 1991).

Vitex trifolia L. var. *trifolia*: Small tree or shrub with leaves 3- or 5-foliolate, the central leaflets are petiolulate, the blades pubescent on both surfaces and oblong-elliptic to ovate-lanceolate. Flowers sessile; grayish to white, 2-4 mm long, 1.5-3 mm broad (Smith 1991).

Ranges

Phaleria nisidai Kaneh.: Southeastern Asia and Ceylon through Malaysia to Micronesia, Australia, and eastward in the Pacific to Samoa and Tonga (Smith 1981). In Palau, it grows in volcanic lowland forest and in freshwater swamp forest (Hillmann Kitalong, DeMeo & Holm 2008).

Scaevola taccada (Gaertn.) Roxb.: Widespread in the Indo-Pacific, usually restricted to open sandy beaches or rocky coasts on most islands and continental shores from East Africa northward to Ceylon, India, and southern Japan, and eastward through Malaysia to tropical Australia and into eastern Polynesia and Hawaii (Smith 1991). In Palau, found growing in freshwater swamp forests and in limestone forests, atolls, and strand vegetation along the coasts (Hillmann Kitalong, DeMeo & Holm 2008).

Vitex trifolia L. var. *trifolia*: Southeastern Asia to southern Africa and Indian Ocean islands and eastward through Malaysia and northern Australia to Polynesia (Smith 1991). Introduced to Palau and found growing in areas that typically have cultivated landscape with ornamental plants (Hillmann Kitalong, DeMeo & Holm 2008).

Traditional uses

General tonic. Four leaves of *Phaleria nisidai* (*ongael*), 1 handful of the branch tips (leaves, flowers, fruits, small branches) of *Vitex trifolia* (*kelsechedui*) and 4 leaves of *Scaevola taccada* (*kirrai*) are boiled in a 1 gal pot for 3 min until water is a dark brown color like dark tea. Drink 1 cup, hot, 3-4 times/day. If you have extra left over, put in refrigerator and you can drink it cold. Stimulates appetite, is a diuretic, and gives you energy. Drink during farm work instead of water, promotes sweat and you feel good. Women can drink it as well.

Pharmacological properties

Phaleria nisidai Kaneh.: A crude ethanolic extract of *Phaleria nisidai* inhibited a tumor-induced reduction of immunostimulatory cytokines and decreased tumor size in carcinoma-bearing mice (Matsuda *et al.*, 2005a). A crude ethanolic extract of *P. nisidai* increased the phagocytic activity of isolated RAW 264.7 macrophages *in vitro* (Matsuda *et al.*, 2005b). Oral administration of a crude ethanol extract of *P. nisidai* leaves decreased blood glucose levels and inhibited body weight gain in an obese-type non-insulin dependent diabetic mouse model. The crude ethanol extract, as well as mangiferin, isolated from this extract, inhibited rise of blood glucose levels in sucrose-loaded healthy mice and inhibited α-glucosidase (Matsuda *et al.*, 2004). A crude ethanolic extract of *P. nisidai* and mangiferin isolated from this extract increased immunostimtulatory cytokines in an immunocompromised diabetic mouse model (Tokunaga *et al.*, 2006).

Scaevola taccada (Gaertn.) Roxb.: Hydroethanolic extracts of the related species, *Scaevola plumieri*, demonstrated antifungal activity against *Candida albicans* (Kpemissi *et al.*, 2003). Another related species, *Scaevola sericea*, on the other hand, showed only moderate anti-fungal activity (Locher *et al.*, 1995). Extracts of *S. spinescens* were active against human cytomegalovirus (Semple *et al.*, 1998). Methanolic extracts of the leaves of *S. frutescens* showed significant anti-inflammatory and antipyretic effects comparable to paracetamol and indomethacin (Umadevi, Mohanta & Manavalan 2005). *Scaevola balansae* bark extracted in methanol was active against the protozoa, *Leishmania donovani* (IC$_{50}$ ranged from 5-10 µg/ml) but showed weak activity against *Trichomonas vaginalis*, another protozoa (Desrivot *et al.*, 2007).

Vitex trifolia L. var. *trifolia*: Carbon tetrachloride-induced hepatic injury was reversed by a single oral dose of an ethanolic extract of *Vitex trifolia* flowers in rats (Anandan *et al.*, 2009). An aqueous extract of the leaves of *V. trifolia* inhibited inflammatory cytokine expression and increased levels of the inflammatory regulator cytokine IL-10 in RAW 264.7 macrophages (Matsui *et al.*, 2009). A methanol extract of *V. trifolia* showed antiviral activity against Herpes simplex and mouse corona virus, a surrogate for human SARS (Vimalanathan, Ignacimuthu & Hudson 2009). Mono- and diterpenes isolated form *V. trifolia* fruit were cytotoxic against a human cervical cancer cell line (Wu *et al.*, 2009) and compounds isolated from this plant have caused cell cycle inhibition (Li *et al.*, 2009) and apoptosis (Wang *et al.*, 2005) in cancer cells. Vitexicarpin, isolated from

the hexane extract of this plant, was able to block the effects of histamine released from sensitized mast cells in isolated guinea pig trachea (Alam *et al.*, 2002). Diterpenoids in *V. trifolia* were active against *Trypanosoma cruzi* epimastigotes (Kiuchi *et al.*, 2004).

Toxicology

Phaleria nisidai Kaneh.: No reports of toxicity were identified.

Scaevola taccada (Gaertn.) Roxb.: An acetonitrile extract of *S. taccada* was toxic to some human cells at a high *in vitro* concentration 1,000 µg/mL (Locher *et al.*, 1995). Oral and interperitoneal administration of 2,000 mg/kg of a methanolic extract of *S. taccada* showed toxicity in rats (Umadevi, Mohanta & Manavalan 2006).

Vitex trifolia L. var. *trifolia*: No reports of toxicity were identified.

NOTES

CHAPTER ELEVEN:
COLDS AND FLU

The common cold is a viral infection of the lining of the nose, sinuses, throat, and large airways. Many different viruses cause colds, but rhinoviruses (of which there are 100 subtypes) are implicated more often than others. Colds caused by rhinoviruses occur more commonly during seasonal changes (i.e. spring and fall, or rainy to dry). Different viruses cause colds during other times of the year. Despite lingering myths, feeling cold, going outside with wet hair, having wet feet, or getting chilled do not cause colds or flu.

Bodily secretions contain cold viruses. Cold and flu viruses are easily transmitted from one person to the next. They are generally spread by direct contact with an infected person such as kissing, handshakes, or from touching a contaminated surface, such as a doorknob, telephone, coins, or cash. When people touch their mouth, nose, or eyes, the viruses gain entry to the body causing the infection that results in a cold. Less often, colds are spread when people breathe air containing droplets that were coughed or sneezed out by an infected person. A cold is most contagious during the first few days after symptoms develop.

Symptoms and Diagnosis

Symptoms of a cold usually start one to three days after infection. Generally, the first symptom is a scratchy or sore throat or discomfort in the nose. A later stage of the cold develops into sneezing, runny nose, and a mild ill feeling. High fever is not common with a cold, but a mild fever may occur at the beginning of the cold. At first, secretions from the nose are watery and clear and can be annoyingly copious. Eventually the fluids become thicker, opaque, yellow-green, and less plentiful. Many people also develop a mild cough. Symptoms usually disappear in four to ten days, although a dry cough can often last into the second week.

Complications or weak immune systems may prolong the disease. Rhinovirus infection often triggers asthma attacks in people with asthma. Some people develop bacterial infections of the middle ear (otitis media) or the sinuses. These infections develop because congestion in the nose blocks the normal drainage of those areas, allowing bacteria to grow in collections of blocked secretions. Other people develop bacterial infections of the lower airways (secondary bronchitis or pneumonia).

Cold versus Flu

By differentiating symptoms, it is relatively easy to distinguish between a cold and flu. While both conditions have symptoms in common, the additional symptoms associated with influenza ("the flu" for short) make it unmistakable. A common cold can last anywhere between two to fourteen days. The sufferer will have nasal congestion and sneezing. A sore throat and dry cough may also accompany the cold, as well as general aches, mild fatigue, and a slight fever.

Unlike colds, flu is commonly associated with fever (sometimes a high fever), intense muscle aches, chills, headaches, and fatigue. After the initial acute stage, flu symptoms can linger for up to two weeks, with some sufferers experiencing fatigue for several weeks. Nasal congestion, sneezing, and sore throat also accompany this illness, but the cough is usually deeper than with a cold.

A cold is usually diagnosed by its typical symptoms. The following symptoms suggest that the infection is not (just) a simple cold: a high fever, severe headaches, rash, difficulty breathing, or chest pain.

Laboratory tests usually are not needed to diagnose a cold. If complications are suspected, doctors may order blood tests and chest x-rays. Remember, serious conditions can masquerade as the common cold; patients who have severe symptoms, feel worse with each passing day, or suffer repeated colds should seek medical care to rule out more serious illnesses.

Prevention of the Flu

The flu vaccine can protect patients against the infection. On February 24, 2010, vaccine experts voted that everyone 6 months and older should get a flu vaccine each year starting with the 2010-2011 influenza season. People at increased risk for complications or are prone to the flu, such as patients with respiratory problems (i.e. asthma, COPD, and cystic fibrosis), those who are immunocompromised, children, the elderly, and those who care for children or the elderly, should especially consider this preventive measure.

Since so many different viruses cause colds and because each virus changes slightly over time, an effective vaccine for colds has not yet been developed. The best preventive measure is practicing good hygiene. Because many cold viruses are spread through direct contact with the secretions of an infected person, people with cold symptoms and people in their household and office should wash their hands frequently. Sneezing and coughing should be done into tissues, which should then be carefully disposed. When possible, people with symptoms should sleep in a separate room. People who are coughing or sneezing because of a cold should not go to work or school where they might infect others. Cleaning shared objects and surfaces with a disinfectant can also help reduce the spread of common cold viruses.

Treatment of Colds

For all of the recommendations used in the treatment of the common cold, it is best to start them at the first sign of symptoms for optimal benefit, because the virus does the majority of replication within the first 48 hrs of the illness.

People with a cold should rest, stay warm, and try to avoid spreading the infection to others. Anyone with a fever or severe symptoms should rest at home. Drinking fluids and inhaling steam or mist from a vaporizer may help to keep secretions loose and easier to expel. Currently available antiviral and antibiotic drugs are not effective against colds even when the nose or cough produces thick or green-colored mucus.

Several popular nonprescription (over-the-counter) remedies can be effective to alleviate cold symptoms. Since those medications do not cure the infection, which usually resolves after a week regardless of treatments, doctors feel that their use is optional, depending on the severity of the cold. Several different types of drugs are used:

- Decongestants: which help open clogged nasal passages
- Antihistamines: which help dry a runny nose
- Cough syrups: which may make coughing easier by thinning secretions or suppressing cough (however, the latest evidence shows that honey is just as, if not more, effective as cough syrups (Oduwole *et al.*, 2010).

These drugs are most often sold as combinations, but can also be obtained individually. For relieving nasal congestion, inhaled decongestants are better than forms taken by mouth. However taking inhaled forms for more than three to five days and then stopping may make congestion worse than it was originally.

It is important to note that the symptoms that patients experience are part of the natural healing process, evidence that the immune system is battling illness. For instance, a fever is the body's way to kill viruses by heating up the internal environment to where viruses cannot thrive. A fever's hot environment also makes germ-killing proteins in the blood circulate more quickly and effectively. Thus, by enduring a moderate fever for a day or two, patients may actually get healthy faster. Coughing is another productive symptom; it clears breathing passages of thick mucus that can carry germs to the lungs and the rest of the body. Even a stuffy nose is best treated mildly or not at all. A decongestant, like Sudafed®, restricts flow to the blood vessels in the nose and throat. But often increased blood flow is desired because it warms the infected area and helps secretions carry germs out of your body.

Salt-water rinsing helps break-up nasal congestion, while also removing virus particles and bacteria from the nose. A popular recipe is below [not to be used with children]:

- Mix ¼ teaspoon salt and ¼ teaspoon baking soda in 8 oz of warm water
- Use a bulb syringe to squirt water into the nose. Hold one nostril closed by applying light finger pressure while squirting the salt mixture into the other nostril
- Let it drain
- Repeat 2-3 times, and then repeat with the other nostril

Staying warm and resting when patients first come down with a cold or the flu helps the body direct its energy toward the immune battle.

Gargling can moisten a sore throat and bring temporary relief. Patients can try ½ teaspoon of salt dissolved in ½ cup of warm water, four times daily. To reduce the tickle in their throat, they can also try an astringent gargle, such as tea that contains tannin, such as black tea, to tighten the membranes. Or they can use a thick, viscous gargle made with honey, popular in North American folk medicine.

Hydration

Maintaining appropriate hydration is the most important action patients can do to help their body recover from a viral infection. They should drink enough water so they are urinating at least three to four times a day. Hot liquids relieve nasal congestion, prevent dehydration, and soothe inflamed membranes that line the nose and throat. If patients are so congested that they cannot sleep at night a hot toddy, an age-old remedy, can be very effective for sleep. To make an herbal toddy, add 1 tsp of honey and 1 small shot (about 1 oz) of whiskey or bourbon. This drink should be limited to one, as too much alcohol can inflame mucus membranes and is therefore counterproductive. Patients can also drink hot soup. If patients take antibiotics, miso soup can help restore healthy bacteria back into the body, post-treatment.

Taking a Steam Shower

Steam showers can moisturize patients' nasal passages and relax them. If patients feel dizzy from the flu, they can run a steamy shower while they sit on a chair nearby and take a sponge bath.

Using Salve Under the Nose

A small dab of mentholated salve under your nose can open breathing passages and help restore the irritated skin at the base of the nose. Menthol, eucalyptus, and camphor all have mild numbing ingredients that may help relieve the pain of a nose rubbed raw. Use caution however, as this practice has been associated with severe adverse outcomes with infants and toddlers.

Infection-fighting foods
The following foods can help fight off a cold or flu:

- Bananas: Soothe upset stomach
- Carrots: Loaded with beta-carotenes, which help boost the immune system
- Chili peppers: Open sinuses and help break up mucus in the lungs
- Rice: Curbs diarrhea
- Tea: Black and green tea (not herbals) contain catechin, a phytochemical purported to have natural antibiotic and anti-diarrhea effects

Chapter Eleven discusses two different plant remedies reported to treat the common cold and flu in Palau. If you have a cold or flu, consult with a plant expert or healer before taking these remedies.

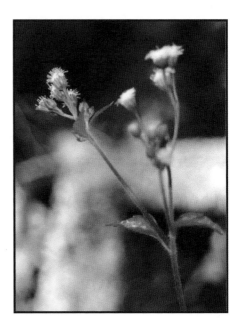

Figure 113. *Ageratum conyzoides* flowers. [RL]

Local name: *ngmak* (Palauan); goatweed, whiteweed (English)
Scientific name: *Ageratum conyzoides* L.
Family: Asteraceae (Daisy Family)

Description
Coarse herb 0.2-1 m high; opposite and simple leaves commonly subacute or obtuse to round at base; the corolla lobes and styles are white to pale lavender. Flowering heads usually 5-8 mm in diameter with 60-75 flowers. Flowering and fruiting seen throughout the year (Smith 1991).

Range
Mexico and the West Indies to South America, now often cultivated and established as an adventive in most warm countries. It was probably an early European introduction into the Pacific Islands as an ornamental (Smith 1991). Introduced to Palau and found growing in savanna grasslands and in areas that typically have cultivated landscape and ornamental plants (Hillmann Kitalong, DeMeo & Holm 2008).

Traditional Uses
Medicine for fever and pneumonia. Decoction of leaves, dosage not specified (Del Rosario & Esguerra 2003).

Pharmacological Properties
Oral administration of an ethanolic leaf extract of *Ageratum conyzoides* for 90 days reduced subchronic and chronic inflammation in rats (Moura *et al.*, 2005).

Toxicology
No hepatotoxicity was observed with oral doses up to 500 mg/kg/day for 90 days in rats (Moura *et al.*, 2005).

COMBINATION THERAPY

a)

b)

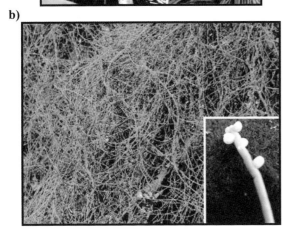

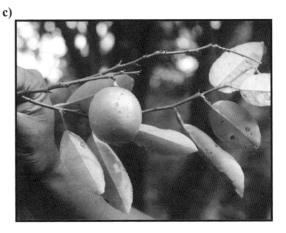

Figure 114. a) *Areca catechu* flowers, fruits, and a dried, fallen leaf. [AK]; **b)** *Cassytha filiformis* with inset showing flowers. [MB]; **c)** *Citrus aurantiifolia* leaves and fruit. [WL]

Local and Scientific names:
buuch (Palauan); betel nut (English) - *Areca catechu* L. (Arecaceae)
techellachull (Palauan); laurel dodder (English) - *Cassytha filiformis* L. (Lauraceae)
malchianged (Palauan); bitter orange (English) - *Citrus aurantiifolia* (Christm.) Swingle (Rutaceae)

Descriptions
Areca catechu L.: Small palm tree with solitary, green, and prominently ringed stem, about 10-30 m high, dbh 15-20 cm. Leaves about 2 m long with 12 pinnae on each side, and usually 2-3 ribbed. Inflorescence with staminate and pistillate flowers with small sepals. The fruit is oblong to ovoid in shape 4-5 cm long, dull orange to red (Smith 1979).
Cassytha filiformis L.: Herbaceous parasitic vine. In Palau it is found growing in savanna grassland and freshwater swamp forest (Hillmann Kitalong, DeMeo & Holm 2008). Tepals are white and the immature fruit is green, becoming yellow and at length white (Smith 1981).
Citrus aurantiifolia (Christm.) Swingle: A tree, 4-8 m tall, usually with many short

169

spines; petioles narrowly winged, leaf blades ovate-elliptic, 4-12 × 2-7 cm. Flowers are small, 2-2.5 cm in diameter, have pale pink to white petals, and the fruits are ovoid, 3-6 cm in diameter and greenish-yellow when ripe, with thin, adherent peel and greenish, very acid fruit (Smith 1985).

Ranges

Areca catechu L.: The origin of *Areca catechu* is uncertain. It is distributed across India and Sri Lanka to southeastern Asia, Indonesia, and the Philippines. It is widely cultivated in the Asiatic tropics, including Pohnpei Island (Smith 1979).

Cassytha filiformis L.: Cosmopolitan in tropical areas, occurring abundantly in most Pacific archipelagos (Smith 1981). It is native to Palau (Hillmann Kitalong, DeMeo & Holm 2008).

Citrus aurantiifolia (Christm.) Swingle: Probably indigenous to Malaysia, and has spread throughout the tropics and subtropics (Smith 1985).

Traditional Uses

Medicine used for colds or flu. Take very end of the leaves of *Areca catechu* (*buuch*), a handful of the vine *Cassytha filiformis* (*techellachull*)—a handful is about the size of a grapefruit—and 2 to 3 roots of *Areca catechu* (*buuch*) (about 5 inch long pieces). Put leaves and vine bundle in a pot of water, boil, and then cover the patient with a blanket and instruct them to inhale the steam [Flora Wasisang].

Pharmacological Properties

Areca catechu L.: Oral administration of an ethanolic extract of *Areca catechu* seed demonstrated anti-inflammatory effects in rat models (Bhandare *et al.*, 2010).

Cassytha filiformis L.: No pharmacological reports relevant to this use were identified.

Citrus aurantiifolia (Christm.) Swingle: Essential oil and terpenes from orange (unspecified related *Citrus* spp.) demonstrated antimicrobial activity against *Salmonella* spp. *in vitro* (O'Bryan *et al.*, 2008). The juice and peel of *Citrus aurantiifolia* contain ascorbic acid (vitamin C) and dehydroascorbic acid (Guimarães *et al.*, 2010). Ascorbic acid (vitamin C) and dehydroascorbic acid showed weak and strong antiviral activity, respectively, against influenza virus type A *in vitro* (Furuya *et al.*, 2008). A prospective, controlled study found that daily megadose of ascorbic acid administered before or after the apperance of cold and flu symptoms relieved and prevented symptoms compared with a control group (Gorton & Jarvis 1999).

Toxicology

Areca catechu L.: No toxicological reports regarding the use of *Areca catechu* leaves were identified.

Cassytha filiformis L.: A toxicological assessment of an aqueous extract of the stems and leaves revealed that a daily oral dose of 250-1,000 mg/kg for 28 days decreased levels of alkaline phosphatase and increased levels of serum cholesterol in rats. A decrease in relative weights of the heart and lung was also observed. The oral LD_{50} was determined to be greater than 500 mg/kg (Babayi *et al.*, 2007).

Citrus aurantiifolia (Christm.) Swingle: Flavonoids found in *Citrus aurantiifolia* have been shown to inhibit cytochrome P450 3A4 isotype (CYP3A4). Compounds that inhibit this enzyme can increase the bioavailability of drugs metabolized by this enzyme *in vivo*, such as warfarin and many other pharmaceuticals (Adepoju & Adeyemi 2010).

CHAPTER TWELVE: EAR, NOSE, AND THROAT

Ear, nose, and throat (ENT) disorders may be affected by inflammation, infection, trauma, tumors, and several miscellaneous conditions. They rarely prove fatal [except for those resulting from neoplasms (tumors), epiglottitis, and neck trauma], but they may cause serious social, cosmetic, and communication problems. Untreated hearing loss or deafness can drastically impair ability to interact with society. Ear disorders also have the ability to impair equilibrium. Nasal disorders can cause changes in facial features and interfere with breathing and tasting. Diseases arising in the throat may threaten airway patency and interfere with speech. In addition, these disorders can cause considerable discomfort and pain for the patient and require thorough assessment and prompt treatment.

Epistaxis

Epistaxis is bleeding from the nostril. Most cases of epistaxis comes from a blood vessel located in the front of the nasal septum (nasal partition) and can be treated in the field. Bleeds coming from further back in the nasal cavity require medical attention. **Recurrent nosebleed and nosebleeds that do not stop with basic measures can rarely signify a systemic medical problem or a posterior bleed and require evaluation by a physician**. Most anterior bleeds can be treated by sitting the patient up, tilting their head downward, and pinching their nose (have the patient keep an open mouth and breathe). Additionally it may help to place ice on the neck or forehead.

Tonsillitis

Tonsillitis refers to inflammation of the pharyngeal tonsils. Individuals with acute tonsillitis present with fever, sore throat, foul breath, dysphagia (difficulty swallowing), odynophagia (painful swallowing), and tender cervical lymph nodes. Most cases of tonsillitis are caused by viruses including: Epstein-Barr virus, cytomegalovirus, herpes viruses, adenovirus, and the measles virus. **Individuals with white exudate on their tonsils, accompanied by sore throat, fever, and enlarged lymph nodes should be evaluated by a doctor to rule out the possibility of Strep throat (a bacterial infection caused by Group A ß hemolytic strep)**. This infection requires an antibiotic to prevent possible spread to other organs (rheumatic fever).

Otitis Media

The scientific name for an ear infection is otitis media (OM). An ear infection is an inflammation of the middle ear, usually caused by bacteria, that occurs when fluid builds up behind the eardrum. Anyone can get an ear infection, but children get them more often than adults. Three out of four children will have at least one ear infection by their third birthday. In fact, ear infections are the most common reason parents bring their child to a doctor.

Severe infections and infections in small children may require an antibiotic, such as amoxicillin, to be taken over 7-10 days. Supportive care includes over-the-counter pain relievers such as acetaminophen or ibuprofen, or eardrops, to help with fever and pain. Because aspirin is considered a major preventable risk factor for Reye's syndrome, a child who has a fever or other flu-like symptoms should not be given aspirin.

If a child does not have severe ear pain or a fever, it may be prudent to wait a day to see if the earache goes away. Sometimes ear pain is not caused by infection, and some ear infections may get better without antibiotics. Relative contraindications to observation include vomiting, three or more antibiotic courses in the current year, antibiotic course within the last two weeks, and/or ear discharge. Using antibiotics cautiously and with good reason helps prevent the development of bacteria that become resistant to antibiotics.

Chapter Twelve discusses seven botanical treatments for ear, nose, and throat conditions in Palau.

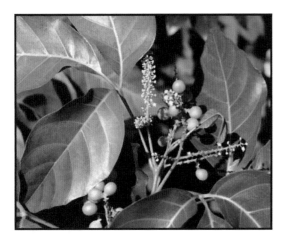

Figure 115. *Allophylus timoriensis* leaves, flowers, and fruits. [CT]

Local name: *chebeludes* (Palauan)
Scientific name: *Allophylus timoriensis* (DC.) Blume
Family: Sapindaceae (Soapberry Family)

Description
Small, sprawling tree 5 m tall with a narrow trunk. The alternate leaves are three parted, 4-19 cm long. The flowers are small and white, borne in clusters, up to 13 cm long. Fruits are red (Smith 1985).

Range
Allophylus timoriensis is widespread throughout the Pacific Islands, from Timor, Malaysia to Tonga and New Guinea. It is found growing mostly at sea level in dense forests, limestone forests, and in thickets (Smith 1985).

Traditional Uses
Medicine used for eye. Rinse mouth with seawater and chew the leaves and plants and use a *lild,* a thin bamboo grass (*Schizostachyum lima*), like a straw and blow the spray to the eyes. This can be applied in the morning, noon and night time [Gloria Emesiochel].

Pharmacological Properties
No pharmacological reports relevant to this use were identified.

Toxicology
No reports of toxicity were identified.

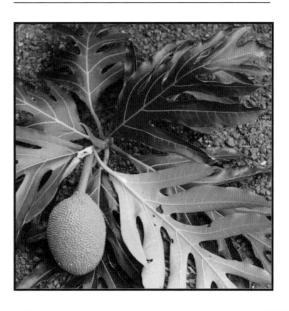

Figure 116. *Artocarpus atilis* leaves and fruit. [AK]

Local name: *meduu* (Palauan); breadfruit (English)
Scientific name: *Artocarpus atilis* (Parkinson) Fosb.
Family: Moraceae (Mulberry Family)

Description
Tree growing to 15-35 m in height. The leaves are large, glossy and dark green with abundant latex. The fruits are yellow-green to yellow-brown when mature. They are found throughout the year, but are principally ripe in March and April (Smith 1981).

Range
Indigenous to New Guinea, the Maluku Islands (Indonesia), western Melanesia, and Micronesia, *Artocarpus altilis* is cultivated abundantly throughout the tropics (Smith 1981).

Traditional Uses
Medicine used for earaches. Collect and pound 3 sheaths of new leaf (*okeok*) of *meduu* (*Artocarpus altilis*) and boil with ¼ cup coconut oil, until oil turns brown, but do not overboil or burn it. Use finger to dip in oil and drop in ear. Use 1 drop maximum, twice daily [Clarence Kitalong, Alfonsa Bintorio, Maria Kim, Nona Luii, Eriko Singeo, Hinako Takeo]. Fallen leaves of *meduu* (*Artocarpus altilis*) are collected and crushed, juice is collected and poured into ear [Gloria Emesiochel].

Pharmacological Properties
No pharmacological reports relevant to this use were identified.

Toxicology
No reports of toxicity were identified.

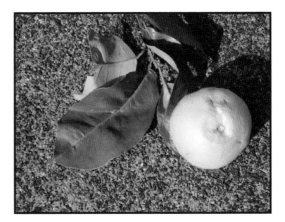

Figure 117. *Citrus sinensis* leaves and fruit. [DL]

Local name: *meradel* (Palauan)
Scientific name: *Citrus* spp.
Family: Rutaceae (Citrus Family)

Traditional uses
Medicine used for sore throat. Squeeze juice of *meradel* (*Citrus* spp.) type locally known as lemons, either green or yellow, into one cup of boiling water. Add sugar or honey to taste and drink until throat feels better. The fruit can also be peeled, and segments can be dipped in salt and eaten throughout the day until the throat feels better [Clarence Kitalong].

Pharmacological Properties
Essential oil and terpenes from orange (unspecified related *Citrus* spp.) demonstrated antimicrobial activity against *Salmonella* spp. *in vitro* (O'Bryan *et al.*, 2008). The juice and peel of *Citrus aurantiifolia* contain ascorbic acid (vitamin C) and dehydroascorbic acid (Guimarães *et al.*, 2010). Ascorbic acid (vitamin C) and dehydroascorbic acid showed weak and strong antiviral activity, respectively, against influenza virus type A *in vitro* (Furuya *et al.*, 2008). A prospective, controlled study found that a daily megadose of ascorbic acid administered before or after the appearance

of cold and flu symptoms relieved and prevented symptoms compared with control group (Gorton & Jarvis 1999).

Toxicology
Flavonoids found in *Citrus aurantiifolia* have been shown to inhibit cytochrome P450 3A4 isotype (CYP3A4). Compounds that inhibit this enzyme can increase the bioavailability of drugs metabolized by this enzyme *in vivo*, such as warfarin and many other pharmaceuticals (Adepoju & Adeyemi 2010).

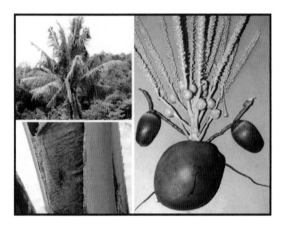

Figure 118. *Cocos nucifera* leaves, husk, and fruits. [DL & WL]

Local name: *lius* (Palauan); coconut (English)
Scientific name: *Cocos nucifera* L.
Family: Arecaceae (Palm Family)

Description
Cocos nucifera is a tall palm, reaching heights of 20-30 m. It bears a terminal crown of leaves. The trunk is grayish brown in color and is 20-40 cm in diameter. The fruits are green, yellow or red depending on the variety. This species may live up to 80-100 years (Purseglove 1988; Smith 1979).

Range
A pantropical species, *Cocos nucifera* is native to the Old World tropics, most likely the Pacific Islands (*Cocos nucifera*, TRAMIL 2008). It has been cultivated extensively throughout the tropics as an important economic crop. Due to its wide distribution, commonness, and unwieldy size, few voucher collections are made of this species (Smith 1979).

Traditional uses
Medicine used for water in the ear after swimming. Drip coconut oil into ear. When you feel the oil enter the ear canal, tilt head and let the oil drip out. This should relieve the problem immediately [Clarence Kitalong].

Pharmacological Properties
The crude water extract and low molecular weight fractions of *Cocos nucifera* inhibited histamine- and serotonin-induced rat paw edema (Rinaldi *et al.*, 2009).

Toxicology
No reports of toxicity were identified.

COMBINATION THERAPIES

a)

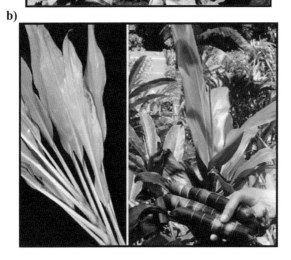

b)

c)

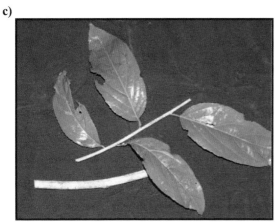

Figure 119. a) *Carica papaya* leaves, flowers, and fruits. [AK]; **b)** *Cordyline fruticosa* leaves are also used to wrap food. [MB & WL]; **c)** *Lophopyxis maingayi.* [MB]

Local and Scientific names:

bobai (Palauan); papaya (English) - *Carica papaya* L. (Caricaceae)

sis (Palauan); ti plant, good luck plant (English) - *Cordyline fruticosa* L. Chev. (Laxamanniaceae)

iuetekill (Palauan) - *Lophopyxis maingayi* Hook. f.: (Lophophyxidaceae)

Descriptions

Carica papaya L.: *Carica papaya* is a fast growing tree, reaching 2-10 m in height. The trunk is soft and fibrous with large leaf scars. The fruit is a fleshy berry, weighing up to 9 kg. The skin may be yellow or green when ripe and the flesh is orange. The seeds are numerous, black and wrinkled (Smith 1981).

Cordyline fruticosa L. Chev.: *Cordyline fruticosa* is a shrub growing 2-4 m in height. The leaves are oppositely arranged, leathery and shaped like a knife blade. They range from 30-50 cm in length and may be red or green in color. The flower is a raceme of small white, purple or red flowers. The fruits are red, fleshy berries (Burkill 1935; Lee Ling 1998).

Lophopyxis maingayi Hook. f.: A climbing liana up to 30 m long; the stem is up to 7 cm in diameter; it has tendrils that can be strong and woody; leaves are spirally arranged, simple, ovate to oblong; inflorescences are axillary or terminal spike-like, pendant raceme; bracts at base transform into tendrils; petals of flowers are white, male flowers with free stamens, female flowers with a superior ovary; the fruit is an obovoid or ellipsoid 5-winged samara (Lemmens & Bunyapraphatsara 2003).

Ranges

Carica papaya L.: *Carica papaya* probably originated from Central America and spread to other tropical regions during the European colonial period. Currently, it is cultivated extensively throughout the tropical regions for its edible fruit (Smith 1981).

Cordyline fruticosa L. Chev.: *Cordyline fruticosa* is indigenous to the Himalayas, Southeast Asia, Malaysia and northern Australia and has become naturalized in the Pacific Islands (Smith 1991). Throughout its range, *C. fruticosa* has been widely cultivated as an ornamental for its colorful leaves (Burkill 1935).

Lophopyxis maingayi Hook. f.: Found from Malaysia and Indonesia to the Solomon and Caroline Islands (Lemmens & Bunyapraphatsara 2003). It is native to Palau and grows in volcanic lowland forests, and areas that typically have cultivated landscape and ornamental plants (Hillmann Kitalong, DeMeo & Holm 2008).

Traditional uses

Medicine used for sinus problems. Pound male *bobai* (*Carica papaya*) flowers and mix with *iuetekill* (*Lophopyxis maingayi*) leaves. Wrap mixture with *sis* (*Cordyline fruticosa*) leaf and snort vapor through papaya stem [Clarence Kitalong].

Pharmacological Properties

Carica papaya L.: Contains antioxidant and anti-inflammatory properties which can reduce the severity of local inflammation (Mikhal'chick *et al.*, 2004) as well as antimicrobials (Dawkins *et al.*, 2003; Starley *et al.*, 1999).

Cordyline fruticosa L. Chev.: No pharmacological reports relevant to this use were identified.

Lophopyxis maingayi Hook. f.: No pharmacological reports relevant to this use were identified.

Toxicology

Carica papaya L.: Allergic reactions to *Carica papaya* are common, with anaphylaxis occuring in 1% of the patients studied (Iwu 1993). People allergic to latex may have an allergic reaction to papain, an enzyme that degrades polypeptides (Quarre *et al.*, 1995).

Cordyline fruticosa L. Chev.: No reports of toxicity were identified.

Lophopyxis maingayi Hook. f.: No reports of toxicity were identified.

a)

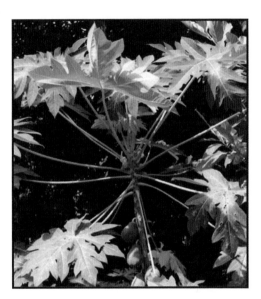

b)

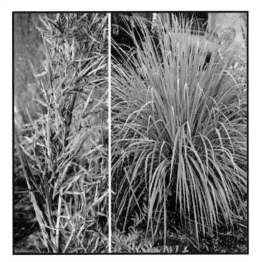

c)

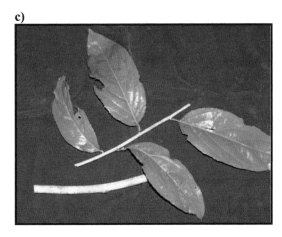

Figure 120. a) *Carica papaya* leaves, flowers, and fruits. [AK]; **b)** *Cymbopogon citratus* showing close-up of panicle, and leaf blades. [AK]; **c)** *Lophopyxis maingayi*. [MB]

Local and Scientific names:
bobai (Palauan); papaya (English) - *Carica papaya* L. (Caricaceae)
keskus (Palauan); lemon grass (English) - *Cymbopogon citratus* (DC. ex Nees) Stapf (Poaceae)
iuetekill (Palauan) - *Lophopyxis maingayi* Hook. f.: (Lophophyxidaceae)

Descriptions
Carica papaya L.: See earlier in this chapter.

Cymbopogon citratus (DC. ex Nees) Stapf: Perennial, shortly rhizomatous. Culms tufted, robust, up to 2 m tall, about 4 mm in diameter. Leaf sheaths glabrous, greenish inside; leaf blades glaucous, 30-90 × 0.5-2 cm. Spathate compound panicle large, lax, up to 50 cm; racemes 1.5-2 cm; rachis internodes and pedicels 2.5-4 mm, loosely villous on margins. Sessile spikelet linear-lanceolate, 5-6 × 0.7 mm; lower glume flat or slightly concave toward base, sharply 2-keeled, keels wingless (Wu & Raven 1994).
Lophopyxis maingayi Hook. f.: See earlier in this chapter.

Ranges
Carica papaya L.: See earlier in this chapter.
Cymbopogon citratus (DC. ex Nees) Stapf: The origin of this plant is Southeast Asia. It has been widely cultivated in tropical Asia and South America (Smith 1979). Introduced and cultivated in Palau (Hillmann Kitalong, DeMeo & Holm 2008).
Lophopyxis maingayi Hook. f.: See earlier in this chapter.

Traditional uses
Medicine used for sinus problems. Use *Lophopyxis maingayi* (*iuetekill*), with *Cymbopogon citratus* (*keskus*) and snort up the nose with a *Carica papaya* stem (*bobai*) like a straw [Clarence Kitalong].

Pharmacological Properties
Carica papaya L.: No pharmacological reports relevant to this use were identified.
Cymbopogon citratus (DC. ex Nees) Stapf: The aqueous leaf extract of *C. citratus* (1g/mL) showed anti-inflammatory activity in a murine *in vitro* assay (Francisco *et al.*, 2011).
Lophopyxis maingayi Hook. f.: No pharmacological reports relevant to this use were identified.

Toxicology

Carica papaya L.: Allergic reactions to *C. papaya* are common, with anaphylaxis occuring in 1% of the patients studied (Iwu 1993). People allergic to latex may have an allergic reaction to papain, an enzyme that degrades polypeptides (Quarre *et al.*, 1995).

Cymbopogon citratus (DC. ex Nees) Stapf: The essential oil of the leaves have the following main components: citral A (32%), citral B (34%), myrcene (20%), and terpinen-4-ol (3%). A complete dose-dependent toxicology profile of this oil was examined *in vivo* and in postmortem histological analyses in rats; results showed that consumption of the oil was safe at doses lower than 1500mg/kg body weight, since significant functional damages to stomach and liver did occur at higher doses. It was concluded that the oil is safe for humans at low recommended concentrations (Fandohan *et al.*, 2008). The no observed adverse effect level for rat embryo-foetotoxicity is 0.5 g myrcene/kg body weight (Delgado *et al.*, 1993).

Lophopyxis maingayi Hook. f.: No reports of toxicity were identified.

b)

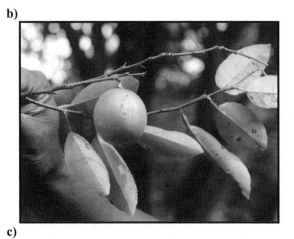

c)

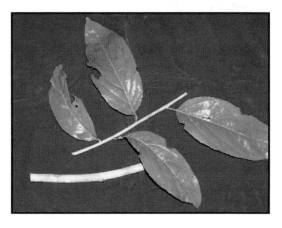

Figure 121. a) *Carica papaya* leaves, flowers, and fruits. [AK]; **b)** *Citrus aurantiifolia* leaves and fruit. [WL]; **c)** *Lophopyxis maingayi.* [MB]

Local and Scientific names:

bobai (Palauan); papaya (English) - *Carica papaya* L. (Caricaceae)

malchianged (Palauan); bitter orange (English) - *Citrus aurantiifolia* (Christm.) Swingle (Rutaceae)

iuetekill (Palauan) - *Lophopyxis maingayi* Hook. f.: (Lophophyxidaceae)

Descriptions

Carica papaya L.: See earlier in this chapter.

Citrus aurantiifolia (Christm.) Swingle: A tree, 4-8 m tall, usually with many short spines; petioles narrowly winged, leaf blades ovate-elliptic, 4-12 × 2-7 cm. Flowers are

a)

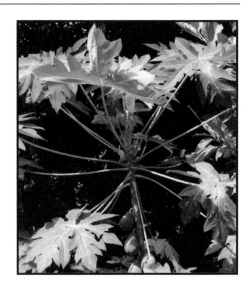

small, 2-2.5 cm in diameter, have pale pink to white petals, and the fruits are ovoid, 3-6 cm in diameter and greenish yellow when ripe, with thin, adherent peel and greenish, very acid fruit (Smith 1985).

Lophopyxis maingayi Hook. f.: See earlier in this chapter.

Ranges

Carica papaya L.: See earlier in this chapter.

Citrus aurantiifolia (Christm.) Swingle: Probably indigenous to Malaysia, and has spread throughout the tropics and subtropics (Smith 1985).

Lophopyxis maingayi Hook. f.: See earlier in this chapter.

Traditional Uses

Medicine used for sinus headaches.

Lophopyxis maingayi (*iuetekill*) leaves are picked and combined with young leaves of *Citrus aurantiifolia* (*malchianged*). They are pounded together and placed in the mouth. While chewing the leaves, dive into a stream or river. (Today people may go under a cool shower instead of diving into a stream or river.) This will relieve headaches, and sinus discomfort. If there is no river nearby, leaves can be chewed while drinking water. Some people combine *iuetekill* leaves with *bobai* (*Carica papaya*) leaves for the same purpose [Dirraklang Merei Ngirametuker]. Young leaves of *iuetekill* are pounded along with young leaves of *malchianged* and chewed and swallowed as you immerse yourself into the river, being sure to have your face in the water, and blow air out of your nose. Can also just be chewed and swallowed but drink lots of water [Tadashi Belchal, Scott Yano].

Pharmacological Properties

Carica papaya L.: Contains antioxidant and anti-inflammatory properties which can reduce the severity of local inflammation (Mikha'chick *et al.*, 2004) as well as antimicrobials (Dawkins *et al.*, 2003; Starley *et al.*, 1999).

Citrus aurantiifolia (Christm.) Swingle: The dried methanolic extract of the related species, *Citrus sinensis*, demonstrated significant analgesic activity when administered orally to mice in the writhing reflux assay (Anbu *et al.*, 2008).

Lophopyxis maingayi Hook. f.: No pharmacological reports relevant to this use were identified.

Toxicology

Carica papaya L.: Due to the powerful effects of some of the compounds in *Carica papaya*, oral use should be avoided by young children and pregnant women. Use of *C. papaya* should also be limited to no more than 7 consecutive days (Germosen-Robineau 1998). *Carica papaya* may possess abortifacient activity (Anuar *et al.*, 2008). Allergic reactions to *C. papaya* are common, with anaphylaxis occuring in 1% of the patients studied (Iwu 1993). People allergic to latex may have an allergic reaction to papain, an enzyme that degrades polypeptides (Quarre *et al.*, 1995). Change in the structure or function of the esophagus in humans may occur with an oral dose of 71 mg/kg (Davis, Thomas & Guice 1987).

Citrus aurantiifolia (Christm.) Swingle: Flavonoids found in *Citrus aurantiifolia* have been shown to inhibit cytochrome P450 3A4 isotype (CYP3A4). Compounds that inhibit this enzyme can increase the bioavailability of drugs metabolized by this enzyme *in vivo*, such as warfarin and many other pharmaceuticals (Adepoju & Adeyemi 2010).

Lophophyxis maingayi Hook. F.: No reports of toxicity were identified.

GLOSSARY OF BOTANICAL AND MEDICAL TERMINOLOGY

Abraded: worn down by friction; eroded

Abscess: a circumscribed collection of pus appearing in an acute or chronic localized infection, and associated with tissue destruction and, frequently, swelling

Aerial or prop roots: roots occurring above ground

Aggregate fruit: usually applied to a cluster or group of small fleshy fruits originating from a number of separate pistils in a single flower, as in the clustered drupelets of the raspberry

Alkaloid: a naturally occurring chemical compound that is a nitrogen-containing base in which at least one nitrogen is part of a ring, i.e. caffeine, nicotine

Analgesic: a compound/substance that relieves pain

Anthelmintic: destroys or expels intestinal worms; also called vermifuge or vermicide

Antigen: any substance that the body regards as foreign or potentially dangerous

Antileishmanial: preventing the spread of leishmania, a disease usually transmitted by sand flies, which result in skin sores and eventual damage to the liver and spleen

Antineoplastic: preventing the spread of neoplastic cells (tumor)

Antinociceptive: pain reliever

Antioxidant: an agent that inhibits cellular oxidation and thus deterioration through oxidative processes

Antiplasmodial: preventing the spread of plasmodium (blood parasites such as malaria)

Antipyretic: fever-reducing

Anxiolytic: a substance or drug that when taken, reduces feeling of anxiety

Aril: fleshy tissue that partially or completely covers the seed

Axil: point of the upper angle formed between the stem and any part (usually a leaf) arising from it

Axillary: positioned in or arising in an axil

Bract: a reduced leaf or leaf-like structure at the base of a flower

Calyx: collectively, all the sepals in a flower

Capillary: hair-like; very slender and fine

Carcinogenic: cancer-inducing

Catatonia: a syndrome of psychomotor disturbances characterized by periods of physical rigidity, negativism, excitement, and stupor

Conjunctivitis: inflammation of the conjunctiva characterized by redness and often accompanied by a discharge; also known as "pinkeye"

Corm: swollen portion of a stem, most of which is underground, looking like a bulb, as in the corm of a taro plant

Cormels: small corms that grow on the main corm

Corolla: collective name for all the petals of a flower

Cultivar: a form of plant originating under cultivation

Cyme: a flat or round-topped determinate inflorescence in which the terminal flower blooms first

Cytotoxic: detrimental or destructive to cells

Defibrinating: removing fibrin from the blood, usually by means of constant agitation

Dermatitis: inflammation of the skin

Dioecious: imperfect flowers, the male and female flowers borne on different plants

Decoction: a liquid preparation made by boiling plant parts in water

Dysentery: intestinal inflammation characterized by painful diarrhea with bloody, mucous feces

Edema: an accumulation of an excessive amount of watery fluid in cells, tissues, or serous cavities

Emollient: soothes and softens skin

Endemic: prevalent in or peculiar to a particular locality, region, or people

Epiphyte: a plant which grows on another plant but does not draw food or water from it

Febrile: denoting or relating to fever

Fibrin: a protein that is involved in the action of clotting blood over a wound

Frond: leaf of a fern

Genotoxic: damaging to DNA, and thereby may cause mutation or cancer

Glabrous: smooth; hairless

Gram-negative (pink)/Gram-positive (purple-black): a method (developed by Danish bacteriologist Hans C.J. Gram) for differential staining of bacteria, indicating fundamental differences in cell wall structure

Hyphae: a hypha (plural form is hyphae) is a long and filamentous type of cell of a fungus that is the primary node of vegetative growth

Hypoglycemic: low blood-sugar level

Imperfect flower: a flower with either pistils or stamens but not both

Inflorescence: the flowering part of a plant

Intraperitoneal: within the peritoneal cavity (membrane lining abdominal cavity)

Ischemic-reperfusion: damage to tissue due to a restriction (mainly arterial narrowing) in blood supply

Lamina: the expanded portion or blade of a leaf or petal

Latex: a milky sap

Liana: a woody, climbing vine

Littoral: growing along the shore

Microbicidal: destructive to microbes

Mycelium: the mass of hyphae making up a colony of fungi

Myocardial ischemic reperfusion injury: compression of the arteries

Neurochemicals: organic plant molecules that when consumed have an affect on the human brain

Node: position on the stem where leaves or branches originate

Non-teratogenic: does not cause abnormal fetal development

Palmate: from a common point, like the fingers of a hand

Panicle: a branched, racemose inflorescence with flowers maturing from the bottom upwards

Papule: pimple

Pedicel: stalk of a single flower in an inflorescence, or of a grass spikelet (pedicellate means the flower is with a pedicel)

Peduncle: the stalk of a solitary flower or inflorescence

Peltate: leaf shaped like a shield

Perineum: the region between the anus and testicles

Petiole: leaf stalk

Piloerection: hair that stands up on end

Pinnae: leaflet of a compound leaf, as in a palm leaf with many pinnae that make up the leaf

Pistil: female reproductive organ of a flower

Phenolic acid: a chemical compound that has antiseptic properties and has been used in the production of prescription drugs

Pneumatophores: specialized structures that stick out of the soil in order to take in air like a straw

Poultice: also cataplasm; soft moist mass, often heated and medicated, that is spread over the skin to treat an inflamed, aching, or painful part of the body

Raceme: an unbranched, elongated inflorescence with pedicellate flowers maturing from the bottom upwards

Rhinitis: inflammation of the nasal mucus membrane

Rhizome: an underground, horizontal stem

Saponin: glycosides of plant origin characterized by foaming in water (soap-forming)

Scape: a leafless peduncle arising from the ground level

Sepal: a segment of the calyx, usually green and lying under the petals of a flower

Serrate: saw like; with the sharp teeth pointing forward on the edge of a leaf

Sessile: attached directly, without a supporting stalk, as a leaf without a petiole

Sorus (plural form is sori): an area of spore production on the underside of a fern leaf

Spadix: a spike with a thick and fleshy axis, usually densely packed with imperfect flowers

Spike: an inflorescence in which the flowers are attached to the main stem without stalks

Stamen: male reproductive organ of a flower

Steroidogenic: steroid-producing

Stolons: an elongate, horizontal stem creeping along the ground and rooting at the nodes or at the tip and giving rise to a new plant

Taproot: a prominent root with few branches, sometimes swollen to store food

Tinea versicolor: a chronic non-inflammatory infection of the skin caused by a fungus (*Pityrosporum orbiculare*, syn. *Melassezia furfur*). Irregular patches on skin appear lighter than the surrounding area.

Tuber: thickened portion of a rhizome (underground stem) bearing nodes and bud, modified for food storage (potato)

Tumor: any abnormal swelling in or on a part of the body

Umbel: a flat-topped or convex inflorescence with the pedicels arising more or less from a common point, like the struts of an umbrella

Vasomotor: causing dilation or constriction of blood vessels

Whorl: a ring-like arrangement of similar parts arising from a common point or node

Yaws: chronic infection affecting the skin, bones and joints caused by a spiral shaped bacteria, *Treponema pallidum*

BIBLIOGRAPHY

Aburjai, T., and F. Natcheh. 2003. Plants used in cosmetics. *Phytother Res* 17(9): 987-1000.

Adedapo, A.A., M.O. Abatan, S.O. Idowu, and O.O. Olorunsogo. 2005. Toxic effects of chromatographic fractions of *Phyllanthus amarus* on the serum biochemistry of rats. *Phytother Res* 19(9): 812-815.

Adedapo, A.A., A.Y. Adegbayibi, and B.O. Emikpe. 2005. Some clinico-pathological changes associated with the aqueous extract of the leaves of *Phyllanthus amarus* in rats. *Phytother Res* 19(11): 971-976.

Adepoju, G., and T. Adeyemi. 2010. Evaluation of the effect of lime fruit juice on the anticoagulant effect of warfarin. *J Young Pharm* 2(3): 269-72.

Adeyemi, O.O., S.O. Okpo, and O.O. Ogunti. 2002. Analgesic and anti-inflammatory effects of the aqueous extract of leaves of *Persea americana* Mill (Lauraceae). *Fitoterapia* 73(5): 375-380.

Adhikary, P., J. Banerji, D. Chowdhury, A.K. Das, C.C. Deb, S.R. Mukherjee, and A. Chatterjee. 1989. Antifertility effect of *Piper betle* Linn. extract on ovary and testis of albino rats. *Indian J Exp Biol* 27(10): 868-870.

Ajayi, I.A., R.A. Oderinde, V.O. Taiwo, and E.O. Agbedana. 2008. Short-term toxicological evaluation of *Terminalia catappa*, *Pentaclethra macrophylla* and *Calophyllum inophyllum* seed oils in rats. *Food Chem* 106(2): 458-465.

Alam, G., S. Wahyuono, I.G. Ganjar, L. Hakim, H. Timmerman, and R. Verpoorte. 2002. Tracheospasmolytic activity of viteosin-A and vitexicarpin isolated from *Vitex trifolia*. *Planta Med* 68(11): 1047-1049.

Ali, I., F.G. Khan, K.A. Suri, B.D. Gupta, N.K. Satti, P. Dutt, F. Afrin, G.N. Qazi, and I.A. Khan. 2010. *In vitro* antifungal activity of hydroxychavicol isolated from *Piper betle* (L.). *Ann Clin Microbiol Antimicrob* 9: 7.

Allen, M.L., M.H. Mellow, M.G. Robinson, and W.C. Orr. 1990 The effect of raw onions on acid reflux and reflux symptoms. *Am J Gastroenterol* 85(4): 377-380.

Ambili, S., A. Subramoniam, and N.S. Nagarajan. 2009. Studies on the antihyperlipidemic properties of *Averrhoa bilimbi* fruit in rats. *Planta Med* 75(1): 55-58.

Anandan, R., B. Jayakar, B. Karar, S. Babuji, R. Manavalanm, and R.S. Kumar. 2009. Effect of ethanol extract of flowers of *Vitex trifolia* Linn. on CCL4 induced hepatic injury in rats. *Pak J Pharm Sci* 22(4): 391-394.

Anbu, J., R. Vasuki, P. Shanmugasundaram, S. George, and M.V. Aanandhi. 2008. Analgesic, antipyretic and wound healing properties of *Citrus sinensis* peel extract. *Biomedicine* 28: 117-120.

Ancuceanu, R.V., and V. Istudor. 2004. Pharmacologically active natural compounds for lung cancer. *Altern Med Rev* 9(4): 402-419.

Anitha, P., and M. Indira. 2006. Impact of feeding ethanolic extract of root bark of *Cananga odorata* (Lam) on reproductive functions in male rats. *Indian J Exp Biol* 44: 976-980.

Anuar, N.S., S.S. Zahari, I.A. Taib, and M.T. Rahman. 2008. Effect of green and ripe *Carica papaya* epicarp extracts on wound healing and during pregnancy. *Food Chem Toxicol* 46: 2384-2389.

Anukam, K.C., and G. Reid. 2009. *In vitro* evaluation of the viability of vaginal cells (VK2/E6E7) and probiotic *Lactobacillus* species in lemon juice. *Sex Health* 6(1): 67-74.

Arora, R.B., C.N. Mathur, and S.D. Seth. 1962. Calophyllolide, a complex coumarin anticoagulant from *Calophyllum inophyllum* Linn. *J Pharm Pharmacol* 14:534-535.

Arvigo, R., and M.J. Balick. 1998. *Rainforest remedies: One hundred healing herbs of Belize.* Twin Lakes, WI: Lotus Press. 283 pp.

Awasthy, K.S., O.P. Chaurasia, S.P. Sinha, and P.K. Khan. 2000. Differential genotoxicity of the crude leaf extract of a medicinal plant, *Casearia tomentosa. Biomed Environ Sci* 13(1): 12-18.

Aziba, P.I., A. Adedeji, M. Ekor, and O. Adeyemi. 2001. Analgesic activity of *Peperomia pellucida* aerial parts in mice. *Fitoterapia* 72(1): 57-58.

Babayi, H., J.J. Udeme, J.A. Abalaka, J.I. Okogun, O.A. Salawu, D.D. Akumka, G.U. Adamu, S.S. Zarma, B.B. Adzu, S.S. Abdulmumuni, K. Ibrahime, B.B. Elisha, S.S. Zakariys, and U.S. Inyang. 2007. Effect of oral adminstration of aqueous whole extract of *Cassytha filiformis* on haematograms and plasma biochemical parameters in rats. *J Med Toxicol* 3(4): 146-151.

Badami, S., R. Aneesh, S. Sankar, M.N. Sathishkumar, B. Suresh, and S. Rajan. 2003. Antifertility activity of *Derris brevipes* variety *coriacea. J Ethnopharmacol* 84(1): 99-104.

Balick, M.J., ed. 2009. *Ethnobotany of Pohnpei: Plants, people, and island culture.* New York/Honolulu: The New York Botanical Garden Press/University of Hawai'i Press. 585 pp.

Banana. 2011. Wikipedia. Accessed on 7 September 2011 at: http://en.wikipedia.org/wiki/banana.

Bani, S., A. Kaul, B. Khan, S.F. Ahmad, K.A. Suri, B.D. Gupta, N.K. Satti, and G.N. Qazi. 2006. Suppression of T lymphocyte activity by lupeol isolated from *Crateva religiosa. Phytother Res* 20(4): 279-287.

Basile, A.C., J.A. Sertie, S. Panizza, T.T. Oshiro, and C.A. Azzolini. 1990. Pharmacological assay of *Casearia sylvestris.* I: Preventive anti-ulcer activity and toxicity of the leaf crude extract. *J Ethnopharmacol* 30(2): 185-197.

Beers, M.H., R.S. Porter, and T.V. Jones, eds. 2003. *The Merck Manual of Medical Information.* 2nd Home Edition. Pp. 1681-7. Whitehouse Station, NJ: Merck Research Laboratories.

Bhalla, T.N., R.C. Saxena, S.K. Nigam, G. Misra, and K.P. Bhargava. 1980. Calophyllolide—a new non-steroidal anti-inflammatory agent. *Indian J Med Res* 72: 762-5.

Bhandare, A.M., A.D. Kshirsagar, N.S. Vyawahare, A.A. Hadambar, and V.S. Thorve. 2010. Potential analgesic, anti-inflammatory, and antioxidant activities of hydroalcoholic extract of *Areca catechu* L. nut. *Food Chem Toxicol* 48: 3412-3417.

Biller, A., M. Boppré, L. Witte, and T. Hartmann. 1994. Pyrrolizidine alkaloids in *Chromolaena odorata.* Chemical and chemoecological aspects. *Phytochemistry* 35(3): 615-619.

bin Jantan, I., J. Jalil, and N.M.A. Warif. 2001. Platelet-activating factor (PAF) antagonistic activities of compounds isolated from *Guttiferae* species. *Pharm Bio* 39(4): 243-246.

Black, P.W. 1968. Notes on Medicinal Plants of Tobi. Unpublished manuscript. 7pp.

Borges, M.H., A.M. Soares, V.M. Rodrigues, S.H. Andriao-Escarso, H. Diniz, A. Hamaguchi, A. Quintero, S. Lizano, J.M. Gutierrez, J.R. Giglio, M.I. Homsi-Brandeburgo. 2000. Effects of aqueous extract of *Casearia sylvestris* (Flacourtiaceae) on actions of snake and bee venoms and on activity of phospholipases A2. *Comp Biochem Physiol B Biochem Mol Biol* 127(1): 21-30.

Bourdy, G., C. Francois, C. Andary, and M. Boucard. 1996. Maternity and medicinal plants in Vanuatu II. Pharmacological screening of five selected species. *J Ethnopharmacol* 52(3): 139-143.

Bradacs, G., L. Maes, and J. Heilmann. 2010. *In vitro* cytotoxic, antiprotozoal, and antimicrobial activities of medicinal plants from Vanuatu. *Phytother Res* 24(6): 800-809.

Buenz, E.J., B.A. Bauer, D.J. Schnepple, D.L. Wahner-Roedler, A.G. Vandell, and C.L. Howe. 2007. A randomized Phase I study of *Atuna racemosa*: A potential new anti-MRSA natural product extract. *J Ethnophramacol* 114(3): 371-376.

Burdock, G.A., and I.G. Carabin. 2008. Safety assessment of Ylang-Ylang (*Cananga* spp.) as a food ingredient. *Food Chem Toxicol* 46(2): 433-445.

Burkill, I. 1935. *A Dictionary of the Economic Products of the Malay Peninsula.* London: Crown Printers.

Cambie, R.C., and L.R. Ferguson. 2003. Potential functional foods in the traditional Maori Diet. *Mutat. Res./ Fundamental and Molecular Mechanisms of Mutagenesis* 523-524: 109-117.

Canfield, J., D. Herbst, and L. Stemmerman. 1992. Rapid ecological assessment of areas in Palau considered for conservation: Ngeremeduu Bay Drainage Area (Draft), U.S. Fish and Wildlife Service, Pacific Islands Office.

Caparros-Lefebvre, D., and A. Elbaz. 1999. Possible relation of atypical Parkinsonism in the French West Indies with consumption of tropical plants: A case-control study. Caribbean Parkinsonism study group. *Lancet* 354(9175): 281-286.

Catanese, B., N. Interdonato, and G. Barillari. 1979. A study of the serum concentrations of ibuprofen and guaiacol in rats after oral administration of ibuprofen, guaiacol, and AF2259. *Boll Chim Farm* 118: 232.

Chah, K.F., C.A. Eze, C.E. Emuelosi, and C.O. Esimone. 2006. Antibacterial and wound healing properties of methanolic extracts of some Nigerian medicinal plants. *J Ethnopharmacol* 104(1-2): 164-167.

Champy, P., G.U. Hoglinger, J. Feger, C. Gleye, R. Hocquemiller, A. Laurens, V. Guerineau, O. Laprevote, F. Medja, A. Lombes, P.P. Michel, A. Lannuzel, E.C. Hirsch, and M. Ruberg. 2004. Annonacin, a lipophilic inhibitor of mitochondrial complex I, induces nigral and striatal neurodegeneration in rats: Possible relevance for atypical Parkinsonism in Guadeloupe. *J Neurochem* 88(1): 63-69.

Chan, L.W., E.L. Cheah, C.L. Saw, W. Weng, and P.W. Heng. 2008. Antimicrobial and antioxidant activities of *Cortex Magnoliae Officinalis* and some other medicinal plants commonly used in South-East Asia. *Chin Med* 3: 15.

Chang, F.R., Y.C. Chao, C.M. Teng, and Y.C. Wu. 1998. Chemical constituents from *Cassytha filiformis* II. *J Nat Prod* 61(7): 863-866.

Chatterjee, A., and S. Deb. 1999. Genotoxic effect of arecoline given either by the peritoneal or oral route in murine bone marrow cells and the influence of N-acetylcysteine. *Cancer Lett* 139(1): 23-31.

Cheenpracha, S., C. Karalai, Y. Rat-A-pa, C. Ponglimanont, and K. Chantrapromma. 2004. New cytotoxic cardenolide glycoside from the seeds of *Cerbera manghas*. *Chem Pharm Bull* 52(8): 1023-1025.

Chen, G., Z. Yin, and X. Zheng. 2010. Effect and mechanism of total flavonoids of orange peel on rat adjuvant arthritis. *Zhongguo Zhongyao Zazhi* 35(10): 1298-1301.

Chen, I.S., H.F. Chen, M.J. Cheng, Y.L. Chang, C.M. Tang, I. Tsutomu, J.J. Chen, and I.L. Tsai. 2001. Quinoline alkaloids and other constituents of *Melicope semecarpifolia* with antiplatelet aggregation activity. *J Nat Prod* 64(9): 1143-1147.

Chen, K.S., Y.L. Chang, C.M. Teng, C.F. Chen, and Y.C. Wu. 2000. Furoquinolines with antiplatelet aggregation activity from leaves of *Melicope confusa*. *Planta Med* 66(1): 80-81.

Chen, Z., M. Duser, A. Flagge, S. Maryska, I. Sander, M. Raulf-Heimsoth, and X. Baur. 2000. Identification and characterization of cross-reactive natural rubber latex and *Ficus benjamina* allergens. *Int Arch Allergy Immunol* 123(4): 291-298.

Chew, F.T., S.H. Lim, H.S. Shang, M.D. Dahlia, D.Y. Goh, B.W. Lee, H.T. Tan, and T.K. Tan. 2000. Evaluation of the allergenicity of tropical pollen and airborne spores in Singapore. *Allergy* 55: 340-347.

Chin, Y.W., W.P. Jones, Q. Mi, I. Rachman, S. Riswan, L.B. Kardono, H.B. Chai, N.R. Farnsworth, G.A. Cordell, S.M. Swanson, J.M. Cassady, A.D. Kinghorn. 2006. Cytotoxic clerodane diterpenoids from the leaves of *Premna tomentosa*. *Phytochemistry* 67(12):1243-8.

Cho, J.Y., S.C. Park, T.W. Kim, K.S. Kim, J.C. Song, S.K. Kim, H.M. Lee, H.J. Sung, H.J. Park, Y.B. Song, E.S. Yoo, C.H. Lee, and M.H. Rhee. 2006. Radical scavenging and anti-inflammatory activity of extracts from *Opuntia humifusa* Raf. *J Pharm Pharmacol* 58: 113-119.

Chou, H.C., J.J. Chen, C.Y. Duh, T.F. Huang, and I.S. Chen. 2005. Cytotoxic and anti-platelet aggregation constituents from the root wood of *Melicope semecarpifolia*. *Planta Med* 71(11): 1078-1081.

Choudhary, D., and R.K. Kale. 2002. Antioxidant and non-toxic properties of *Piper betle* leaf extract: *In vitro* and *in vivo* studies. *Phytother Res* 16: 461-466.

Clayton, G. D., and F. E. Clayton, eds. 1981-1982. *Patty's Industrial Hygiene and Toxicology*. New York: John Wiley Sons. 2528 pp.

Cocos nucifera. 1998. TRAMIL Medicinal Plant Database. Accessed on 20 August 2008 at: http://www.funredes.org/tramil/english/plantdata.html/ref_id/746.

Cole, T.G., M.C. Falanruw, C.D. MacLean, C.D. Whitesell, and A.H. Ambacher. 1987. Vegetation survey of the Republic of Palau. *Pacific Southwest Forest and Range Experiment Station Resource Bulletin* PSW-22, Berkeley, California.

Colegate, S.M., P.R. Dorling, and C.R. Huxtable. 1986. Dianellidin, stypandrol and dianellinone: An oxidation-related series from *Dianella revoluta*. *Phytochemistry* 25: 1245-1247.

Colegate, S.M., P.R. Dorling, and C.R. Huxtable. 1987. Stypandrone: A toxic naphthalene-14-quinone from *Stypandra imbricata* and *Dianella revoluta*. *Phytochemistry* 26: 979-981.

Costion, C., and A. Kitalong. 2006. *Babeldaob forest survey*. Palau: Belau National Museum and The Nature Conservancy. 60 pp.

Council, N.R. 1977. *Drinking Water & Health*. Washington, DC: National Academy Press.

Davis, M., L.C. Thomas, and K.S. Guice. 1987. Esophagitis after papain. *Journal of Clinical Gastroenterology* 9: 127-130.

Davvamani, S.N., J. Gowrishankar, G. Anhuganapathi, K. Srinivasan, D. Natarajan, G. Perumal, C. Mohanasundari, and K. Moorthy. 2005. Studies on antimicrobial activties of certain medicinal ferns against selected dermatophytes. *Indian Fern Journal* 22: 191-195.

Dawkins, G., H. Hewitt, Y. Wint, P.C. Obiefuna, and B. Wint. 2003. Antibacterial effects of *Carica papaya* fruit on common wound organisms. *The West Indian Medical Journal* 52: 290-292.

de Cock, P.A., H. Vorwerk, and D.P. Bruynzeel. 1998. Hand dermatitis caused by ferns. *Contact Dermatitis* 39: 324.

de Fatima Arrigoni-Blank, M., E.G. Dmitrieva, E.M. Franzotti, A.R. Antoniolli, M.R. Andrade, and M. Marchioro. 2004. Anti-inflammatory and analgesic activity of *Peperomia pellucida* (L.) HBK (Piperaceae). *J Ethnopharmacol* 91(2-3): 215-218.

DeFilipps, R.A., S.L. Maina, and L.A Pray. 1988. The Palauan and Yap Medicinal Plant Studies of Masayoshi Okabe, 1941-43. Atoll Research Buletin No.317. National Museum of Natural History, Smithsonian Institution, Washington, D.C.

Delbourg, M.F., D.A. Moneret-Vautrin, L. Guillous, and G. Ville. 1995. Hypersensitivity to latex and *Ficus benjamina* allergens. *Ann Allerg Asthma Immunol* 75(6): 496-500.

Delgado, I.F., R.R. Carvalho, A.C.M. de Almeida Noguiera, A.P. Mattos, L.H. Figueiredo, S.H.P. Oliveira, I. Chahoud, and F.J.R. Paumgartten. 1993. Study on embryo-foetotoxicity of β-myrcene in the rat. *Food Chem Toxicol* 31: 31-35.

Del Rosario, A.G., and N.M. Esguerra. 2003. *Medicinal Plants in Palau*. Vol. 1. Koror, Republic of Palau: Palau Community College, Cooperative Research and Extension.

de Mattos, E.S., M.J.S. Frederico, T.D. Colle, D.V. de Pieri, R.R. Peters, and A.P. Piovezan. 2007. Evaluation of antinociceptive activity of *Casearia sylvestris* and possible mechanism of action. *J Ethnopharmacol* 112(1): 1-6.

de Melo, N.I., L.G. Magalhaes, C.E. de Carvalho, K.A. Wakabayashi, G. de P. Aguiar, R.C. Ramos, A.L. Mantovani, I.C. Turatti, V. Rodrigues, M. Groppo, W.R. Cunha, R.C. Veneziani, and A.E. Crotti. 2011. Schistosomicidal activity of the essential oil of *Ageratum conyzoides* L. (Asteraceae) against adult *Schistosoma mansoni* worms. *Molecules* 16: 762-763.

Desrivot, J., J. Waikedre, P. Cabalion, C. Herrenknecht, C. Bories, R. Hocquemiller, and A. Fournet. 2007. Antiparasitic activity of some New Caledonian medicinal plants. *J Ethnopharmacol* 112: 7-12.

Dever, G.J., and S.A. Finau. 1995. The Yanuca Island declaration: Pacific health in the twenty-first century. *Pacific Health Dialog* 2(2): 70-74.

Devi, K.P., M. Sreepriya, T. Devaki, and K. Balakrishna. 2003. Antinociceptive and hypnotic effects of *Premna tomentosa* L. (Verbenaceae) in experimental animals. *Pharmacol Biochem Behav* 75(2): 261-264.

Dharmani, P., P.K. Mishra, R. Maurya, V. Singh Chauhan, and G. Palit. 2005. *Allophylus serratus*: A plant with potential anti-ulcerogenic activity. *J Ethnopharmacol* 99(3):361-366.

Dias, D.A., C.A. Silva, and S. Urban. 2009. Naphthalene aglycones and glycosides from the Australian medicinal plant, *Dianella callicarpa*. *Planta Med* 75(13): 1442-7.

Donnegan, J.A., S.L. Butler, O. Kuegler, B.J. Stroud, B.A. Hiserote, and K. Rengulbai. 2007. Palau's Forest Resources, 2003. Resource Bull. PNW-RB-252. Portland, OR: U.S. Department of Agriculture, Forest Service, Pacific Northwest Research Station. 52 pp.

Dorne, M., and T. Friedman. 1940. *Derris* root dermatitis. *JAMA* 115(15): 1268-1270.

Eddleston, M., and S. Haggalla. 2008. Fatal injury in eastern Sri Lanka, with special reference to cardenolide self-poisoning with *Cerbera manghas* fruits. *Clin Toxicol* 46(8): 745-748.

Egashira, K., H. Ohtani, S. Itoh, N. Koyabu, M. Tsujimoto, H. Murakami, and Y. Sawada. 2004. Inhibitory effects of pomelo on the metabolism of tacrolimus and the activities of CYP3A4 and p-glycoprotein. *Drug Metab Dispos* 32(8): 828-833.

Englberger, L., A. Lorens, A. Levendusky, J. Daniells. 2009. Banana: An essential traditional crop on Pohnpei. pp. 89-131. In: M.J. Balick, ed. *Ethnobotany of Pohnpei: Plants, people and island culture.* New York/Honolulu: The New York Botanical Garden Press/University of Hawai'i Press.

Esteves, I., I.R. Souza, M. Rodrigues, L.G. Cardoso, L.S. Santos, J.A. Sertie, F.F. Perazzo, L.M. Lima, J.M. Schneedorf, J.K. Bastos, and J.C. Carvalho. 2005. Gastric antiulcer and anti-inflammatory activities of the essential oil from *Casearia sylvestris* Sw. *J Ethnopharmacol* 101(1-3): 191-196.

Fandohan, P., B. Gnonlonfin, A. Laleye, J.D. Gbenou, R. Darboux, and M. Moudachirou. 2008. Toxicity and gastric tolerante of essential oils from *Cymbopogon citratus*, *Ocimum gratissimum* and *Ocimum basilicum* in Wistar rats. *Food Chem Toxicol* 46: 2493-2497.

Fang, S.-H., Y.K. Rao, and Y.-M. Tzeng. 2008. Anti-oxidant and inflammatory mediator's growth inhibitory effects of compounds isolated from *Phyllanthus urinaria*. *J Ethnopharmacol* 116: 333-340.

Feinsilver, J.M. 1993. *Healing the masses: Cuban health politics at home and abroad.* Berkeley: University of California Press.

Fletcher, P.S., S.J. Harman, A.R. Boothe, G.F. Doncel, and R.J. Shattock. 2008. Preclinical evaluation of lime juice as a topical microbicide candidate. *Retrovirology* 5: 3.

Fosberg, F.R. 1946. *Botanical report on Micronesia.* Honolulu, HI: U.S. Commercial Company Economic Survey. 323 pp.

Fosberg, F.R. 1947. Micronesian mangroves. *J NYBG* 4(570): 125-148.

Fosberg, F.R. 1953. Vegetation of the Oceanic province of the Pacific. In: Proceedings of the Eighth Pacific Science Congress 1957. National Research Council of the Philippines: University of the Philippines. pp. 48-55.

Fosberg, F.R. 1960. The vegetation of Micronesia I. General descriptions, the vegetation of the Marianas Islands, and a detailed consideration of the vegetation of Guam. *Bull Am Museum Nat Hist* 119(1): 1-75.

Fosberg, F.R., D. Otobed, M.H. Sachet, and R.L. Oliver, D.A. Powell, and J.E. Canfield. 1980. *Vascular plants of Palau with vernacular names.* Washington, D.C.: Department of Botany, Smithsonian Institution. 43p.

Fosberg, F.R., and L. Raulerson. 1990. New and Noteworthy Micronesian Plants. *Micronesica* 23(2):150.

Fosberg, F.R., and M.H. Sachet. 1975a. Flora of Micronesia, 1: Gymnospermae. *Sm C Bot* 20: 1-15.

Fosberg, F.R., and M.H. Sachet. 1975b. Flora of Micronesia, 2: Casuarinaceae, Piperaceae, and Myricaceae. *Sm C Bot* 24: 1-28.

Fosberg, F.R., and M.H. Sachet. 1977. Flora of Micronesia, 3: Convolvulaceae. *Sm C Bot* 36: 1-33.

Fosberg, F.R., and M.H. Sachet. 1979. *Maesa* (Myrsinaceae) in Micronesia. *Phytologia* 44(1): 363-369.

Fosberg, F.R., and M.H. Sachet. 1980a. Flora of Micronesia, 4: Caprifoliaceae-Compositae. *Sm C Bot* 46: 1-71.

Fosberg, F. R., and M.H. Sachet. 1980b. Systematic studies of Micronesian plants. *Sm C Bot* 45: 1-44.

Fosberg, F.R., and M.H. Sachet. 1980c. Systematic studies of Micronesian plants. Washington, D.C.: Department of Botany, Smithsonian Institution. 40p

Fosberg, F.R., and M.H. Sachet. 1981. Nomenclatural Notes on Micronesian Ferns. *American Fern Journal* 71(3): 82-84

Fosberg, F.R., and M.H. Sachet. 1984. Micronesian Poaceae: Critical and Distributional Notes. Washington, D.C.: Department of Botany, Smithsonian Institution. 102p

Fosberg, F.R., and M.H. Sachet. 1987. The Genus *Timonius* (Rubiaceae) in the Palau Islands. *Micronesica* 20 (1-2):157-164.

Fosberg, F.R., and M.H. Sachet. 1991. Studies in Indo-Pacific Rubiaceae. *Allertonia* 6 (3): 191-278

Fosberg, F.R., M.H. Sachet, and R.L. Oliver. 1979. A geographical checklist of the Micronesian dicotyledonae. *Micronesica* 15(1-2): 41-298.

Fosberg, F.R., M.H. Sachet, and R.L. Oliver. 1982. A Geographical Checklist of the Micronesian Pteridophytes and Gymnosperms. Botany Department, Smithsonian Institution, Washington, D.C. *Micronesica* 18 (1):23-82.

Fosberg, F.R., M.H. Sachet, and R.L. Oliver. 1987. A Geographical Checklist of the Micronesian Monocotyledoneae. Botany Department, Smithsonian Institution, Washington, D. C. *Micronesica* 20 (1-2):19-129.

Fosberg. F.R., M.H. Sachet, and R.L. Oliver. 1993. Flora of Micronesia, 5: Bignoniaceae-Rubiaceae. *Smithsonian Contributions to Botany* 81:1-135

Francisco, V., A. Figueirinha, B.M. Neves, C. García Rodríguez, M.C. Lopes, M.T. Cruz, and M.T. Batista. 2011. *Cymbopogon citratus* as source of new and safe anti-inflammatory drugs: bio-guided assay using lipopolysaccharide-stimulated macrophages. *J Ethnopharmacol* 133(2): 818-827.

Friend, N., and N. Tabak. 1995. *Medicinal Plants of Ngaraard*. Ngaraard State, Republic of Palau: Center for Island Management Studies, School for Field Studies. 40pp

Furuya, A., M. Uozaki, H. Yamasaki, T. Arakawa, M. Arita, and A.H. Koyama. 2008. Antiviral effects of ascorbic and dehydroascorbic acids *in vitro*. *Int J Mol Med* 22(4): 541-545.

Ganguly, S., S. Mula, S. Chattopadhyay, and M. Chatterjee. 2007. An ethanol extract of *Piper betle* Linn. mediates its anti-inflammatory activity via down-regulation of nitric oxide. *Journal of Pharmacy & Pharmacology* 59: 711-718.

Ghazanfar, S.A. 1994. *Handbook of Arabian Medicinal Plants*. CRC Press. Boca Raton, FL.

Geetha, T., and P. Varalakshmi. 1999. Anticomplement activity of triterpenes from *Crateva nurvala* stem bark in adjuvant arthritis in rats. *General Pharmacology* 32(4): 495-497.

Geller-Bernstein, C., N. Keynan, A. Bejarano, A. Shomer-Ilan, and Y. Waisel. 1987. Positive skin tests to fern spore extracts in atopic patients. *Ann Allergy* 58: 125-127.

Germosen-Robineau, L., ed. 1998. *Farmacopea vegetal Caribena* (TRAMIL). Santo Domingo: Enda-caribe.

Gills, J. 2004. *God's prescription for healing: Five divine gifts of healing.* Lake Mary, FL: Siloam Press. 256 pp.

Gladman, A.C. 2006. Toxicodendron dermatitis: Poison ivy, oak, and sumac. *Wilderness Environ Med* 17: 120-128.

Gopi, S., and O.H. Setty. 2010. Protective effect of *Phyllanthus fraternus* against bromobenzene induced mitochondrial dysfunction in rat liver mitochondria. *Food Chem Toxicol* 48(8-9): 2170-2175.

Gorton, H.C., and K. Jarvis. 1999. The effectiveness of vitamin C in preventing and relieving the symptoms of virus-induced respiratory infections. *J Manipulative Physiol Ther* 22(8): 530-533.

Goskowicz, M.O., S.F. Friedlander, and F. Lawrence. 1994. Endemic "lime" disease: Phytophotodermatitis in San Diego County. *Pediatrics* 3: 828-830.

Goun, E., G. Cunningham, D. Chu, C. Nguyen, and D. Miles. 2003. Antibacterial and antifungal activity of Indonesian ethnomedical plants. *Fitoterapia* 74(6): 592-596.

Gowri, P.M., S.V.S. Radhakrishnan, S.J. Basha, A.V.S. Sarma, and J.M Rao. 2009. Oleanane-type isomeric triterpenoids from *Barringtonia racemosa. J Nat Prod* 72: 791-795.

Grant, R., P.A. Basson, H.H. Booker, J.B. Hofherr, and M. Anthonissen. 1991. Cardiomyopathy caused by avocado (*Persea americana* Mill) leaves. *J S Afr Vet Assoc* 62(1): 21-2.

Grenier, J., C. Fradette, G. Morelli, G.J. Merritt, M. Vanderick, and M.P. Ducharme. 2006. Pomelo juice, but not cranberry juice, affects the pharmacokinetics of cyclosporine in humans. *Clin Pharmacol Ther* 79(3): 255-262.

Grosvenor, P.W., A. Supriono, and D.O. Gray. 1995. Medicinal plants from Riau province, Sumatra, Indonesia. Part 2: Antibacterial and antifungal activity. *J Ethnopharmacol* 45: 97-111.

Guimarães, R., L. Barros, J.C. Barreira, M.J. Sousa, A.M. Carvalho, and I.C. Ferreira. 2010. Targeting excessive free radicals with peels and juices of citrus fruits: grapefruit, lemon, lime and orange. *Food Chem Toxicol* 48(1): 99-106.

Habtemariam, S., A.I. Gray, G.W. Halbert, and P.G. Waterman. 1990. A novel antibacterial diterpene from *Premna schimperi. Planta Med* 56: 187-189.

Habtemariam, S., A.I. Gray, and P.G. Waterman. 1992. Antibacterial diterpenes from the aerial parts of *Premna oligotricha. Planta Med* 58: 109-110.

Hanley, M.J., P. Cancalon, W.W. Widmer, and D.J. Greenblatt. 2011. The effect of grapefruit juice on drug dispostion. *Expert Opin Drug Metab Toxicol* 7(3): 267-286.

Hardman, J.G., P.B.L.E. Limbird, and A.G. Gilman. 2001. *Goodman and Gilman's The Pharmacological Basis of Therapeutics.* 10th ed. New York, NY: McGraw-Hill. p. 1245.

Hausen, B.M., and K.H. Schulz. 1977. Occupational contact dermatitis due to croton (*Codiaeum variegatum* (L.) A. Juss var. *pictum* (Lodd.) Muell. Arg.). Sensitization by plants of the Euphorbiaceae. *Contact Dermatitis* 3(6): 289-292.

Hayes, W.J., and E.R. Laws, eds. 1991. *Handbook of Pesticide Toxicology, Volume 2, Classes of Pesticides.* Academic Press, NY.

Hennebelle T., B. Weniger, H. Joseph, S. Sahpaz, and F. Bailleul. 2009. *Senna alata. Fitoterapia* 80: 385-393.

Henson, S. 2008. Coconut palm's health benefits dicussed. *HerbClip*. Accessed on 23 August 2011 at: http://cms.herbalgram.org/herbclip/355/review030382-355.html.

Henty, E.E. 1980. Harmful plants in Papua New Guinea. *Bot Bull* 12: 64.

Hiên, T.T., C. Navarro-Delmasure, and T. Vy. 1991. Toxicity and effects on the central nervous system of a *Cerbera odollam* leaf extract. *J Ethnopharmacol* 34(2-3): 201-206.

Hillmann Kitalong, A. 2008. Forests of Palau: A long term perspective. *Micronesica* 40 (1/2): 9-31.

Hillmann Kitalong, A., M.J. Balick, F. Rehuher, M. Besebes, S. Hanser, K. Soaladaob, G. Ngirchobong, F. Wasisang, W. Law, R. Lee, V.R. Tadao, C. Kitalong, C.U. Kitalong. 2011. Plants, people, and culture in the villages of Oikull and Ibobang, Republic of Palau. pp. 63-84. In: J. Liston, J.G. Clark, and D. Alexander, eds. *Pacific Island Heritage: Archeology, Identity & Community*. Terra Australis 35. Canberra: Australian National University.

Hillmann Kitalong, A., R.A. DeMeo, and T. Holm. 2008. *Native Trees of Palau: A Field Guide.* The Environment Inc. Koror, Palau. 249 pp.

Hillmann Kitalong, A., and T. Holm. 2004. Forest Habitat Assessment Project. Report for the Palau Conservation Society. 17 pp.

Hooker, J.D. 1875. *The flora of British India.* By J. D. Hooker assisted by various botanists. Published under the authority of the secretary of state for India in council. L. Reeve, London.

Hoshizaki, B.J., and R.C. Moran. 2001. *Fern Grower's Manual*. Portland: Timber Press. 624 pp.

Hussain, F., M.A. Abdulla, S.M. Noor, S. Ismail, and H.M. Al. 2008. Gastroprotective effects of *Melastoma malabathricum* aqueous leaf extract against ethanol-induced gastric ulcer in rats. *American Journal of Biochemistry and Biotechnology* 4(4): 438-441.

Hyland, B.P.M., T. Whiffin, and F.A. Zich. 2010. *Australian Tropical Rainforest Plants Edition 6* (*RFK6*). Accessed on 6 August 2011 at: http://keys.trin.org.au:8080/key-server/data/0e0f0504-0103-430d-8004-060d07080d04/media/Html/index.html.

Irobi, O.N. 1992. Activities of *Chromolaena odorata* (Compositae) leaf extract against *Pseudomonas aeruginosa* and *Streptococcus faecalis*. *J Ethnopharmacol* 37(1): 81-83.

Irobi, O.N. 1997. Antibiotic properties of ethanol extract of *Chromolaena odorata* (Asteraceae). *Int J Pharmacogn* 35(2): 111-115.

Itoigawa, M., C. Ito, H.T. Tan, M. Kuchide, H. Tozuda, H. Nishino, and H. Furukawa. 2001. Cancer chemopreventive agents, 4-phenylcoumarins from *Calophyllum inophyllum*. *Cancer Letters* 169(1): 15-19.

Iwu, M.M. 1993. *Handbook of African medicinal plants*. Boca Raton: CRC Press Inc.

Javed, R.A., K. Marrero, M. Rafique, M.U. Khan, D. Jamarai, and J. Vieira. 2007. Life-threatening hyperkalaemia developing following excessive ingestion of orange juice in a patient with baseline normal renal function. *Singapore Med J* 48(11): e293-e295.

Jones, W.H.S., trans 1923. *Hippocrates, On Ancient Medicine.* Loeb Classical Library. No. 147. Cambridge, MA: Harvard University Press. 432 pp.

Joseph, J.M., K. Sowndhararajan, and S. Manian. 2010a. Protective effects of methanolic extract of *Hedyotis puberula* (G. Don) R. Br. ex Arn. against experimentally induced gastric ulcers in rat. *J Ethnopharmacol* 131(1): 216-219.

Joseph, J.M., K. Sowndhararajan, and S. Manian. 2010b. Evaluation of analgesic and anti-inflammatory potential of *Hedyotis puberula* (G. Don) R. Br. ex Arn. in experimental animal models. *Food Chem Toxicol* 48(7): 1876-1880.

Joshi, J., S. Ghaisas, A. Vaidya, R. Vaidya, D.V. Kamat, A.N. Bhagwat, and S. Bhide. 2003. Early human safety study of turmeric oil (*Curcuma longa* oil) administered orally in healthy volunteers. *J Assoc Physicians India* 51: 1055-1060.

Kagawa, Y., G.J. Dever, C.T. Otto, P. Charupoonphol, S. Supannatas, Y. Yanagisawa, M. Sakuma, and K. Hasegawa. 2003. Single nucleotide polymorphism and lifestyle-related diseases in the Asia-Pacific region: Comparative study in Okinawa, Palau and Thailand. *Asia Pac J Public Health* 15 Suppl: S10-4.

Kamiya, K., Y. Tanaka, H. Endang, M. Umar, and T. Satake. 2005. New anthraquinone and iridoid from the fruits of *Morinda citrifolia*. *Chem Pharm Bull* 53: 1597-1599.

Kanehira, R. 1933. Flora Micronesia. *Bot Mag Tokyo* 248: 675.

Kashman, Y., K.R. Gustafon, R.W. Fuller, J.H. Cardellina, J.B. McMahon, M.J. Currens, R.W. Buckheit, S.H. Hughes, G.M. Cragg, and M.R. Boyd. 1992. The calanolides, a novel HIV-inhibitory class of coumarin derivatives from the tropical rainforest tree, *Calophyllum lanigerum*. *J Med Chem* 35(15): 2735-2743.

Kassuya, C.A.L., A. Silvestre, O. Menezes-de-Lima Jr., D.M. Marotta, V.L.G. Rehder, and J.B. Calixto. 2006. Antiinflammatory and antiallodynic actions of the lignan niranthin isolated from *Phyllanthus amarus*: Evidence for interaction with platelet activating factor receptor. *Eur J Pharmacol* 546: 182-188.

Khan, M.R., A.D. Omoloso, and Y. Barewai. 2006. Antimicrobial activity of the *Derris elliptica*, *Derris indica* and *Derris trifoliata* extractives. *Fitoterapia* 77(4): 327-330.

Khan, S., A. Jabbar, C.M. Hasan, and M.A. Rashid. 2001. Antibacterial activity of *Barringtonia racemosa*. *Fitoterapia* 72: 162-164.

Kiemer, A.K., T. Hartung, C. Huber, and A.M. Vollmar. 2003. *Phyllanthus amarus* has anti-inflammatory potential by inhibition of iNOS, COX-2, and cytokines via the NF-κB pathway. *Journal of Hepatology* 38: 289-297.

Kim, Y.J., H.C. Kim, H. Ko, E.C. Amor, J.W. Lee, and H.O. Yang. 2011. Stercurensin inhibits nuclear factor-κB-dependent inflammatory signals through attenuation of TAK1-TAB1 complex formation. *J Cell Biochem* 112(2): 548-558.

Kiuchi, F., K. Matsuo, M. Ito, T.K. Qui, and G. Honda. 2004. New norditerpenoids with trypanocidal activity from *Vitex trifolia*. *Chem Pharm Bull* 52(12): 1492-1494.

Klimpel, S., F. Abdel-Ghaffar, K.A. Al-Rasheid, G. Aksu, K. Fischer, B. Strassen, and H. Mehlhorn. 2011. The effects of different plant extracts on nematodes. *Parasitol Res* 108(4): 1047-1054.

Kloucek, P., Z. Polesny, B. Svobodova, E. Vlkova, and L. Kokoska. 2005. Antibacterial screening of some Peruvian medicinal plants used in Callería District. *J Ethnopharmacol* 99(2): 309-312.

Kpemissi, E.A., K. Batawila, K. Kokou, K. Koumaglo, C. de Souza, P. Bouchet, and K. Akpagana. 2003. Antimicrobial properties of three threatened sand dune species from the Togolese littoral. *Acta Botanica Gallica* 150: 107-115.

Kulkarni, P., R. Paul, and N. Ganesh. 2010. *In vitro* evaluation of genotoxicity of avocado (*Persea americana*) fruit and leaf extracts in human peripheral lymphocytes. *J Environ Sci Health C Environ Carcinog Ecotoxicol Rev* 28(3): 172-87.

Kuo, S.C., C.M. Teng, L.G. Lee, T.H. Chiu, T.S. Wu, S.C. Huang, J.B. Wu, T.Y. Shieh, R.J. Chang, and T.C. Chou. 1991. 6-Pentadecylsalicylic acid: An antithrombin component isolated from the stem of *Rhus semialata* var. *roxburghii*. *Planta Med* 57: 247-249.

Lai, C.-H., S.-H. Fang, Y.K. Rao, M. Geethangili, C.-H. Tang, Y.-J. Lin, C.-H. Hung, W.-C. Wang, and Y.-M. Tzeng. 2008. Inhibition of *Helicobacter pylori*-induced inflammation in human gastric epithelial AGS cells by *Phyllanthus urinaria* extracts. *J Ethnopharmacol* 118: 522-526.

Lai, H.Y., Y.Y. Lim, and S.P. Tan. 2009. Antioxidative, tyrosinase inhibiting and antibacterial activities of leaf extracts from medicinal ferns. *Biosci Biotechnol Biochem* 73: 1362-1366.

Lampe, K.F. 1986. Dermatitis-producing plants of south Florida and Hawaii. *Clinics in Dermatology* 4(2): 83-93.

Lannuzel, A., P.P. Michel, G.U. Hoglinger, P. Champy, A. Jousset, F. Medja , A. Lombes, F. Darios, C. Gleye, A. Laurens, R. Hocquemiller, E.C. Hirsch, and M. Ruberg. 2003. The mitochondrial complex I inhibitor annonacin is toxic to mesencephalic dopaminergic neurons by impairment of energy metabolism. *Neuroscience* 121(2): 287-296.

Lannuzel, A., M. Ruberg, and P.P. Michel. 2008. Atypical Parkinsonism in the Caribbean island of Guadeloupe: Etiological role of the mitochondrial complex I inhibitor annonacin. *Mov Disord* 23(15): 2122-2128.

Le Coz, C.J. 2004. Allergic contact dermatitis from tamanu oil (*Calophyllum inophyllum, Calophyllum tacamahaca*). *Contact Dermatitis* 51(4): 216-7.

Lee, C.-Y., W.-H. Peng, H.-Y. Cheng, F.-N. Chen, M.-T. Lai, and T.-H. Chiu. 2006. Hepatoprotective effect of *Phyllanthus* in Taiwan on acute liver damage induced by carbon tetrachloride. *American Journal of Chinese Medicine* 34: 471-482.

Lee, K.K., J.H. Kim, J.J. Cho, and J.D. Choi. 1999. Inhibitory effects of 150 plant extracts on elastase activity, and their anti-inflammatory effects. *Int J Cosm Sci* 21(2): 71-82.

Lee, R., N. Shere, M.J. Balick, F. Sohl, A.S. Roberts, K. Herrera, S. Dahmer, M. Lieskovsky, A. Dores, W. Raynor, P. Raynor, E. Albert, M. Hunt, C. Trauernicht, L. Offringa, I. Adam, and W. Law. 2010. *Pohnpei primary health care manual. Health care in Pohnpei, Micronesia: Traditional uses of plants for health and healing.* Charleston, SC: CreateSpace. 178 pp.

Lee Ling, D. 1998. *Cordyline fruticosa.* College of Micronesia-FSM. Accessed on 10 November 2010 at: http://www.comfsm.fm/~dleeling/botany/1998/vhp/cordyline_fruticosa.html.

Leeya, Y., M.J. Mulvany, E.F. Queiroz, A. Marston, K. Hostettmann, and C. Jansakul. 2010. Hypotensive activity of an n-butanol extract and their purified compounds from leaves of *Phyllanthus acidus* (L.) Skeels in rats. *Eur J Pharmacol* 649(1-3): 301-313.

Lemmens, R.H.M.J., and N. Bunyapraphatsara, eds. 2003. *Prosea: Plant resources of South-East Asia: Medicinal poisonous plants* 12(3): 1-661.

Lewis, W.H., and M.P.F. Elvin-Lewis. 2003. *Medical botany: Plants affecting human health.* 2nd ed. Hoboken, NJ: John Wiley & Sons, Inc.

Li, X., L. Xu, P. Wu, H. Xie, Z. Huang, W. Ye, and X. Wei. 2009. Prenylflavonols from the leaves of *Macaranga sampsonii*. *Chem Pharm Bull* 57: 495-498.

Lim, T.Y., Y.Y. Lim, and C.M. Yule. 2009. Evaluation of antioxidant, antibacterial and anti-tyrosinase activities of four *Macaranga* species. *Food Chem* 114: 594-599.

Lin, J., Y. Chen, L. Wei, X. Chen, W. Xu, Z. Hong, T.J. Sferra, and J. Peng. 2010. *Hedyotis diffusa* Willd extract induces apoptosis via activation of the mitochondrion-dependent pathway in human colon carcinoma cells. *Int J Oncol* 37(5): 1331-1338.

Lin, S.-Y., C.-C. Wang, Y.-L. Lu, W.-C. Wu, and W.-C. Hou. 2008. Antioxidant, anti-semicarbazide-sensitive amine oxidase, and anti-hypertensive activities of geraniin isolated from *Phyllanthus urinaria*. *Food Chem Toxicol* 46: 2485-2492.

Locher, C.P., M.T. Burch, H.F. Mower, J. Berestecky, H. Davis, B. Van Poel, A. Lasure, D.A. Vanden Berghe, and A.J. Vlietinck. 1995. Anti-microbial activity and anti-complement activity of extracts obtained from selected Hawaiian medicinal plants. *J Ethnopharmacol* 49(1):23-32.

Lohezic-Le Devehat, F., A. Bakhtiar, C. Bezivin, M. Amoros, and J. Boustie. 2002. Antiviral and cytotoxic activities of some Indonesian plants. *Fitoterapia* 73: 400-405.

Lopez-Lazaro, M., C. Martin-Cordero, A. Bermejo, D. Cortes, and M.J. Ayuso. 2001. Cytotoxic compounds from Annonaceus species as DNA topoisomerase I poisons. *Anticancer Res* 21(5): 3493-3497.

Lyte, M. 1997. Induction of Gram-negative bacterial growth by neurochemical containing banana (*Musa paradisiaca*) extracts. *FEMS Microbiol Lett* 154: 245-250.

Machiko, A. 2002. *Modekngei: A New Religion in Belau, Micronesia*. Tokyo, Japan: Shinsensha Press. 378p.

Mackeen, M.M., A.M. Ali, S.H. El-Sharkawy, M.Y. Manap, K.M. Salleh, N.H. Lajis, and K. Kawazu. 1997. Antimicrobial and cytotoxic properties of some Malaysian traditional vegetables (Ulam). *Int J Pharmacog* 35(3): 174-178.

Macpherson, C., and L. Macpherson. 1990. *Samoan medical belief and practice*. Auckland, New Zealand: University of Auckland Press. 279 pp.

Madan, S., G.N. Singh, K. Coolí, M. Ali, Y. Kumat, R.M. Singh, and O. Prakash. 2009. Isoflavonoids from *Flemingia strobilifera* (L.) R. Br. Roots. *Acta Pol Pharm* 66(3): 297-303.

Malaraijan, P., G. Gopalakrishanan, S. Narasimhan, and K.J.K. Veni. 2006. Analgesic activity of some Indian medicinal plants. *J Ethnopharmacol* 106(3): 425-428.

Martini, L.H., F. Jung, F.A. Soares, L.N. Rotta, D.A. Vendite, M.E. dos Santos Frizzo, R.A. Yunes, J.B. Calixto, S. Wofchuk, and D.O. Souza. 2007. Naturally occurring compounds affect glutamatergic neurotransmission in rat brain. *Neurochem Res* 32: 1950-1956.

Mathivanan, N., G. Surendiran, K. Srinivasan, and K. Malarvizhi. 2006. *Morinda pubescens* J.E. Smith (*Morinda tinctoria* Roxb.) fruit extract accelerates wound healing in rats. *Journal of Medicinal Food* 9(4): 591-593.

Matsuda, H., M. Tokunaga, N. Hirata, H. Iwahashi, S. Naruto, and M. Kubo. 2004. Studies on Palauan medicinal herbs. I. Antidiabetic effect of Ongael, leaves of *Phaleria nisidai* (Meisn.) F. Vill. *Nat Med* 58(6): 278-283.

Matsuda, H., M. Tokunaga, H. Iwahashi, S. Naruto, H. Yagi, T. Masuko, and M. Kubo. 2005a. Studies on Palauan medicinal herbs. III. Antitumor and immunostimulatory activities of Ongael, leaves of *Phaleria cumingii* (Meisn.) F. Vill. *J Trad Med* 22: 314-320.

Matsuda, H., M. Tokunaga, H. Iwahashi, S. Naruto, H. Yagi, T. Masuko, and M. Kubo. 2005b. Studies on Palauan Medicinal Herbs. II. Activation of Mouse Macrophages RAW 264.7 by Ongael, Leaves of *Phaleria cumingii* (Meisn.) F. Vill. and its acylglucosylsterols. *Biol Pharm Bull* 28(5): 929-933.

Matsui, M., S. Kumar-Roine, H.T. Darius, M. Chinain, D. Laurent, and S. Pauillac. 2009. Characterisation of the anti-inflammatory potential of *Vitex trifolia* L. (Labiatae), a multipurpose plant of the Pacific traditional medicine. *J Ethnopharmacol* 126(3): 427-433.

Mazura, M.P., D. Susanti, and M.A. Rasadah. 2007. Anti-inflammatory action of components from *Melastoma malabathricum*. *Pharm Biol* 45: 372-375.

McCutcheon, A.R., S.M. Ellis, R.E. Hancock, and G.H. Towers. 1994. Antifungal screening of medicinal plants of British Columbian native peoples. *J Ethnopharmacol* 44: 157-169.

McKenzie, R.A., and O.P. Brown. 1991. Avocado (*Persea americana*) poisoning of horses. *Aust Vet J* 68(2): 77-8.

McLaren, D.S., and M. Frigg. 2001. Sight and life manual on vitamin A deficiency disorders (VADD). 2nd ed. Basel, Switzerland: Task Force Sight and Life.

Mendonça-Filho, R.R., I.A. Rodrigues, D.S. Alivano, A.L. Santos, C.S. Alviano, A.H. Lopes, and S.M. Rosa. 2004. Leishmanicidal activity of polyphenolic-rich extract from husk fiber of *Cocos nucifera* Linn. (Palmae). *Res Microbiol* 155(3): 136-143.

Merlin, M., D. Jano, W. Raynor, T. Keene, J. Juvik, and B. Sebastian. 1992. *Tuhke en Pohnpei (Plants of Pohnpei)*. Honolulu, HI: East-West Center.

Millonig, G., S. Stadelmann, and W. Vogel. 2005. Herbal hepatoxocity: Acute hepatitis caused by a Noni preparation. *Eur J Gastroenterol Hepatol* 17(4): 445-447.

Mikhal'chick, E.V., A.V. Ivanova, M.V. Anurov, S.M. Titkova, L.Y. Pen'kov, Z.F. Kharaeva, and L.G. Korkina. 2004. Wound-healing effect of papaya-based preparation in experimental thermal trauma. *Bull Exp Biol Med* 137: 560-562.

Ministry of Health, Republic of Palau. 2009. *Annual report 2009: Healthy Palau in a healthful environment.* Koror, Palau: Ministry of Health Palau. 45 pp.

Mishra, U.S., P.N. Murthy, P.K. Choudhury, G. Panigrahi, S. Mohapatra, and D. Pradhan. 2010. Antibacterial and analgesic effects of the stem barks of *Callophylum inophyllum*. *Int J ChemTech Res* 2(2): 973-979.

Moreno-Ancillo, Á., C. Domínguez-Noche, A.C. Gil-Adrados, and P.M. Cosmes. 2004. Allergy to banana in a 5-month-old infant. *Pediatr Allergy Immu* 15: 284-5.

Morton, J. 1987. *Fruits of warm climates*. Miami: Florida Flair Books. 505 pp.

Moura, A.C., E.L. Silva, M.C. Fraga, A.G. Wanderley, P. Afiatpour, and M.B. Maia. 2005. Antiinflammatory and chronic toxicity study of the leaves of *Ageratum conyzoides* L. in rats. *Phytomedicine* 12: 138-142.

Mukhopadhyay, A., N. Basu, and N. Ghatak. 1982. Anti-inflammatory and irritant activities of curcumin analogues in rats. *Agents Actions* 12: 508-515.

Murthy, M.M., M. Subramanyam, K.V. Giridhar, and A. Jeetty. 2006. Antimicrobial activities of bharangin from *Premna herbaceae* Roxb. and bharangin monoacetate. *J Ethnopharmacol* 104(1-2): 290-292.

Naaz, F., S. Javed, and M.Z. Abdin. 2007. Hepatoprotective effect of ethanolic extract of *Phyllanthus amarus* Schum. et Thonn. on aflatoxin B1-induced liver damage in mice. *J Ethnopharmacol* 113: 503-509.

Nayak, B.S., J.R. Marshall, G. Isitor, and A. Adogwa. 2011. Hypoglycemic and hepatoprotective activity of fermented fruit juice of *Morinda citrifolia* (Noni) in diabetic rats. *Evid Based Complement Alternat Med* [Epub ahead of print]. Accessed on 27 August 2011 at: http://www.ncbi.nlm.nih.gov/pubmed/20981320.

Nayak, B.S., S. Sandiford, and A. Maxwell. 2009. Evaluation of the wound-healing activity of ethanolic extract of *Morinda citrifolia* L. leaf. *Evid Based Complement Alternat Med* 6(3): 351-356.

Nelson, L.R., R.D. Shih, and M.J. Balick. 2007. *Handbook of poisonous and injurious plants*. 2nd ed. New York: Springer/The New York Botanical Garden.

Ngamkitidechakul, C., K. Jaijoy, P. Hansakul, N. Soonthornchareonnon, and S. Sireeratawong. 2010. Antitumor effects of *Phyllanthus emblica* L.: Induction of cancer cell apoptosis and inhibition of *in vivo* tumour promotion and *in vitro* invastion of human cancer cells. *Phytotherapy Research* 24(9): 1405-1413.

Ngono Ngane, A., R. Ebelle Etame, F. Ndifor, L. Biyiti, P.H. Amvam Zollo, and P. Bouchet. 2006. Antifungal Activity of *Chromolaena odorata* (L.) King & Robinson (Asteraceae) of Cameroon. *Chemotherapy* 52(2): 103-106.

Nonato, F.R., T.M.O. Nogueira, T.A.A. Barros, A.M. Lucchese, C.E.C. Oliveira, R.R. dos Santos, M.B.P. Soares, and C.F. Villarreal. 2010. Antinociceptive and anti-inflammatory activities of *Adiantum latifolium* Lam.: evidence for a role of IL-1B inhibition. *J Ethnopharmacol* In press. Corrected proof available online June 8, 2010.

Norhanom, A.W., and M. Yadav. 1995. Tumour promoter activity in Malaysian Euphorbiaceae. *Brit J Cancer* 71(4): 776-779.

Nualsanit, T., P. Rojanapanthu, W. Gritsanapan, S.H. Lee, D. Lawson, and S.J. Baek. 2011. Damnacanthal, a noni component, exhibits antitumorigenic activity in human colorectal cancer cells. *J Nutr Biochem* [Epub ahead of print]. Accessed on 27 August 2011 at: http://www.ncbi.nlm.nih.gov/pubmed/21852088.

Nworu, C.S., P.A. Akah, F.B. Okoye, and C.O. Esimone. 2010. Aqueous extract of *Phyllanthus niruri* (Euphorbiaceae) enhances the phenotypic and functional maturation of bone marrow-derived dendritic cells and their antigen-presentation function. *Immunopharmacol Immunotoxicol* 32(3): 393-401.

Oben, J., E. Enonchong, S. Kothari, W. Chambliss, R. Garrison, and D. Dolnick. 2009. *Philodendron* and *Citrus* extracts benefit joint health in osteoarthritis patients: A pilot, double-blind, placebo-controlled study. *Nutr J* 8: 38.

O'Bryan, C.A., P.G. Crandall, V.I. Chalova, and S.C. Ricke. 2008. Orange essential oils antimicrobial activities against *Salmonella* spp. *J Food Sci* 73(6): M264-267.

Oduwole, O., M.M. Meremikwu, A. Oyo-Ita, and E.E. Udoh. 2010. Honey for acute cough in children. *Cochrane Database Sys Rev* (1) CD007094.

Okabe, M. 1941. Folk Medicines of the Palau Islander. *Journal of Anthropological Society of Nippon* (56): 413-426. H. Takeda, trans. 1953. Military Geology Branch U.S. Geological Survey for Intelligence Division. Office of the Engineer Headquarters, Far East Command. Tokyo, Japan.

Oku, H., Y. Ueda, M. Linuma, and K. Ishiguro. 2005. Inhibitory effects of xanthones from Guttiferae plants on PAF-induced hypotension in mice. *Planta Med* 71: 90-92.

Oladejo, O.W., I.O. Imosemi, F.C. Osuagwu, O.O. Oyedele, O.O. Oluwadara, O.E. Ekpo, A. Aiku, O. Adewoyin, and E.E. Akang. 2003. A comparative study of the wound healing properties of honey and *Ageratum conyzoides*. *Afr J Med Med Sci* 32: 193-196.

Oludare, B.T., O.A. Olajide, O.O. Soyannwo, and J.M. Makinde. 2000. Anti-inflammatory, antipyretic and antispasmodic properties of *Chromolaena odorata*. *Pharm Biol* 38(5): 367-370.

Owoyele, B.V., S.O. Oguntoye, K. Dare, B.A. Ogunbiyi, E.A. Aruboula, and A.O. Soladoye. 2008. Analgesic, anti-inflammatory and antipyretic activities from flavonoid fractions of *Chromolaena odorata*. *J Med Plants Res* 2(9): 219-225.

Owoyele, V.B., J.O. Adediji, and A.O. Soladoye. 2005. Anti-inflammatory activity of aqueous leaf extract of *Chromolaena odorata*. *Inflammopharmacol* 13(5-6): 479-84.

Palau Society of Historians. 2000. *Medicine and Therapy. Traditional and Customary Practices*. English Series 6. Koror, Republic of Palau: Division of Cultural Affairs. 16pp.

Palau Society of Historians. 2001. *Traditional Items and Properties of a Household, Clan, and Village*. English Series 7. Koror, Republic of Palau: Division of Cultural Affairs. 51pp.

Palombo, E.A., and S.J. Semple. 2001. Antibacterial activity of traditional Australian medicinal plants. *J Ethnopharmacol* 77: 151-157.

Pankajakshy, A., and I. Madambath. 2009. Spermatotoxic effects of *Cananga odorata* (Lam): A comparison with gossypol. *Fertil Steril* 91(5 Suppl): 2243-6.

Panossian, A., G. Wikman, and H. Wagner. 1999. Plant adaptogens III. Earlier and more recent aspects and concepts on their mode of action. *Phytomedicine* 6(4): 287-300.

Parmar, H.S., and A. Kar. 2008. Antiperoxidative, antithyroidal, antihyperglycemic, and cardioprotective role of *Citrus sinensis* peel extract in male mice. *Phytother Res* 22: 791-795.

Paulsen, E., P.S. Skov, and K.E. Andersen. 1998. Immediate skin and mucosal symptoms from pot plants and vegetables in gardeners and greenhouse workers. *Contact Dermatitis* 39: 166-170.

Pawlus, A.D., B.N. Su, W.J. Keller, and A.D. Kinghorn. 2005. An anthraquinone with potent quinone reductase-inducing activity and other constituents of the fruits of *Morinda citrifolia* (noni). *J Nat Prod* 68(12): 1720-2.

Phan T.T., J. Allen, M.A. Hughes, G. Cherry, and F. Wojnarowska. 2000. Upregulation of adhesion complex proteins and fibronectin by human keratinocytes treated with an aqueous extract from the leaves of *Chromolaena odorata* (Eupolin). *Eur J Dermatol* 10(7): 522.

Phan, T.T., M.A. Hughes, and G.W. Cherry. 2001. Effects of an aqueous extract from the leaves of *Chromolaena odorata* (Eupolin) on the proliferation of human keratinocytes and on their migration in an *in vitro* model of reepithelialization. *Wound Repair Regen* 9(4): 305-313.

Phan, T.T., M.A. Hughes, G.W. Cherry, T.T. Le, and H.M. Pham. 1996. An aqueous extract of the leaves of *Chromolaena odorata* (formerly *Eupatorium odoratum*) (Eupolin) inhibits hydrated collagen lattice contraction by normal human dermal fibroblasts. *J Altern Complement Med* 2(3): 335-343.

Pomeranz, M.K., and J.K. Karen. 2007. Images in clinical medicine: Phytophotodermatitis and limes. *N Engl J Med* 357(1): e1.

Prayong, P., S. Barusrux, and N. Weerapreeyakul. 2008. Cytotoxic activity screening of some indigenous Thai plants. *Fitoterapia* 79(7-8): 598-601.

Prosperi, J., B.R. Ramesh, P. Grard, L.P. Jayatissa, S. Aravajy, and D. Depommier. 2005. *Checklist of Mangrove species of Southeast India and Sri Lanka.* Accessed on 14 November 2010 at: http://umramap.cirad.fr/amap2/logiciels_amap/Mangrove_web/Mangrove_list.html.

Purseglove, J.W. 1988. *Tropical Crops: Monocotyledons.* New York: Longman Scientific & Technical.

Quarre, J.P., J. Lecomte, D. Lauwers, P. Gilbert, and J. Thiriaux. 1995. Allergy to latex and papain. *J Allergy Clin Immun* 95: 922.

Radford, D.J., A.D. Gillies, J.A. Hinds, and P. Duffy. 1986. Naturally occurring cardiac glycosides. *Med J Aust* 144(10): 540-544.

Ranga Rao, R., A.K. Tiwari, P. Prabhakar Reddy, K. Suresh Babu, A.Z. Ali, K. Madhusudana, and J. Madhusudana Rao. 2009. New furanoflavanoids, intestinal a-glucosidase inhibitory and free-radical (DPPH) scavenging, activity from antihyperglycemic root extract of *Derris indica* (Lam.). *Bioorg Med Chem* 17(14): 5170- 5175.

Rao, M.V., and K.M. Alice. 2001. Contraceptive effects of *Phyllanthus amarus* in female mice. *Phytother Res* 15: 265-267.

Rao, Y.K., S.-H. Fang, and Y.-M. Tzeng. 2006. Anti-inflammatory activities of constituents isolated from *Phyllanthus polyphyllus. J Ethnopharmacol* 103: 181-186.

Rapaport, M., 1999. *The Pacific Islands: Environment & Society.* Honolulu, HI: The Bess Press. 442 pp.

Ratnasooriya, W.D., S.A. Deraniyagala, S.D. Bathige, C.L. Goonasekara, J.R. Jayakody. 2005. Antinociceptive action of aqueous extract of the leaves of *Ixora coccinea. Acta Biol Hung* 56(1-2): 21-34.

Raulerson, L., A.F. Rinehart, M.C. Falanruw, Y. Singeo, S. Slappy, and S. Victor. 1997. A botanical reconnaissance of the proposed compact road alignment on Babeldaob Island, Republic of Palau. *University of Guam Herbarium Contribution* 32. Guam: University of Guam Herbarium.

Recommendations. 2010. U.S. Preventive Services Task Force. Accessed on 28 November 2011 at: http://www.uspreventiveservicestaskforce.org/recommendations.htm.

Rinaldi, S., D.O. Silva, F. Bello, C.S. Alviano, D.S. Alviano, M.E. Matheus, and P.D. Fernandes. 2009. Characterization of the antinociceptive and anti-inflammatory activities of *Cocos nucifera* L. (Palmae). *J Ethnopharmacol* 122(3): 541-546.

Roux, K. 2005. *Microsorum.* South African National Biodiversity Institute. Accessed on 19 April 2011 at: http://www.plantzafrica.com/plantklm/microsorum.html.

Saad, R.J., and W.D. Chey. 2006. Review article: Current and emerging therapies for functional dyspepsia. *Alimentary Pharmacology and Therapeutics* 24: 475-492.

Sadasivan, S., P.G. Latha, J.M. Sasikumar, S. Rajashekaran, S. Shyamal, and V.J. Shine. 2006. Hepatoprotective studies on *Hedyotis corymbosa* (L.) Lam. *J Ethnopharmacol* 106(2): 245-249.

Sagay, A.S., G.E. Imade, V. Onwuliri, D.Z. Egah, M.J. Grigg, J. Musa, T.D. Thacher, J.O. Adisa, M. Potts, and R.V. Short. 2009. Genital tract abnormalities among female sex workers who douche with lemon/lime juice in Nigeria. *Afr J Reprod Health* 13(1): 37-45.

Saleem, M. 2009. Lupeol, a novel anti-inflammatory and anti-cancer dietary triterpene. *Cancer Lett* 285(2): 109-15.

Salsedo, C.A. 1970. The Search for Medicinal Plants of Micronesia. *Micronesian Reporter* 3rd Quarter: 10-17.

Salsedo, C.A., and D.G. Smith. 1987. Medicinal Plants of Palau. *Phytologia* 64(1): 63-77.

Saraswat, A., and B. Kumar. 2005. Anaphylactic reaction to apple, banana and lychee: What is common between botanically disparate plant families? *Int J Dermatol* 44: 996-998.

Sarkar, D., P. Saha, S. Gamre, S. Bhattacharjee, C. Hariharan, S. Ganguly, R. Sen, G. Mandal, S. Chattopadhyay, and S. Majumdar. 2008. Anti-inflammatory effect of allylpyrocatechol in LPS-induced macrophages is mediated by suppression of iNOS and COX-2 via the NF-κB pathway. *Int Immunopharmacol* 8: 1264-1271.

Sarkar, M., P. Gangopadhyay, B. Basak, K. Chakrabarty, J. Banerji, P. Adhikary, and A. Chatterjee. 2000. The reversible antifertility effect of *Piper betle* Linn. on Swiss albino male mice. *Contraception* 62: 271-274.

Schelpe, E.A.C.L.E. 1970. *Flora Zambesiaca*. Accessed on 20 April 2011 at: http://apps.kew.org/efloras/namedetail.do?qry=namelist&flora=fz&taxon=7628&nameid=19154.

Schutz, B.A., A.D. Wright, T. Rali, and O. Sticher. 1995. Prenylated flavanones from leaves of *Macaranga pleiostemona*. *Phytochemistry* 40: 1273-1277.

Semali, L., and J. Kincheloe, eds. 1999. *What is indigenous knowledge? Voices from the Academy*. New York: Garland Publishing. 382 pp.

Semple, S.J., S.M. Pyke, G.D. Reynolds, and R.L. Flower. 2001. *In vitro* antiviral activity of the anthraquinone chrysophanic acid against poliovirus. *Antiviral Res* 49: 169-178.

Semple, S.J., G.D. Reynolds, M.C. O'Leary, and R.L. Flower. 1998. Screening of Australian medicinal plants for antiviral activity. *J Ethnopharmacol* 60: 163-172.

Sen, S., G. Talukder, and A. Sharma. 1989. Betel cytotoxicity. *J Ethnopharmacol* 26: 217-247.

Sengupta, A., P. Adhikary, B.K. Basak, K. Chakrabarti, P. Gangopadhyay, J. Banerji, and A. Chatterjee. 2000. Pre-clinical toxicity evaluation of leaf-stalk extractive of *Piper betle* Linn. in rodents. *Indian J Exp Biol* 38: 338-342.

Shibumon, G., and P.J. Benny. 2010. Antifungal activity of acetonic extract of *Flacourtia inermis* fruit against human opportunistic pathogens. *J Global Pharma Technology* 2(6): 28-34.

Shirwaikar, A., P.M. Bhilegaonkar, S. Malini, and J.S. Kumar. 2003. The gastroprotective activity of the ethanol extract of *Ageratum conyzoides*. *J Ethnopharmacol* 86: 117-121.

Shitut, S., V. Pandit, and B.K. Mehta. 1999. The antimicrobial efficiency of *Piper betle* Linn. leaf (stalk) against human pathogenic bacteria and phytopathogenic fungi. *Cent Eur J Pub Health* 7: 137-139.

Singh, A.K., J. Singh, M. George, and L. Joseph. 2010. Anti-diabetic effect of *Flacourtia jangomas* extract in alloxan-induced diabetic rats. *Pharmacology* 2: 253-259.

Singh, F., R. Shukla, B. Prakash, A. Kumar, S. Singh, P.K. Mishra, and N.K. Dubey. 2010. Chemical profile, antifungal, antiaflatoxigenic and antioxidant activity of *Citrus maxima* Burm. and *Citrus sinensis* (L.) Osbeck essential oils and their cyclic monoterpene, DL-limonene. *Food Chem Toxicol* 48(6): 1734-1740.

Singh, M.M., N. Singh, P.B. Khare, and A.K.S. Rawat. 2008. Antimicrobial activity of some important *Adiantum* species used traditionally in indigenous systems of medicine. *J Ethnopharmacol* 115: 327-329.

Singh, W.R., T.K. Rajkhowa, K.H.V. Chanu, M.A. Ali, C. Lalmuanthanga, P. Mohan, and M.A.A. Shah. 2010. Histopathological changes caused by accidental avocado leaves toxicity in rabbits. *Int J Res Pharm Sci* 1(4): 517-520.

Smith, A.C. 1979, 1981, 1985, 1988, 1991. *Flora of Vitiensis Nova: A Flora of Fiji (Spermatophytes Only)*. Vol. 1-5. Hawaii: Pacific Tropical Botanical Garden.

Society for Ecological Restoration International. 2009. *Traditional Knowledge and the Convention on Biological Diversity*. Article 8(j). Accessed on 17 October 2011 at: http://www.cbd.int/traditional/intro.shtml.

Spino, C., M. Dodier, and S. Sotheeswaran. 1998. Anti-HIV coumarins from *Calophyllum* seed oil. *Bioor Med Chem Lett* 8: 3475-3478.

Stadlbauer, V., P. Fickert, C. Lackner, J. Schmerlaib, P. Krisper, M. Trauner, and R.E. Stauber. 2005. Hepatotoxicity of NONI juice: Report of two cases. *World J Gastroenterol* 11(30): 4758-4760.

Stanghellini, V., R. Giorgio, G. Barbara, R. Cogliandro, C. Tosetti, F. De Ponti, and R. Corinaldesi. 2004. Delayed gastric emptying in functional dyspepsia. *Curr Treat Options Gastroenterol* 7: 259-264.

Starley, I.F., P. Mohammed, G. Schneider, and S.W. Bickler. 1999. The treatment of paediatric burns using topical papaya. *Burns* 25: 636-639.

Stemmermann, L. 1981. *A Guide to Pacific Wetland Plants*. Honolulu, HI: U.S. Army Corps of Engineers, Honolulu District. 118p.

Stévigny, C., S. Block, M.C. De Pauw-Gillet, E. de Hoffmann, G. Llabrès, V. Adjakidjé, and J. Quetin-Leclercq. 2002. Cytotoxic aporphine alkaloids from *Cassytha filiformis*. *Planta Med* 68: 1042-1044.

Stoof, T.J., and D.P. Bruynzeel. 1989. Contact allergy to *Nephrolepis* ferns. *Contact Dermatitis* 20: 234-235.

Suklampoo, L., P. Khongsirisatjatam, R. Ruangsiri, and S. Dechaprakrom. 2010. Antimicrobial activity of crude extracts from pomelo peel of Khao-yai and Thong-dee varieties. Proceedings from Kasetsart University Annual Conference, Bangkok (Thailand). 3-5 Feb.

Suksamrarn, A., A. Chotipong, T. Suavansri, S. Boongird, P. Timsuksai, S. Vimuttipong, and A. Chuaynugul. 2004. Antimycobacterial activity and cytotoxicity of flavonoids from the flowers of *Chromolaena odorata*. *Arch Pharm Res* 27(5): 507-511.

Sulaiman, M.R., A. Mohd Padzil, K. Shaari, S. Khalid, W.M. Shaik Mossadeq, A.S. Mohamad, S. Ahmad, A. Akira, D. Israf, and N. Lajis. 2010. Antinociceptive activity of *Melicope ptelefolia* ethanolic extract in experimental animals. *J Biomed Biotechnol* [Epub 2 January 2011].

Sulaiman, M.R., M.N. Somchit, D.A. Israf, Z. Ahmad, and S. Moin. 2004. Antinociceptive effect of *Melastoma malabathricum* ethanolic extract in mice. *Fitoterapia* 75: 667-672.

Sunilson, J.A.J., A.V. Anandarajagopal, A.V. Kumari, and S. Mohan. 2009. Antidiarrheal activity of leaves of *Melastoma malabathricum* Linn. *Indian J Pharm Sci* 71: 691-695.

Susanti, D., H.M. Sirat, F. Ahmad, R.M. Ali, N. Aimi, and M. Kitajima. 2007. Antioxidant and cytotoxic flavonoids from the flowers of *Melastoma malabathricum* L. *Food Chem* 103: 710-716.

Tafelkruyer, J., and W.G. van Ketel. 1976. Sensitivity to *Codiaeum variegatum*. *Contact Dermatitis* 2(5): 288.

Tao, N., Y. Gao, Y. Liu, and F. Ge. 2010. Carotenoids from the peel of Shatian pummelo (*Citrus grandis* Osbeck) and its antimicrobial acitivity. *Am Eur J Agricul Environ Sci* 7(1): 110-115.

Telmetang, M. 1993. Bai. *Imuul Series* No. 1. Koror, Republic of Palau: The Society of Historians. 37pp.

Temme, E.H., R.P. Mensink, and G. Hornstra. 1997. Effects of medium chain fatty acid (MCFA), myristic acid and oleic acid on serum lipoproteins in healthy subjects. *J Lipid Res* 38: 1746-1754.

Tewari, P.V., C. Chaturvedi, and S.N. Dixit. 1970. Antifertility effect of betal leaf stalk (*Tambul patrabrint*): a preliminary experimental study. *J Res Indian Med* 4: 143-151.

Tewtrakul, S., S. Cheenpracha, and C. Karalai. 2009. Nitric oxide inhibitory principles from *Derris trifoliata* stems. *Phytomedicine* 16(6-7): 568-572.

Thang, P.T., S. Patrick, L.S. Teik, and C.S. Yung. 2001. Anti-oxidant effects of the extracts from the leaves of *Chromolaena odorata* on human dermal fibroblasts and epidermal keratinocytes against hydrogen peroxide and hypoxanthine-xanthine oxidase induced damage. *Burns* 27: 319-327.

Thani, W., O. Vallisuta, P. Siripong, and N. Ruanwises. 2010. Anti-proliferative and antioxidant activities of Thai noni/Yor (*Morinda citrifolia* Linn.) leaf extract. *Southeast Asian J Trop Med Public Health* 41(2): 482-9.

Thatoi, H.N., S.K. Panda, S.K. Rath, and S.K. Dutta. 2008. Antimicrobial activity and ethnomedicinal uses of some medicinal plants from Similipal Biosphere Reserve, Orissa. *Asian J Plant Sci* 7: 260-267.

Thomas, C.L. 1981. *Taber's Cyclopedic Medical Dictionary*. Philadelphia: F.A. Davis Company.

Thomas, T.J., B. Panikkar, A. Subramoniam, M.K. Nair, and K.R. Panikkar. 2002. Antitumour property and toxicity of *Barringtonia racemosa* Roxb seed extract in mice. *J Ethnopharmacol* 82: 223-227.

Thomson, M., M.A. Alnaqeeb, T. Bordia, J. M. Al-Hassan, M. Afzal, and M. Ali. 1998. Effects of aqueous extract of onion on the liver and lung of rats. *J Ethnopharmacol* 61(2): 91-99.

Thomson, M.A., P.W. Preston, L. Prais, and I.S. Foulds. 2007. Lime dermatitis from gin and tonic with a twist of lime. *Contact Dermatitis* 56(2): 114-115.

Tokunaga, M., H. Matsuda, H. Iwahashi, H. Iwahashi, S. Naruto, T. Tsuruoka, H. Yagi, T. Masuko, and M. Kubo. 2006. Studies on Palauan medicinal herbs. IV. Immunopotentiatory activities of Ongael, leaves of *Phaleria cumingii* (Meisn.) F. Vill. in diabetic mice. *J Trad Med* 23: 24-26.

Tona, L., K. Kambu, N. Ngimbi, K. Cimanga, and A.J. Vlietinck. 1998. Antiamoebic and phytochemical screening of some Congolese medicinal plants. *J Ethnopharmacol* 61(1): 57-65.

Tsai, T. H., G.J. Wang, and L.C. Lin. 2008. Vasorelaxing alkaloids and flavonoids from *Cassytha filiformis*. *J Nat Prod* 71(2): 289-291.

Tsai, Y.C., Chen, C.Y., Yang, N.I., and Yang, C.C. 2008. Cardiac glycoside poisoning following suicidal ingestion of *Cerbera manghas*. *Clin Toxicol* 46(4): 340-341.

Tsang, A., M. Von Korff, S. Lee, J. Alonso, E. Karam, M.C. Angermeyer, G.L. Guimaraes Borges, E.J. Bromet, K. Demytteneare, G. De Girolamo, R. De Graaf, O. Gureje, J.-P. Lepine, J.M. Haro, D. Levinson, M.A. Oakley Browne,

J. Posada Villa, S. Seedat, and M. Watanabe. 2008. Common chronic pain conditions in developed and developing countries: Gender and age differences and comorbidity with depression-anxiety disorders. *J Pain* 9(10): 883-891.

Tuntipopipat, S., C. Muangnoi, and M.L. Failla. 2009. Anti-inflammatory activities of extracts of Thai spices and herbs with lipopolysaccharide-activated RAW 264.7 murine macrophages. *J Med Food* 12(6): 1213-1220.

Umadevi, S., G.P. Mohanta, and R. Manavalan. 2006. Screening of folklore claim of *Scaevola frutescens* Krause. *Indian J Tradit Know* 5(4): 531-536.

Umadevi, S., G.P. Mohanta, and R. Manavalan. 2005. Studies on antipyretic and anti-inflammatory activities of *Scaevola frutescens*. *Pharmazie* 60: 398-399.

USDA, ARS, National Genetic Resources Program. *Germplasm Resources Information Network - (GRIN)* [Online Database]. 2011. National Germplasm Resources Laboratory, Beltsville, Maryland. Accessed on 19 April 2011 at: http://www.ars-grin.gov/cgi-bin/npgs/html/taxon.pl?447762.

van Ketel, W.G. 1979. Occupational contact dermatitis due to *Codiaeum variegatum* and possibly to *Aeschynantus pulcher*. *Derm Beruf Umwelt* 27(5): 141-142.

van Steenis, C.G.G.J., and M.J. van Steenis-Kruseman. 1972. Series I. Vol. 6. *Flora Malesiana*. Jakarta, Indonesia: Noordhoff-Kloff.

Vieira, R.H,. D.P. Rodrigues, F.A. Gonçalves, F.G. Menezes, J.S. Aragão, and O.V. Sousa. 2001. Microbicidal effect of medicinal plant extracts (*Psidium guajava* Linn. and *Carica papaya* Linn.) upon bacteria isolated from fish muscle and known to induce diarrhea in children. *Rev Inst Med Trop Sao Paolo* 43(3): 145-148.

Vimalanathan, S., S. Ignacimuthu, and J.B. Hudson. 2009. Medicinal plants from Tamil Nadu (Southern India) are a rich source of antiviral activities. *Pharm Biol* 47(5): 422-429.

Vinutha, B., D. Prashanth, K. Salma, S.L. Sneeja, D. Pratiti, R. Padmaja, S. Radica, A. Amit, K. Venkateshwarlu, and M. Deepak. 2007. Screening of selected Indian medicinal plants for acetylcholinesterase inhibitory activity. *J Ethnopharmacol* 109(2): 359-363.

Wagner, W.L., D.R. Herbst, and S.H. Sohmer. 1990. *Manual of the flowering plants of Hawai'i*. Vols. 1 & 2. Honolulu, HI: University of Hawai'i Press/Bishop Museum Press.

Wang, H.Y., B. Cai, C.-B. Cui, D.Y. Zhang, and B.F. Yang. 2005. Vitexicarpin, a flavonoid from *Vitex trifolia* L., induces apoptosis in K562 cells via mitochondria-controlled apoptotic pathway. *Yao Xue Xue Bao* 40(1): 27-31.

Wang, L.Q., B.S. Min, Y. Li, N. Nakamura, G.W. Qin, C.J. Li, and M. Hattori. Annonaceous acetogenins from the leaves of *Annona montana*. 2002. *Bioorg Med Chem* 10(3): 561-5.

Warshaw, E.M., and K.A. Zug. 1996. Sesquiterpene lactone allergy. *Am J Contact Dermatitis* 7(1): 1-23.

Watson, W.A., T.L. Litovitz, G.C. Rodgers Jr., W. Klein-Schwartz, N. Reid, J. Youniss, A. Flanagan, and K.M. Wruk. 2005. 2004 Annual report of the American Association of Poison Control Centers Toxic Exposure Surveillance System. *Am J Emerg Med* 23: 589-666.

Weil, A. 1983. *Health and healing*. Boston: Houghton Mifflin Company.

Weil, A. 1995. *Natural health, natural medicine: A comprehensive manual for wellness and self-care*. Boston: Houghton Mifflin Company.

Werner, D., C. Thuman, and J. Maxwell. 1992. *Where there is no doctor: A village health care handbook.* Berkeley: Hesperian Foundation.

Westendorf, J., K. Effenberger, H. Iznaguen, and S. Basar. 2007. Toxicological and analytical investigations of noni (*Morinda citrifolia*) fruit juice. *J Agric Food Chem* 55(2): 529-537.

Wiart, C., S. Mogana, S. Khalifah, M. Mahan, S. Ismail, M. Buckle, A.K. Narayana, and M. Sulaiman. 2004. Antimicrobial screening of plants used for traditional medicine in the state of Perak, Peninsular Malaysia. *Fitoterapia* 75(1): 68-73.

Wijesundera G., S. Deraniyagala, and A. Amarasekara. 1996. Antifungal activity of *Barringtonia ceylanica* bark extract: Palankumbura. *J Natl Council Sci Sri Lanka* 24: 279-283.

World Health Organization. 1995. *Yanuca Island Declaration.* Manila, Philippines: Regional Office for the Western Pacific. 12 pp.

World Health Organization.1997. *The Rarotonga agreement: Towards healthy islands.* Manila, Philippines: Regional Office for the Western Pacific. 16 pp.

World Health Organization. 1999. *The Palau action statement: On healthy islands.* Meeting of the Ministers of Health for the Pacific Island Countries Koror. Koror, Republic of Palau. 15 pp.

World Health Organization. 2001. *Apia action plan on traditional medicine in the Pacific Island countries.* Manila, Philippines: Regional Office for the Western Pacific. 119 pp.

World Health Organization. 2002. *WHO traditional medicine strategy 2002-2005.* Geneva, Switzerland. 63 pp.

World Health Organization. 2011. Palau. Accessed on 30 September 2011 at: http://www.who.int/countries/plw/en/.

Wu, J., T. Zhou, S.W. Zhang, X.H. Zhang, and L.J. Xuan. 2009. Cytotoxic terpenoids from the fruits of *Vitex trifolia* L. *Planta Med* 75(4): 367-370.

Wu, Z., and P.H. Raven, eds. 1994—. *Flora of China.* Beijing and St. Louis: Science Press and Missouri Botanical Garden Press. Accessed on 11 April 2011 at: http://flora.huh.havard.edu/china/.

Xu, J., M.L. Go, and L.Y. Lim. 2003. Modulation of digoxin transport across caco-2 cell monolayers by citrus fruit juices: Lime, lemon, grapefruit, and pummelo. *Pharm Res* 20(2): 169-176.

Yadav, R.P., and A. Singh. 2001. Environmentally safe molluscicides from two common Euphorbiales. *Iberus* 19(1): 65-73.

Yagi, S.M., S. El Tigani, and S.E.I. Adam. 1998. Toxicity of *Senna obtusifolia* fresh and fermented leaves (kawal), *Senna alata* leaves and some products from *Senna alata* on rats. *Phytother Res* 12(5): 324-330.

Yakubu, M.T., M.A. Akanji, and A.T. Oladiji. 2007. Evaluation of antiandrogenic potentials of aqueous extract of *Chromolaena odoratum* (L.) K. R. leaves in male rats. *Andrologia* 39: 235-243.

Yuan, S.S., H.L. Chang, H.W. Chen, Y.T. Yeh, Y.H. Kao, K.H. Lin, Y.C. Wu, and J.H. Su. 2003. Annoniacin, a mono-tetrahydrofuran acetogenin, arrests cancer cells at the G1 phase and causes cytotoxicity in a Bax- and caspase-3-related pathway. *Life Sci* 72(25): 2853-61.

Zaidan, M.R.S., A. Noor Rain, A.R.Badrul, A. Adlin, A. Norazah, and L. Zakiah. 2005. *In vitro* screening of five local medicial plants for antibacterial activity using disc diffusion method. *Tropical Biomedicine* 22(2): 165-170.

Zakaria, Z.A., Z.D.F.A. Ghani, R.N.S.R.M. Nor, H.K. Gopalan, M.R. Sulaiman, A.M.M. Jais, M.N. Somchit, A.A. Kader, and J. Ripio. 2008. Antinociceptive, anti-inflammatory, and antipyretic properties of an aqueous extract of *Dicranopteris linearis* leaves in experimental animal models. *J Nat Med* 62: 179-187.

Zakaria, Z.A., R.N.S.R.M. Nor, H.K. Gopalan, Z.D.F.A. Ghani, M.R. Sulaiman, G.R. Devi, A.M.M. Jais, M.N. Somchit, and C.A. Fatimah. 2006. Antinociceptive, anti-inflammatory and antipyretic properties of *Melastoma malabathricum* leaves aqueous extract in experimental animals. *Can J Physiol Pharm* 84: 1291-1299.

Zhang, Z., H.N. ElSohly, M.R. Jacob, D.S. Pasco, L.A. Walker, and A.M. Clark. 2002. Natural products inhibiting *Candida albicans* secreted aspartic proteases from *Lycopodium cernuum*. *J Nat Prod* 65(7): 979-985.

APPENDIX: HERBARIUM SPECIMENS

Herbarium specimens cited as vouchers (references) for the research presented in this book have been deposited in collections of The New York Botanical Garden (NY), the National Tropical Botanical Garden (PTBG), and the Belau National Museum (BNM).

Species	Voucher specimen
Adiantum philippense L.	J. Canfield *BNMH1074*; Y.E.J. Mexia *5504*
Ageratum conyzoides L.	M.J. Balick *4088, 4226*
Aidia racemosa (Cavanilles) Tirvengadum	M.J. Balick *4505*
Allium cepa L.	L. Dunn *499*
Allophylus timorensis (DC.) Blume	M.J. Balick *4531*; S. Perlman *20748, 20757*;
Angiopteris evecta (G. Forst.) G.F. Hoffm.	D.H. Lorence *9018*; K.R. Wood *10476*
Annona muricata L.	M.J. Balick *4429*
Areca catechu L.	D.H. Lorence *8190*
Artocarpus atilis (Parkinson) Fosb.	M.J. Balick *4510*
Atuna racemosa Raf. subsp. *racemosa*	M.J. Balick *3835, 4139*
Averrhoa bilimbi L.	M.J. Balick *4430, 4484*
Barringtonia racemosa (L.) Spreng.	M.J. Balick *4560*; C. Trauernicht *313*
Callicarpa elegans Hayek	M.J. Balick *4492, 4549*
Calophyllum inophyllum L.	M.J. Balick *4374*; R. Kanehira *2343*
Cananga odorata (Lam.) Hook. f. & Thomson	M.J. Balick *3810, 3833*
Carica papaya L.	M.J. Balick *4257*
Casearia hirtella Hosok.	M.J. Balick *4364, 4408*
Cassytha filiformis L.	M.J. Balick *4363*; C. Trauernicht *113*
Casuarina equisetifolia L.	M.J. Balick *4403*; C. Trauernicht *387*
Cerbera manghas L.	M.J. Balick *4362, 4376*
Cheilocostus speciosus (J.Koenig) C.Specht	J.J. Saimon *1*; J.A. Sanney *138*
Chromolaena odorata (L.) R. M. King & H. Rob.	M.J. Balick *3447, 4383*; P. Acevedo-Rodriguez *3873*
Citrus aurantiifolia (Christm.) Swingle	T. Flynn *4281, 5664*
Citrus mitis Blanco	E. Albert *208*
Clerodendrum paniculatum L.	M.J. Balick *3853, 4296*; S. Perlman *20776*
Cocos nucifera L.	A. Dores *60*; B. Ekiek *83*; A. Raynor *124*
Codiaeum variegatum (L.) Blume	M.J. Balick *4387*
Colocasia esculenta L. Schott	M.J. Balick *4465*
Cordyline fruticosa L. Chev.	M.J. Balick *4442*
Crateva religiosa G. Forst.	M.J. Balick *4276*
Curcuma longa L.	M.J. Balick *3850, 4030*
Cymbopogon citratus (DC. ex Nées) Stapf	A. Dores *124*; D.H. Lorence *9773*
Cyrtandra palawensis Schltr.	S. Perlman *20834, 20872*
Decaspermum parviflorum (Lam.) A. J. Scott	M.J. Balick *4369*; T. Flynn *6597*
Derris trifoliata Lour.	M.J. Balick *4427*
Dianella carolinensis Laut.	M.J. Balick *4391*; S. Perlman *20735*; C. Trauernicht *334*
Dicranopteris linearis (Burm. f.) Und. var. *ferruginea* (Blume) Rac.	T. Flynn *6252, 7031*; D.H. Lorence *7764*
Dolichandrone spathacea (L. f.) K. Schum.	M.J. Balick *4433*
Epipremnum pinnatum (L.) Engl.	M.J. Balick *4558*; T. Flynn *7118*; D.H. Lorence *8632*
Eugenia reinwardtiana (Blume) DC.	M.J. Balick *4533*; S. Perlman *20717*
Eurya japonica Thunb. var. *nitida* (Korth.) This.-Dyer	M.J. Balick *4034*; C. Trauernicht *338*
Ficus copiosa Steud.	D.H. Lorence *8297*; S. Perlman *20869*

Flacourtia inermis Roxb.	D.E. Atha *823*
Flacourtia rukam Zoll. & Mor. var. *micronesica* Fosb. & Sach.	C. Costion *115*; T. Flynn *6577*; D.H. Lorence *8759*
Flemingia strobilifera (L.) R. Br.	T. Flynn *6823*; D.H. Lorence *8225*
Glochidion ramiflorum J.R. Forst. & G. Forst.	M.J. Balick *3825, 3924*
Hedyotis korrorensis (Val.) Hosok.	D.H. Lorence *8207*; C. Trauernicht *332*
Heritiera littoralis Dryander	T. Flynn *6642*
Hibiscus rosa-sinensis L. var. *rosa-sinensis*	M.J. Balick *3851*; D.H. Lorence *8103*
Horsfieldia irya (Gaertn.) Warb.	T. Flynn *7222*; D.H. Lorence *8924*
Ixora casei Hance	M.J. Balick *4385*; C. Trauernicht *307*
Limnophila chinensis (Osb.) Merr. subsp. *aromatica* (Lam.) Yamazaki	M.J. Balick *4457*; D.H. Lorence *9655*
Lophopyxis maingayi Hook. f.	M.J. Balick *4556*
Lycopodiella cernua (L.) Pic. Serm	M.J. Balick *4453*; D.H. Lorence *9388*
Macaranga carolinensis Volk.	M.J. Balick *4397*
Melastoma malabathricum L. var. *mariannum* (Naudin) Fosb. & Sach.	M.J. Balick *4395, 4445, 4570*; S. Perlman *20737*
Melicope denhamii (Seem.) T.G. Hartley	T. Flynn *6410*
Microsorum scolopendria (Burm. f.) Copel.	M.J. Balick *4420*
Millettia pinnata (L.) Panigraphi	M.J. Balick *4541*; S. Perlman *20754*
Morinda citrifolia L.	D.H. Lorence *9669*; C. Trauernicht *388*
Musa × *paradisiaca* L.	M.J. Balick *3907*; P. Raynor *142*
Nepenthes mirabilis (Lour.) Druce	M.J. Balick *4390*
Nephrolepis acutifolia (Desv.) Christ	M.J. Balick *4428*; W. Law *194*; C. Trauernicht *283*
Opuntia cochenillifera (L.) Mill.	D.H. Lorence *5144, 5237*
Pandanus tectorius Parkinson ex Du Roi	M.J. Balick *4367, 4368*
Pangium edule Reinw. ex Blume	M.J. Balick *3805*; D.H. Lorence *9646*
Paraderris elliptica (Wall.) Adema	T. Flynn *7337*; J.A. Sanney *103*
Pemphis acidula J. R. Forst.	S. Perlman *20721, 20762*
Peperomia pellucida (L.) Kunth	A. Dores *8, 210*; B. Ekiek *34*
Persea americana Mill.	T. Flynn *2091*; D.H. Lorence *5268*
Phaleria nisidai Kaneh.	S. Perlman *20873*
Phyllanthus palauensis Hosok.	M.J. Balick *4396*; S. Perlman *20742*
Pinanga insignis Becc.	D.H. Lorence *8203*
Piper betle L. f. *densum* (Blume) Fosb.	M.J. Balick *4467*
Piriqueta racemosa (Jacq.) Sweet	A. Kitalong *BNMH2840*
Pouteria obovata (R. Br.) Baehni	M.J. Balick *4361*; D.H. Lorence *9687*
Premna serratafolia L.	M.J. Balick *3853, 3873, 4113, 4288*
Psidium guajava L.	M.J. Balick *3830*; T. Flynn *1611, 2495*
Pyrrosia lanceolata (L.) Farw.	M.J. Balick *4536*; D.H. Lorence *9661*; S. Perlman *20761*; C. Trauernicht *379*
Rhus taitensis Guill.	M.J. Balick *4410*
Scaevola taccada (Gaertn.) Roxb.	M.J. Balick *4548*; R. Lee *1000*
Scyphiphora hydrophyllacea C. F. Gaertn.	T. Flynn *6357*
Semecarpus venenosus Volk.	T. Flynn *5604*; D.H. Lorence *7967*
Senna cf. *obtusifolia* (L.) H.S. Irwin & Barneby	T. Flynn *6906*; P. Raynor *126*; A. Whistler *4790*
Syzygium samarangense (Blume) Merr. & Perry	M.J. Balick *4537*
Terminalia catappa L.	M.J. Balick *3859, 4575*; T. Flynn *2502*
Terminalia crassipes Kaneh. & Hatus.	C. Costion *63, 64, 499*; D.H. Lorence *8226*
Trema sp.	D.H. Lorence *9381*; K.R. Wood *10287*
Vitex trifolia L. var. *trifolia*	T. Flynn *1253, 2528*; J.A. Sanney *154*

INDEX

NOTES

NOTES

NOTES

NOTES

31371576R00124